Health Assessment

made Incredibly Visual!®

Third Edition

9/19

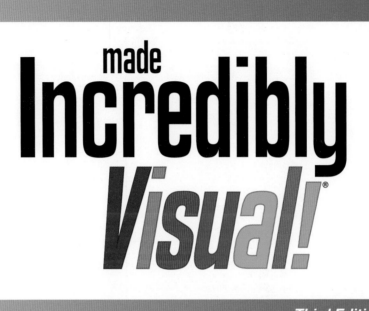

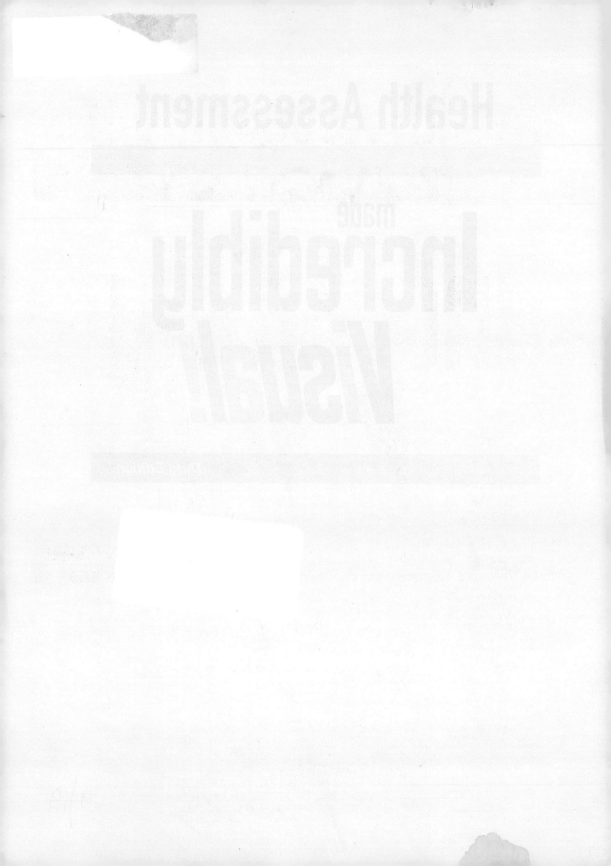

Health Assessment

made Incredibly Visual!®

Third Edition

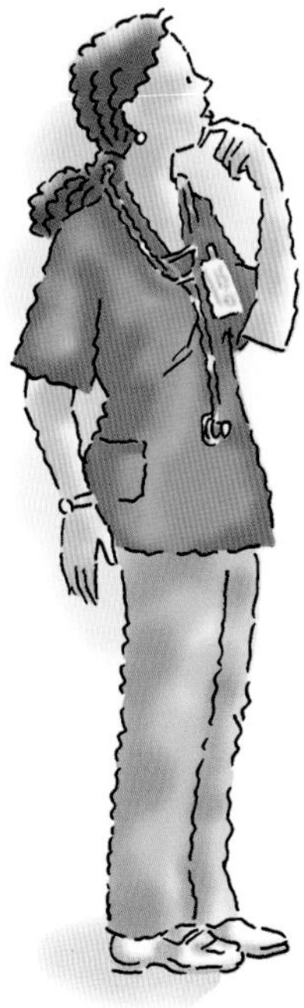

Clinical Editor
Laura M. Willis, DNP, APRN, FNP-C
Family Nurse Practitioner
Urbana Family Medicine and Pediatrics
Urbana, Ohio

Wolters Kluwer

Philadelphia • Baltimore • New York • London
Buenos Aires • Hong Kong • Sydney • Tokyo

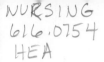

Acquisitions Editor: Nicole Dernoski
Product Development Editor: Maria M. McAvey
Production Project Manager: Cynthia Rudy
Design Coordinator: Elaine Kasmer
Manufacturing Coordinator: Kathleen Brown
Marketing Manager: Linda Wetmore
Prepress Vendor: SPi Global

3rd Edition

9 8 7 6 5 4 3 2

Printed in China

Library of Congress Cataloging-in-Publication Data
Names: Willis, Laura M., 1969- editor.
Title: Health assessment made incredibly visual! / [edited by] Laura M. Willis.
Other titles: Incredibly visual.
Description: 3rd edition. | Philadelphia : Wolters Kluwer, [2017] | Series: Incredibly visual | Includes bibliographical references and index.
Identifiers: LCCN 2016022163 | ISBN 9781496325143
Subjects: | MESH: Nursing Assessment—methods | Physical Examination—methods | Handbooks | Atlases
Classification: LCC RT48 | NLM WY 49 | DDC 616.07/54—dc23 LC record available at https://lccn.loc.gov/2016022163

LWW.com

Dedication

This book is dedicated to students everywhere. My hope is that the information in this book will inspire you to become masters at health assessment.

And this book is dedicated, with gratitude and love, to Andrew, Dan, Steven, and my mom and dad: each of you have inspired me to be better at what I do every single day.

Gratefully,
Laura

Contributors

Nancy Berger, MSN, RN, BC, CNE
Program Coordinator
Charles E. Gregory School of Nursing at Raritan Bay Medical Center
Perth Amboy, New Jersey

Dana Reeves, MSN, RN, NP-BC
Assistant Professor
University of Arkansas Fort Smith (UAFS)
Fort Smith, Arkansas

Tracy Taylor, MSN, RN
Associate Professor, Division of Nursing
Kettering College
Kettering, Ohio

Allison J. Terry, PhD, MSN, RN
Assistant Dean of Clinical Planning
College of Nursing and Health Sciences
Auburn University at Montgomery
Montgomery, Alabama

Leigh Ann Trujillo, MSN, RN
Director, Med-Surgery/Telemetry/Peds/Inpatient Orthopedics
IU Health La Porte
La Porte, Indiana

Rita M. Wick, BSN, RN
Education Specialist
Berkshire Health Systems
Pittsfield, Massachusetts

Sharon E. Wing, PhD(c), RN, CNL
Associate Professor
Coordinator of Medical Surgical Nursing
Nursing Department
Cleveland, Ohio

Previous Edition Contributors

Nancy Berger, MSN, RN, BC, CNE

Marsha L. Conroy, MSN, APN, RN

Roseanne Hanlon Rafter, MSN, GCNS, BC, RN

Dana Reeves, MSN, RN, NP-BC

Denise Stefancyk, BSN, RN, CCRC

Allison J. Terry, PhD, MSN, RN

Leigh Ann Trujillo, BSN, RN

Rita M. Wick, BSN, RN

Sharon E. Wing, PhD(c), RN, CNL

Lisa Wolf, RN, MS, CMSRN

Foreword

The third edition of *Health Assessment Made Incredibly Visual* is a must-have for students, working nurses, and nurses returning to practice. The vividly detailed illustrations and photographs of abnormal findings are definitely "outside the norm." The graphic depictions of best assessment practices that appear throughout in "Skill check" are unique and innovative. And "Take note" captures lifelike charts that illustrate the correct ways to document assessment findings. This is a visually stunning and exciting new work.

Contents

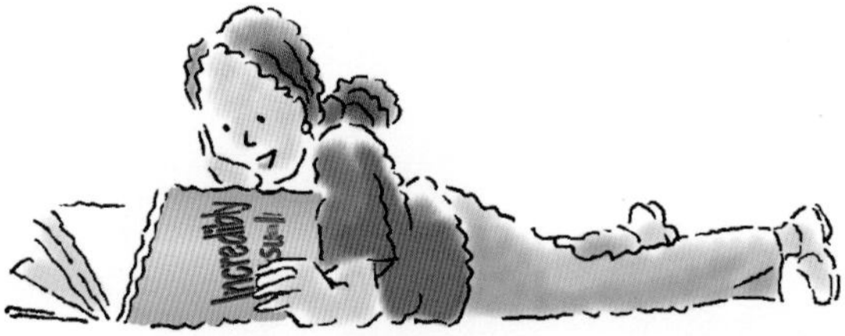

Chapter 1

Fundamentals

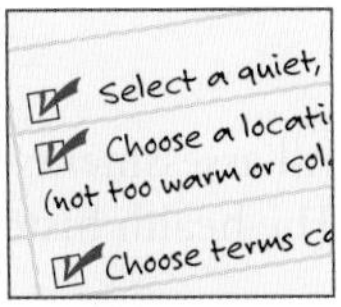
Select a quiet,
Allergies
Food:

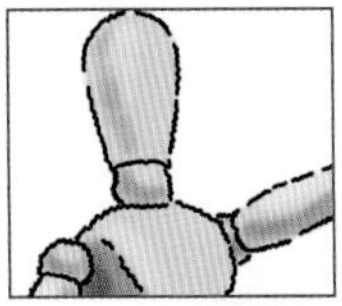

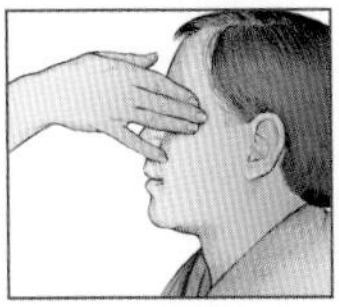

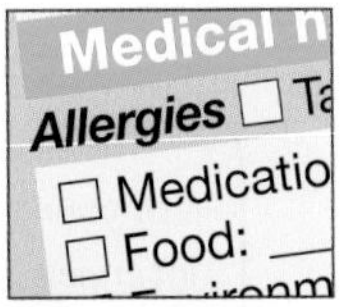

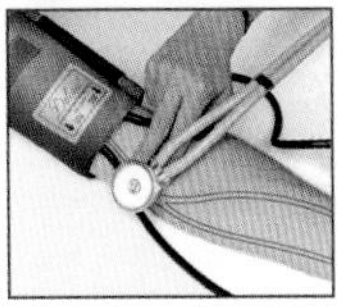

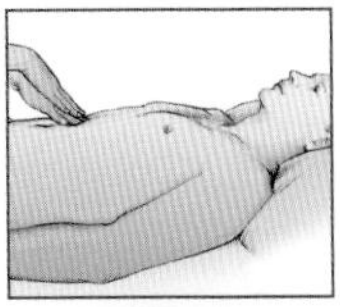

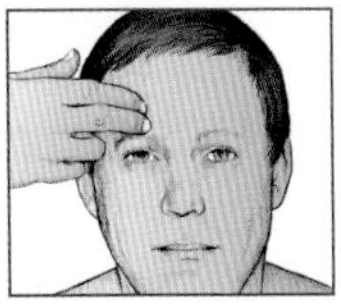

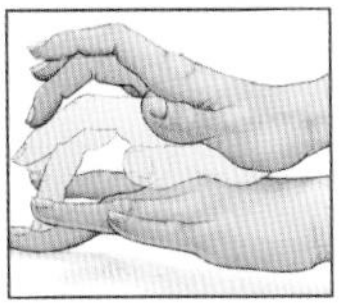

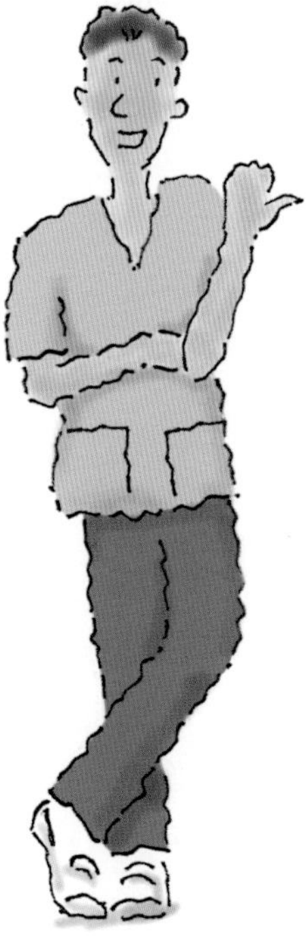

Health history

All assessments involve collecting two kinds of data: ***objective*** and *subjective*. The health history gathers subjective data about the patient.

Objective data (signs)

- Are observed during a physical examination
- Are verifiable
- Include findings such as a red, swollen arm in a patient

Subjective data (symptoms)

- Provided by the patient or "subject"
- Verified only by the patient
- Include statements such as "My head hurts" or "I have trouble sleeping"

Interviewing tips

To make the most of your patient interview, create an environment in which the patient feels comfortable. Also, use the following techniques to ensure effective communication.

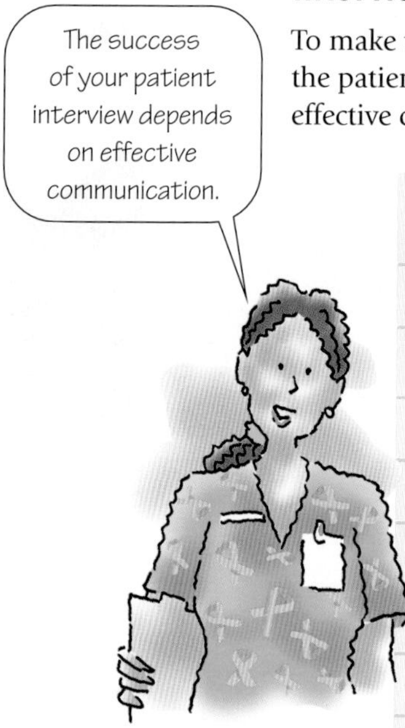
The success of your patient interview depends on effective communication.

- ☑ Select a quiet, private setting.
- ☑ Choose a location where there is a comfortable temperature (not too warm or cold) and adequate lighting.
- ☑ Choose terms carefully and avoid using medical jargon.
- ☑ Speak slowly and clearly.
- ☑ Use effective therapeutic communication techniques, such as silence, facilitation, confirmation, reflection, and clarification.
- ☑ Use open-ended and closed-ended questions as appropriate.
- ☑ Use appropriate body language.
- ☑ Confirm patient statements to avoid misunderstanding.
- ☑ Summarize and conclude with "Is there anything else?"

Components of a complete health history

Biographical data

Name ______________________________
Address ______________________________
Date of birth ______________________________

Advance directive explained: ☐ Yes ☐ No
Copy of Advance Directive on chart: ☐ Yes ☐ No
Preferred Language: ______________________________

Chief complaint

History of present illness (include time frame, signs and symptoms)

____
____

Current medications

MEDICATION, DOSE, ROUTE	FREQUENCY	LAST DOSE	REASON FOR TAKING

> Be sure to include prescription medications, over-the-counter medications, herbal preparations, and vitamins and supplements, birth control pills or implanted birth control, hormone therapy.

Medical histo

Allergies ☐ Tape ☐

☐ Medication: ___
☐ Food: ___
☐ Environmental: ___
☐ Blood reaction: ___
☐ Other: ___

Childhood illnesses

ILLNESS	DATE

Previous hospitalizations
(Illness, accident or injury, surgery, blood transfusion)

LIST ALL	DATE

Health problems	Yes	No
Arthritis	☐	☐
Blood problem (anemia, sickle cell, clotting, bleeding)	☐	☐
Cancer	☐	☐
Diabetes mellitus	☐	☐
Eye problem (cataracts, glaucoma)	☐	☐
Heart disease (heart failure, MI, valve)	☐	☐
Hiatal hernia	☐	☐
HIV/AIDS	☐	☐
Hypertension	☐	☐
Kidney problem	☐	☐
Liver problem	☐	☐
Lung problem (asthma, bronchitis, emphysema, pneumonia, TB, shortness of breath)	☐	☐
Stroke	☐	☐
Thyroid problem	☐	☐
Ulcers (duodenal, peptic)	☐	☐
Psychological disorder (depression, anxiety)	☐	☐

Name and phone numbers of next of kin or support network:

NAME	RELATIONSHIP	PHONE #

Obstetric history (females)

Last menstrual period ___
Gravida ___ Para
Menopause ☐ Yes (Date) ___

> Ask about the patient's feelings of safety to help identify physical, psychological, emotional, and sexual abuse issues

Sexual history (all pat

Do have sex with ☐ men ☐ wo
Preferred pronoun/gende identity ___

Psychosocial history

Coping strategies
____

Feelings of safety
____

Social history

Tobacco Use ☐ No ___ ☐ Yes (# packs/day___ # years ___) (cigarettes, pipe, cigar) ☐ smokeless tobacco (dip, chew) ☐ vapor user
Alcohol ☐ No ☐ Yes (type ___ amount/day ___) (# years)
Illicit drug use ☐ No ☐ Yes (type ___) (# years)

Any recent changes in weight?

Religious and cultural observances

____

Activities of daily living

Diet and exercise regimen ___
Elimination patterns ___
Sleep patterns ___
Bathing and Dressing ___
Sleep/rest patterns ___
Work and leisure activities ___
Use of safety measures (seat belt, bike helmet, sunscreen) ___

> Ask about the patient's family medical history

Health maintenance history

	DA E OF MOST RECENT RESULTS
Colonoscopy	
Dental examination	
Eye examination	
Immunizations	
Mammography	

Family medical history

Health problem	Yes	No	Who (parent, grandparent, sibling)
Arthritis	☐	☐	
Cancer	☐	☐	
Diabetes mellitus	☐	☐	
Heart disease (heart failure, MI, valve disease)	☐	☐	
Hypertension	☐	☐	
Stroke	☐	☐	

Review of structures and systems

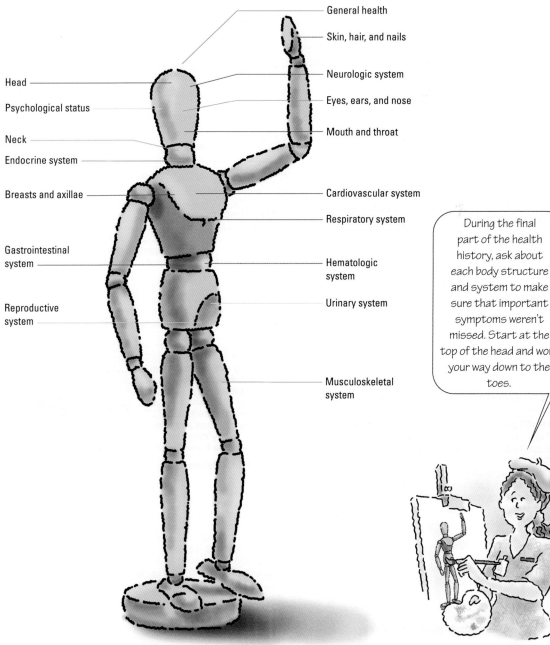

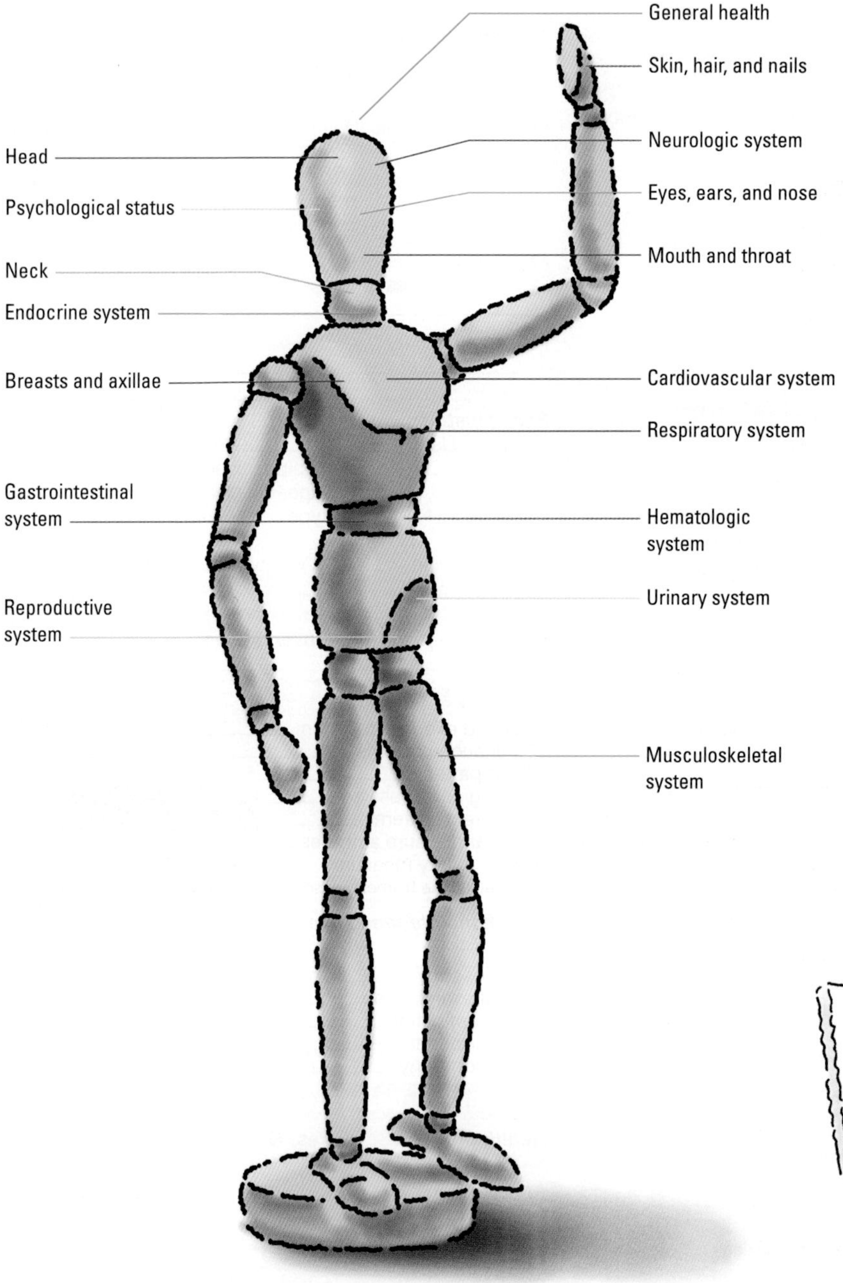
General health
Skin, hair, and nails
Head
Neurologic system
Psychological status
Eyes, ears, and nose
Neck
Mouth and throat
Endocrine system
Breasts and axillae
Cardiovascular system
Respiratory system
Gastrointestinal system
Hematologic system
Urinary system
Reproductive system
Musculoskeletal system

During the final part of the health history, ask about each body structure and system to make sure that important symptoms weren't missed. Start at the top of the head and work your way down to the toes.

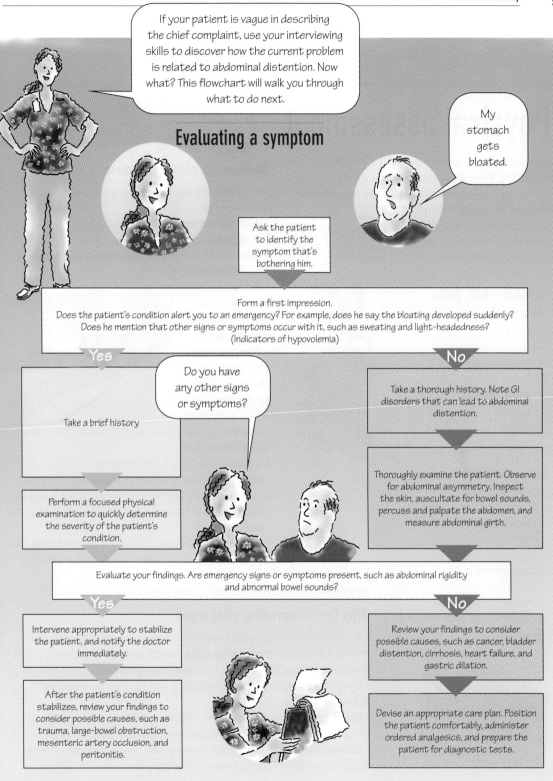

If your patient is vague in describing the chief complaint, use your interviewing skills to discover how the current problem is related to abdominal distention. Now what? This flowchart will walk you through what to do next.

Evaluating a symptom

My stomach gets bloated.

Ask the patient to identify the symptom that's bothering him.

Form a first impression.
Does the patient's condition alert you to an emergency? For example, does he say the bloating developed suddenly? Does he mention that other signs or symptoms occur with it, such as sweating and light-headedness? (Indicators of hypovolemia)

Yes

Take a brief history

Perform a focused physical examination to quickly determine the severity of the patient's condition.

No

Take a thorough history. Note GI disorders that can lead to abdominal distention.

Thoroughly examine the patient. Observe for abdominal asymmetry. Inspect the skin, auscultate for bowel sounds, percuss and palpate the abdomen, and measure abdominal girth.

Do you have any other signs or symptoms?

Evaluate your findings. Are emergency signs or symptoms present, such as abdominal rigidity and abnormal bowel sounds?

Yes

Intervene appropriately to stabilize the patient, and notify the doctor immediately.

After the patient's condition stabilizes, review your findings to consider possible causes, such as trauma, large-bowel obstruction, mesenteric artery occlusion, and peritonitis.

No

Review your findings to consider possible causes, such as cancer, bladder distention, cirrhosis, heart failure, and gastric dilation.

Devise an appropriate care plan. Position the patient comfortably, administer ordered analgesics, and prepare the patient for diagnostic tests.

Physical assessment

Assemble the necessary tools for the physical assessment. Then perform a general survey to form your initial impression of the patient. Obtain baseline data, including height, weight, and vital signs. This information will direct the rest of your assessment.

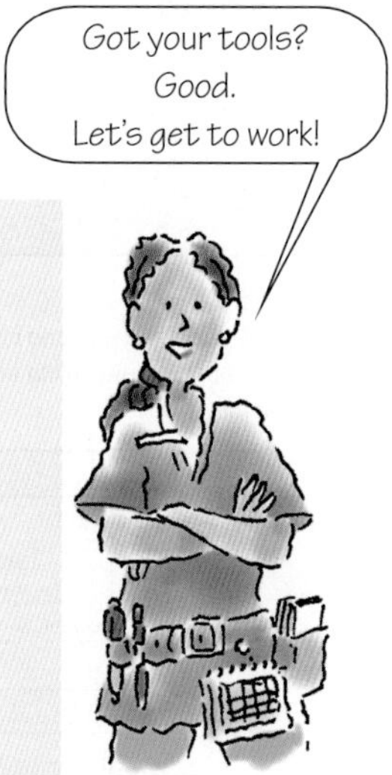
Got your tools?
Good.
Let's get to work!

Assessment tools

- Cotton balls
- Gloves
- Metric ruler (clear)
- Near-vision and visual acuity charts
- Ophthalmoscope
- Otoscope
- Penlight
- Percussion hammer
- Paper clip
- Scale with height measurement
- Skin calipers
- Specula (nasal and vaginal)
- Sphygmomanometer
- Stethoscope
- Tape measure (cloth or paper)
- Thermometer
- Tuning fork
- Wooden tongue blade
- Watch or clock with second hand

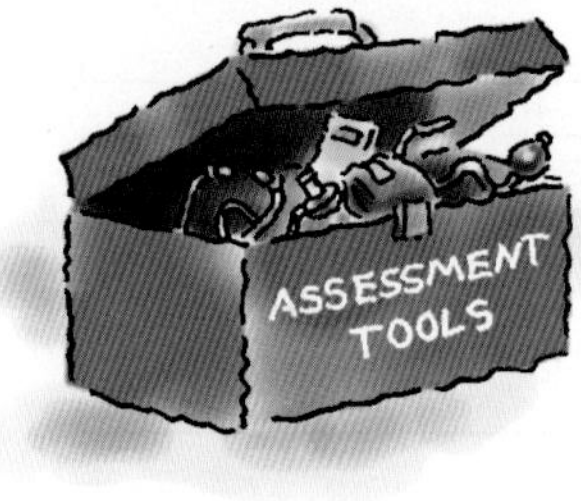
ASSESSMENT
TOOLS

Skill check

Measuring blood pressure

- Position your patient with upper arm at heart level and palm turned up.
- Apply the cuff snugly, 1″ (2.5 cm) above the brachial pulse.
- Position the manometer at your eye level.
- Palpate the brachial or radial pulse with your fingertips while inflating the cuff.
- Inflate the cuff to 30 mm Hg above the point where the pulse disappears.
- Place the bell of your stethoscope over the point where you felt the pulse, as shown in the photo. (Using the bell will help you better hear Korotkoff sounds, which indicate pulse.)

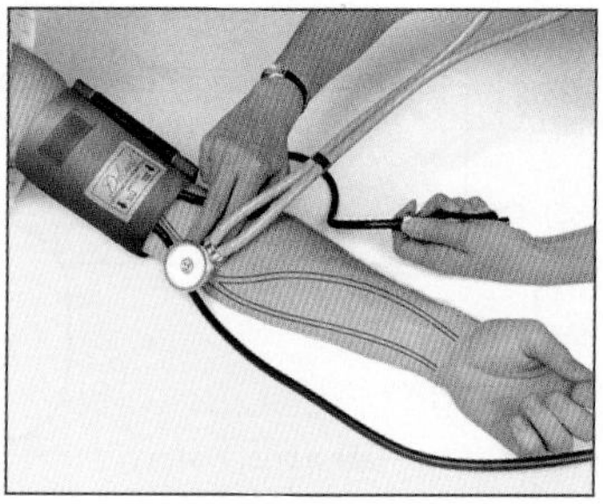

- Release the valve slowly (for example, allow it to drop 2 to 3 mm Hg/second) and note the point at which Korotkoff sounds reappear. The start of the pulse sound indicates the systolic pressure.
- The sounds will become muffled and then disappear. The last Korotkoff sound you hear is the diastolic pressure.

Tips for interpreting vital signs

- Analyze vital signs during the same interaction with the patient. Two or more abnormal values may provide clues to the patient's problem. For example, a rapid, thready pulse along with low blood pressure may signal shock.
- If you obtain an abnormal value, assess the vital sign again to make sure it's accurate.
- Remember that normal readings vary with the patient's age. For example, temperature decreases with age, and respiratory rate can increase with age.
- Remember that an abnormal value for one patient may be a normal value for another, which is why baseline values are so important.

Physical assessment techniques

When you perform the physical assessment, you'll use four techniques: inspection, palpation, percussion, and auscultation. Use these techniques in this sequence except when you perform an abdominal assessment.

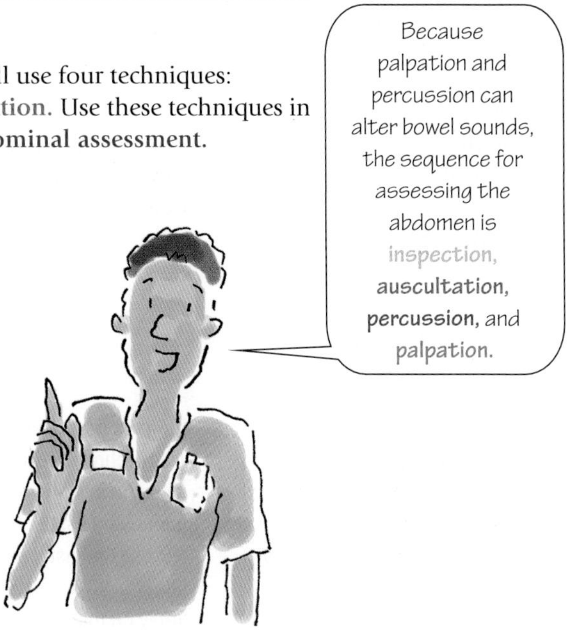
Because palpation and percussion can alter bowel sounds, the sequence for assessing the abdomen is inspection, auscultation, percussion, and palpation.

1 Inspection

Inspect each body system using vision, smell, and hearing to assess normal conditions and deviations. Observe for color, size, location, movement, texture, symmetry, odors, and sounds as you assess each body system.

2 Palpation

Palpation requires you to touch the patient with different parts of your hands, using varying degrees of pressure. Because your hands are your tools, keep your fingernails short and your hands warm. Wear gloves when palpating mucous membranes or areas in contact with body fluids. Palpate tender areas last.

Types of palpation

Light palpation

- Use this technique to feel for surface abnormalities.
- Depress the skin 1/2″ to 3/4″ (1.5 to 2 cm) with your finger pads, using the lightest touch possible.
- Assess for texture, tenderness, temperature, moisture, elasticity, pulsations, superficial organs, and masses.

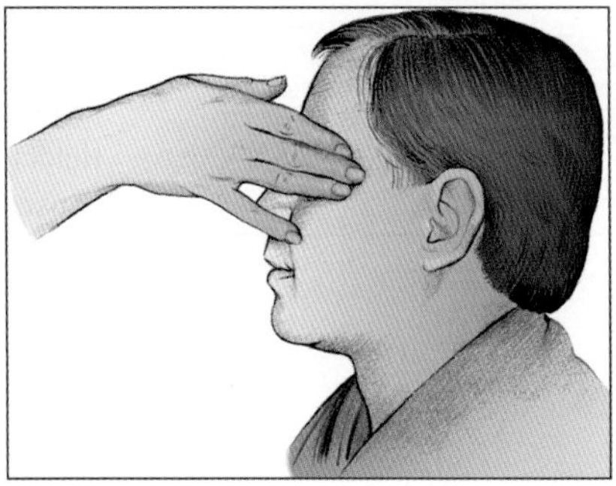

Deep palpation

- Use this technique to feel internal organs and masses for size, shape, tenderness, symmetry, and mobility.
- Depress the skin 1½″ to 2″ (4 to 5 cm) with firm, deep pressure.
- Use one hand on top of the other (bimanual palpation) to exert firmer pressure, if needed.

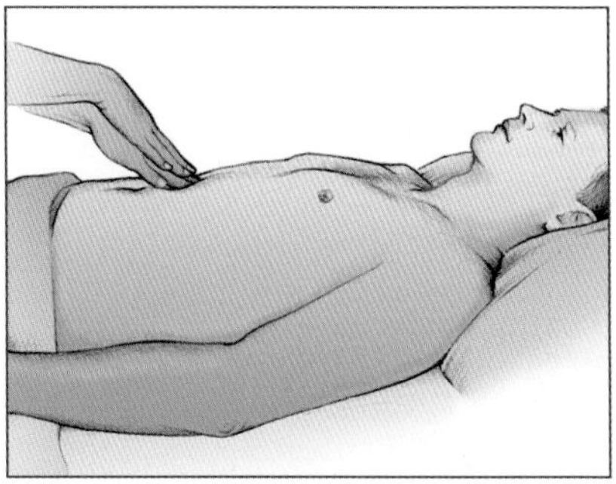

3

Percussion

Percussion involves tapping your fingers or hands quickly and sharply against parts of the patient's body to help you locate organ borders, identify organ shape and position, and determine if an organ is solid or filled with fluid or gas.

4

Auscultation

Auscultation involves listening for various breath, heart, and bowel sounds with a stethoscope.

Types of percussion

Direct percussion

This technique reveals tenderness; it's commonly used to assess an adult patient's sinuses. Here's how to do it:

- Using one or two fingers, tap directly on the body part.
- Ask the patient to tell you which areas are painful, and watching for facial signs of discomfort such as wincing or grimacing.

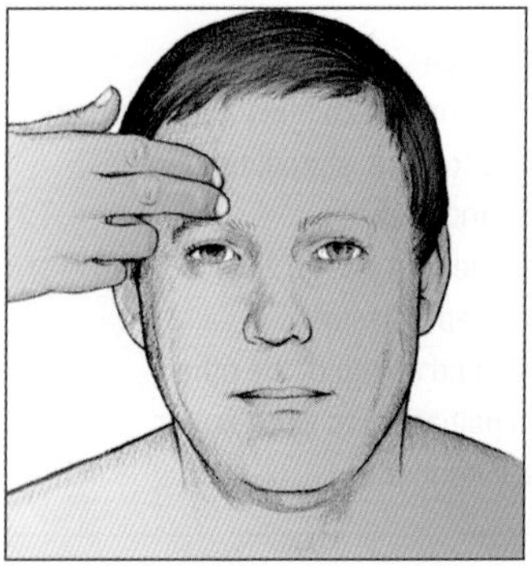

Indirect percussion

This technique elicits sounds that give clues to the makeup of the underlying tissue. Here's how to do it:

- Press the distal part of the middle finger of your nondominant hand firmly on the body part.
- Keep the rest of your hand off the body surface.
- Flex the wrist of your dominant hand.
- Using the middle finger of your dominant hand, tap quickly and directly over the point where your other middle finger touches the patient's skin.
- Listen to the sounds produced.

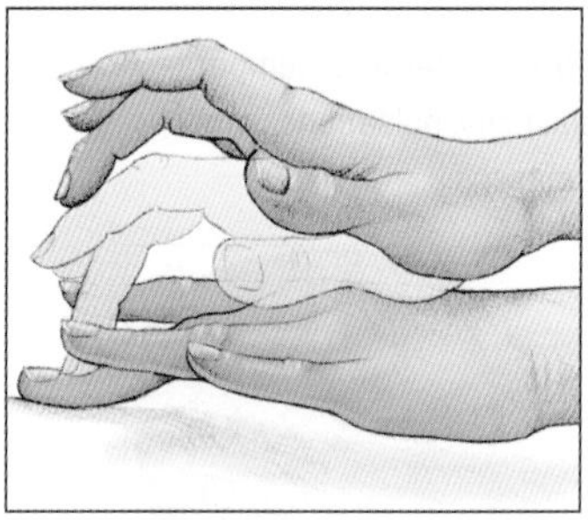

Getting ready

- Provide a quiet environment.
- Make sure the area to be auscultated is exposed. (Auscultating over a gown or bed linens can interfere with sounds.)
- Warm the stethoscope head in your hand.
- Close your eyes to help focus your attention.

How to auscultate

- Use the diaphragm to pick up high-pitched sounds, such as first (S_1) and second (S_2) heart sounds. Hold the diaphragm firmly against the patient's skin, enough to leave a slight ring on the skin afterward.
- Use the bell to pick up low-pitched sounds, such as third (S_3) and fourth (S_4) heart sounds. Hold the bell lightly against the patient's skin, just enough to form a seal. Holding the bell too firmly causes the skin to act as a diaphragm, obliterating low-pitched sounds.
- Listen to and try to identify the characteristics of one sound at a time.

Documentation

Get to know your stethoscope

Your stethoscope should have snug-fitting ear tips, which you'll position toward your nose. The stethoscope should also have tubing no longer than 12″ to 15″ (38.1 cm) with an internal diameter not greater than 1/8″ (0.3 cm). It should have both a diaphragm and bell. The parts of a stethoscope are labeled below.

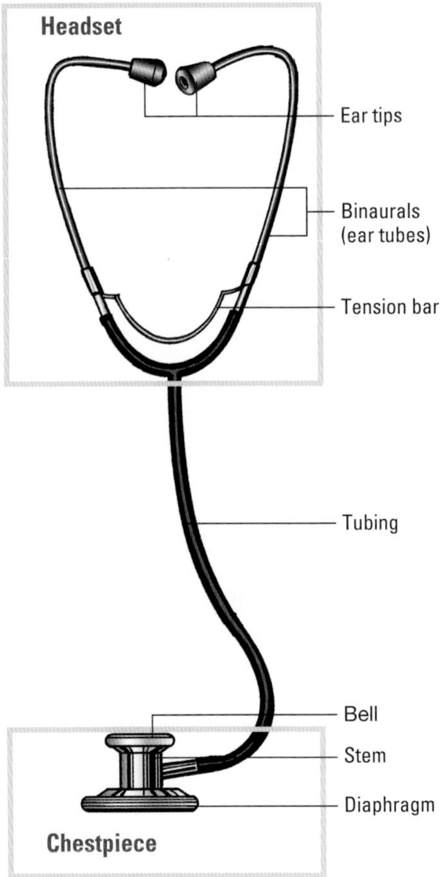
Headset
Ear tips
Binaurals (ear tubes)
Tension bar
Tubing
Bell
Stem
Diaphragm
Chestpiece

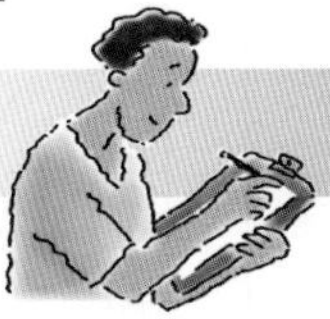

Take note

Documenting initial assessment findings

Here's an example of how to record your findings on an initial assessment form.

General information

Name Henry Gibson

Age 55 Sex M Height 163 cm Weight 57 kg

T 37 °C (oral) P 76 R 14 B/P (R) 150/90 sitting

(L) 148/88 sitting Pain Scale 3/10

Room 328

Admission time 0800

Admission date 4-28-100

Doctor Manzel

Admitting diagnosis: Pneumonia

Patient's stated reason for hospitalization "To get rid of the pneumonia"

Allergies Penicillin-hives, Codeine-nausea

Current medications None

Name	Dosage	Last taken

General survey

In no acute distress. Slender, alert, and well-groomed. Communicates well. Makes eye contact and expresses appropriate concern throughout exam. C. Smith, RN

Q&A

Show and tell

Identify the assessment technique being used in each illustration.

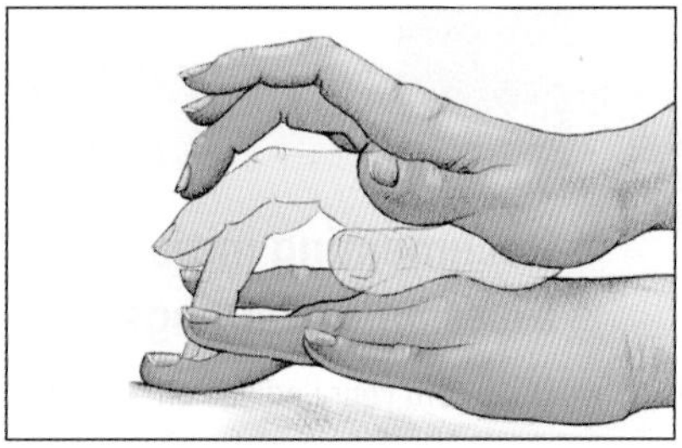

1. ______________________

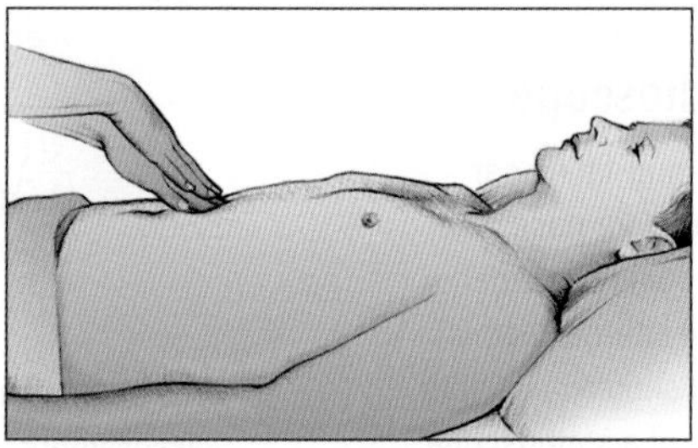

2. ______________________

My word!

Unscramble the words given below to discover terms related to fundamentals of assessment. Then use the circled letters from those words to answer the question posed.

Question: Assessment of which body part does not follow the usual sequence?

1. tunicaastolu ◯ _ _ _ _ _ _ _ _ _ ◯ _
2. divateacub jest _ _ ◯ _ _ _ _ _ _ _ ◯ _ _ _
3. place inchmotif _ _ _ ◯ _ _ _ ◯ _ _ _ _ _ _
4. aplaintop _ _ _ _ _ _ _ _ ◯

Answer: _ _ _ _ _ _ _

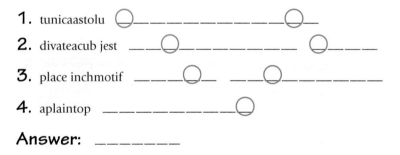

Answers: Show and tell 1. Indirect percussion, 2. Deep palpation; My word! 1. Auscultation, 2. Subjective data, 3. Chief complaint, 4. Palpation; Question: Abdomen

Selected References

Fawcett, T., & Rhynas, S. (2012). Taking a patient history: The role of the nurse. *Nursing Standard, 15*(26), 41–46.

Hinkle, J. L., & Cheever, K. H. (2014). *Brunner and Suddarth's textbook of medical-surgical nursing* (13th ed.). Philadelphia, PA: Lippincott Williams & Wilkins.

Jarvis, C. (2012). *Physical examination and health assessment* (6th ed.). St. Louis, MO: W.B. Saunders.

Jensen, S. (2011). *Nursing health assessment: A best practice approach*. Philadelphia, PA: Lippincott Williams & Wilkins.

The Joint Commission. (2015). Facts about pain management. Retrieved from http://www.jointcommission.org/pain_management/

Taylor, C., Lillis, C., Lynn, P., & LeMone, P. (2015). *Fundamentals of nursing: The art and science of person-centered nursing care* (8th ed.). Philadelphia, PA: Lippincott Williams & Wilkins.

Taylor, L., & LeMone, L. (2014). *Taylor's video guide to clinical nursing skills* (2nd ed.). Philadelphia, PA: Lippincott Williams & Wilkins.

Weber, J. R., & Kelley, J. H. (2014). *Health assessment in nursing* (5th ed.). Philadelphia, PA: Lippincott Williams & Wilkins.

Chapter 2

Skin, hair, and nails

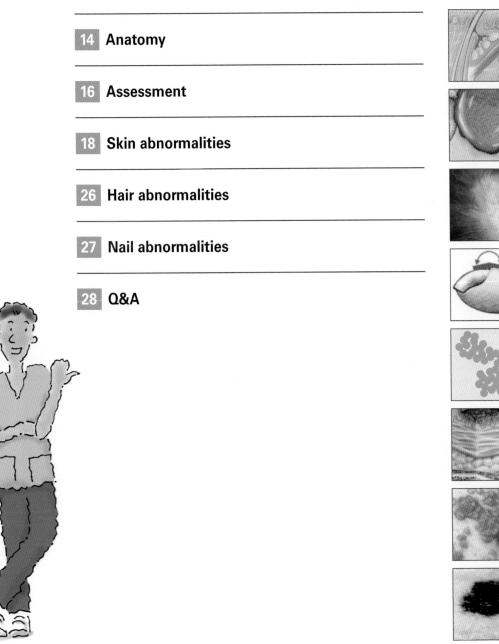

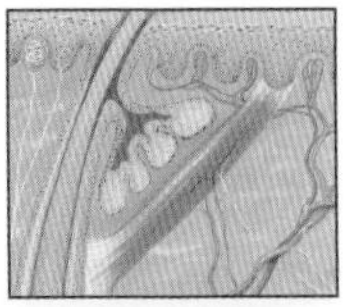

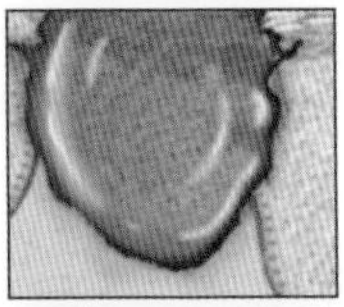

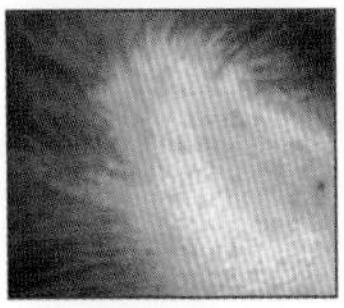

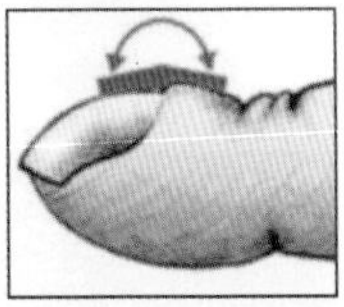

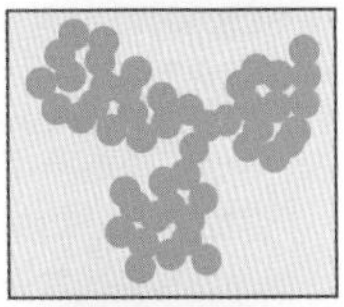

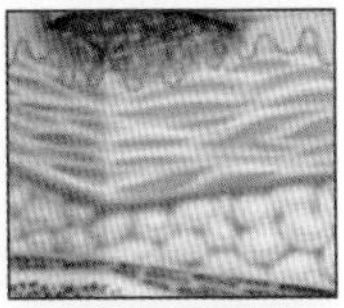

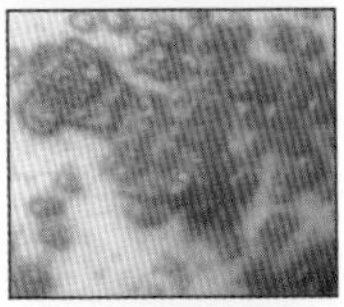

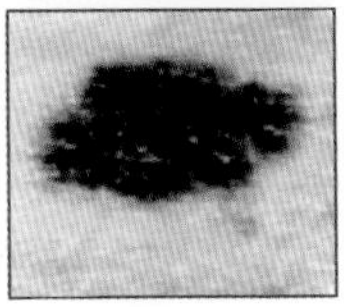

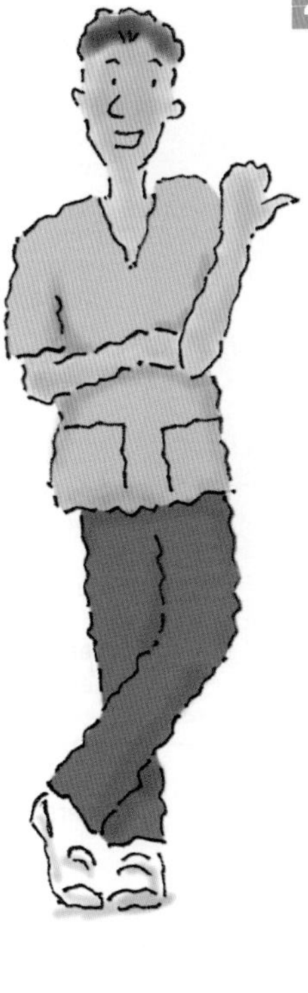

Anatomy

Skin

The skin covers and protects the internal structures of the body. It consists of two distinct layers: the **epidermis** and the **dermis**. **Subcutaneous tissue** lies beneath these layers.

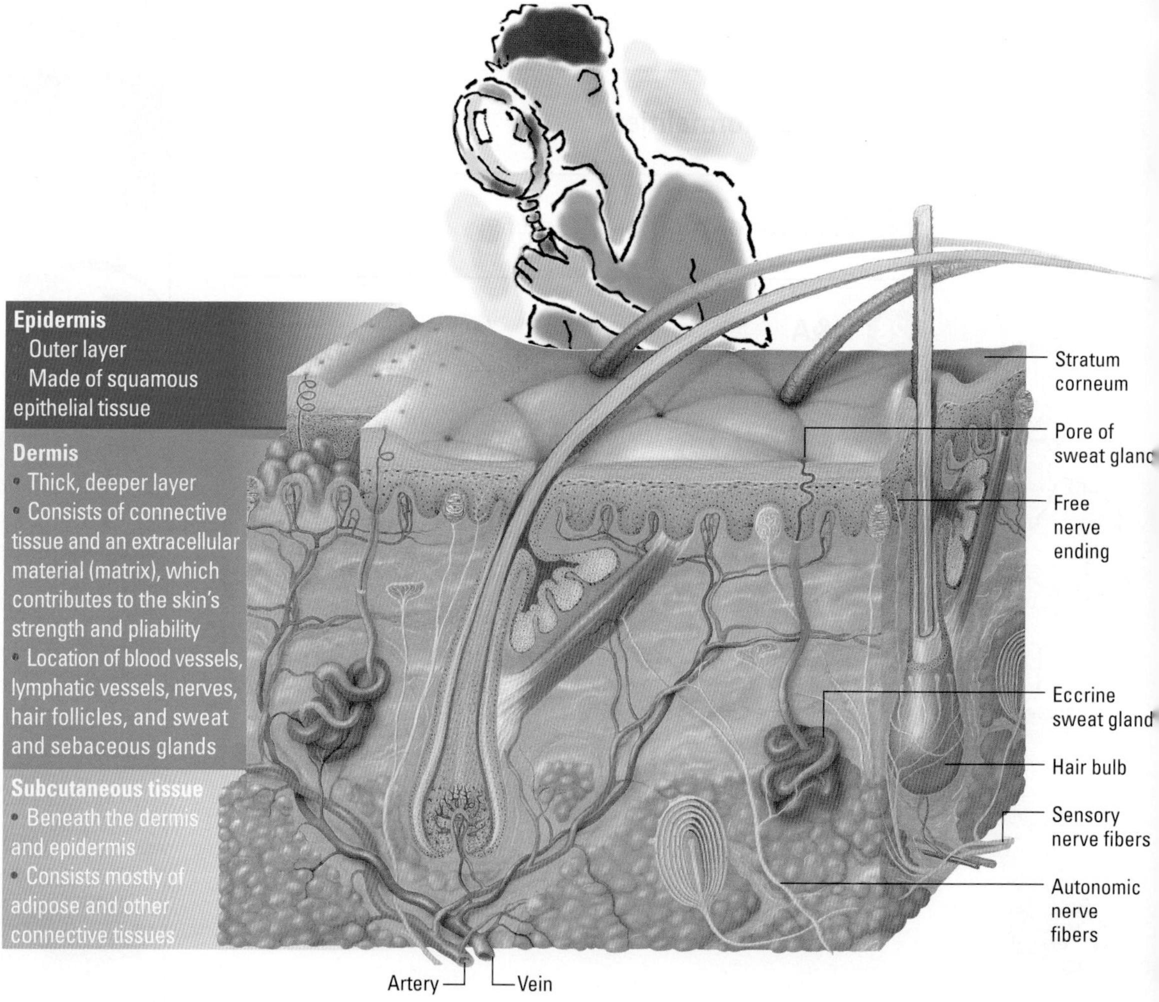
Epidermis
Outer layer
Made of squamous epithelial tissue
Dermis
• Thick, deeper layer
• Consists of connective tissue and an extracellular material (matrix), which contributes to the skin's strength and pliability
• Location of blood vessels, lymphatic vessels, nerves, hair follicles, and sweat and sebaceous glands
Subcutaneous tissue
• Beneath the dermis and epidermis
• Consists mostly of adipose and other connective tissues
Stratum corneum
Pore of sweat glan
Free nerve ending
Eccrine sweat gland
Hair bulb
Sensory nerve fibers
Autonomic nerve fibers
Artery
Vein

Hair

Hair is formed from keratin produced by matrix cells in the dermal layer of the skin. Each hair lies in a hair follicle.

Nails

Nails are formed when epidermal cells are converted into hard plates of keratin.

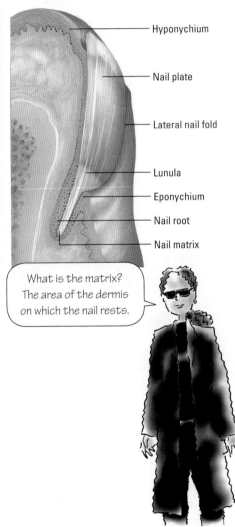

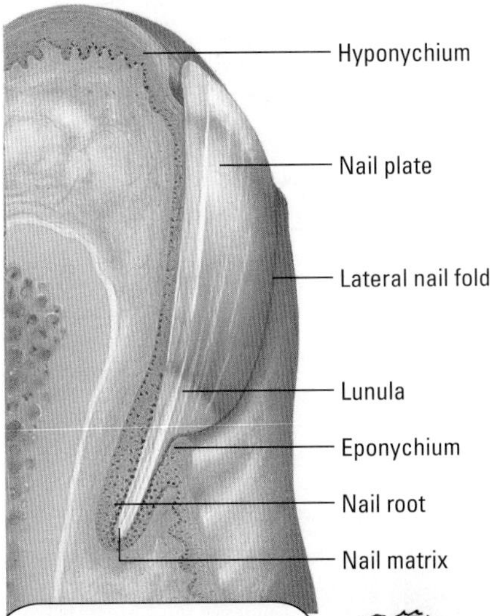
Hyponychium
Nail plate
Lateral nail fold
Lunula
Eponychium
Nail root
Nail matrix

What is the matrix? The area of the dermis on which the nail rests.

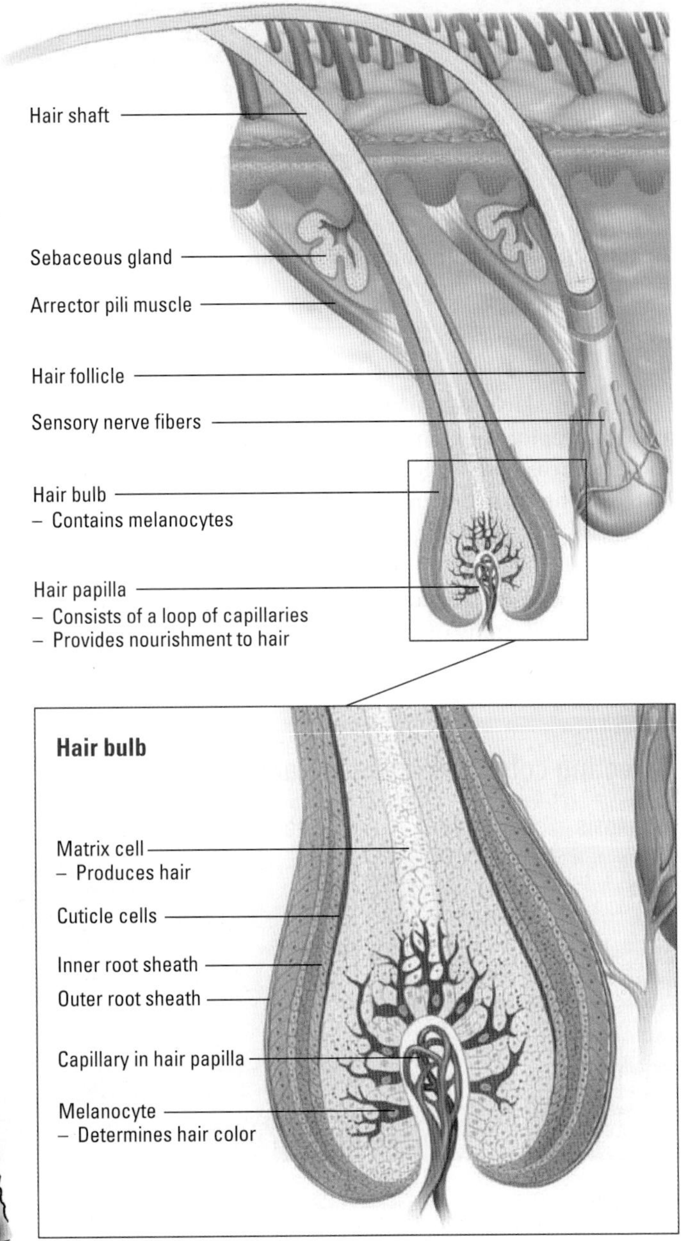
Hair shaft
Sebaceous gland
Arrector pili muscle
Hair follicle
Sensory nerve fibers
Hair bulb
– Contains melanocytes
Hair papilla
– Consists of a loop of capillaries
– Provides nourishment to hair
Hair bulb
Matrix cell
– Produces hair
Cuticle cells
Inner root sheath
Outer root sheath
Capillary in hair papilla
Melanocyte
– Determines hair color

Assessment

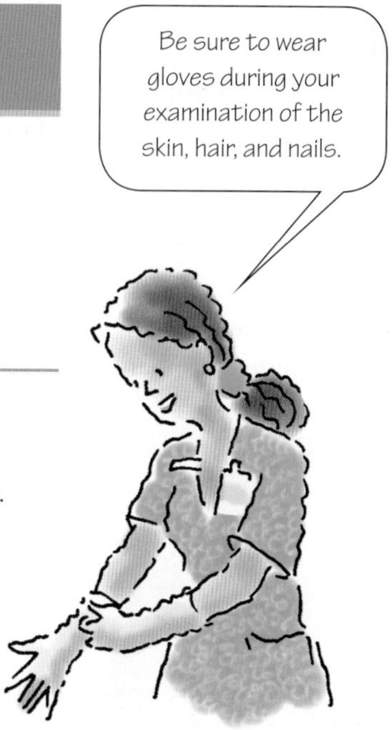
Be sure to wear gloves during your examination of the skin, hair, and nails.

To assess the skin, hair, and nails, use inspection and palpation.

Skin

Observe the skin's overall appearance. Then inspect and palpate the skin area by area, focusing on color, moisture, texture, turgor, and temperature. Look for areas of damage to the skin. Skin that splits or cracks easily increases the chance of **infection!**

Color

Look for localized areas of bruising, cyanosis, pallor, and erythema. Check for uniformity of color and hypopigmented or hyperpigmented areas.

Detecting color variations in dark-skinned people

Cyanosis	Edema	Erythema	Jaundice	Pallor	Petechiae	Rashes
Examine the conjunctivae, palms, soles, buccal mucosa, and tongue. Look for dull, dark, bluish color.	Examine the area for decreased color and palpate for tightness.	Palpate the area for redness and/or warmth.	Examine the sclerae and hard palate in natural, not fluorescent, light if possible. Look for a yellow color.	Examine the sclerae, conjunctivae, buccal mucosa, lips, tongue, nail beds, palms, and soles. Look for an ashen, grayish blue color.	Examine areas of lighter pigmentation such as the abdomen. Look for tiny, purplish red dots.	Palpate the area for skin texture changes.

Moisture

Observe the skin's moisture content. The skin should be relatively dry, with a minimal amount of perspiration.

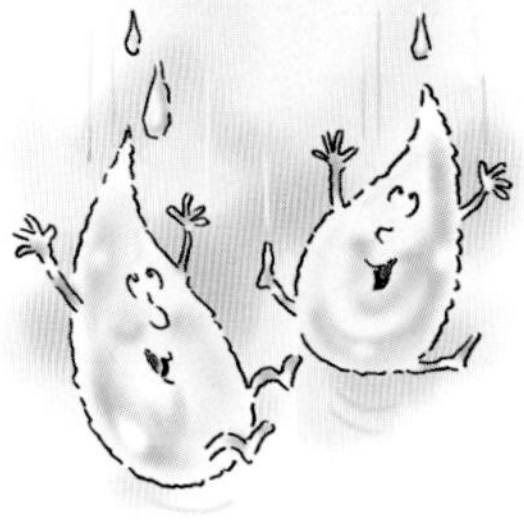

Texture and turgor

Inspect and palpate the skin's texture, noting its thickness and mobility. It should look smooth and be intact.

Skill check

Assessing skin turgor in an adult

Gently squeeze the skin on the forearm or sternal area between your thumb and forefinger, as shown. Due to the decreased elasticity of the skin with age, the best place to check the older adult is the sternal area.

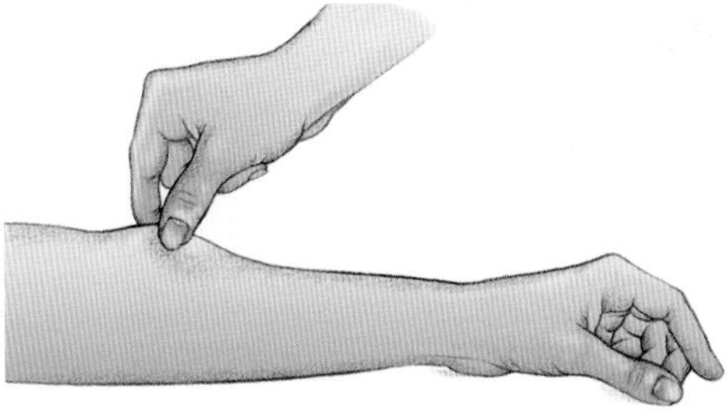

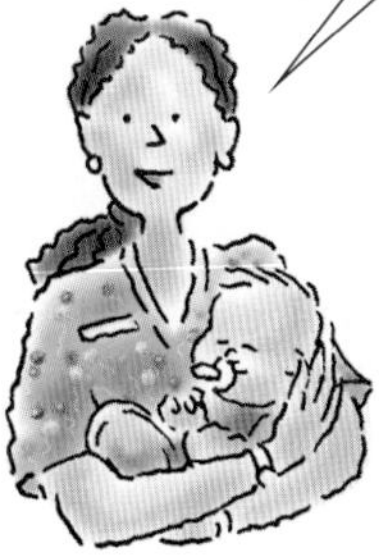
To assess skin turgor in an infant, grasp a fold of loosely adherent abdominal skin between your thumb and forefinger and pull the skin taut. Then release the skin. The skin should quickly return to its normal position. If the skin remains tented, the infant has poor turgor.

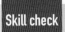

If the skin quickly returns to its original shape, the patient has normal turgor. If it returns to its original shape slowly over 30 seconds or maintains a tented position, as shown, the skin has poor turgor.

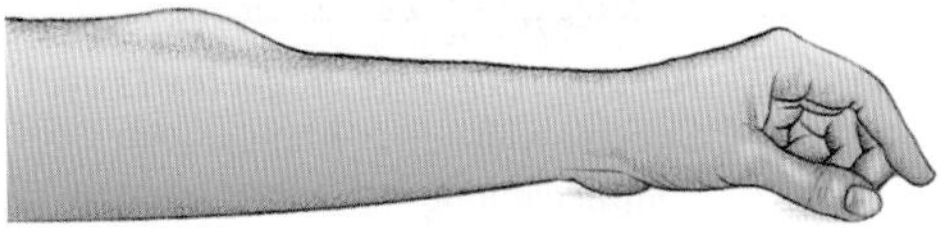

Temperature

Palpate the skin bilaterally for temperature using the dorsal surface of your hands and fingers. The dorsal surface is the most sensitive to temperature changes. Warm skin suggests normal circulation; cool skin suggests a possible underlying disorder.

Normal skin variations

You may see normal variations in the skin's texture and pigmentation. Such variations may include nevi, or moles, and freckles (shown below).

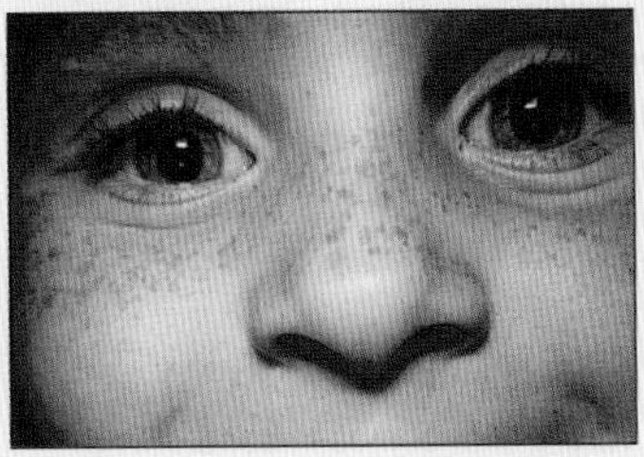

Hair

When assessing the hair, note the distribution, quantity, texture, and color. Hair should be evenly distributed.

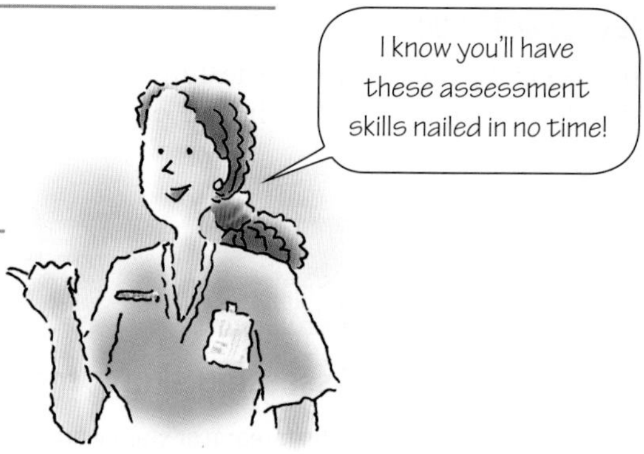
I know you'll have these assessment skills nailed in no time!

Nails

Examine the nails for color, shape, thickness, consistency, and contour. Nail color is pink in light-skinned people and brown in dark-skinned people. The nail surface should be slightly curved or flat and the edges smooth and rounded.

Skin abnormalities

Lesions

When evaluating a lesion, you'll need to classify it as primary (new) or secondary (a change in a primary lesion). Then determine if it's solid or fluid filled and describe its characteristics, pattern, location, and distribution. Include a description of symmetry, borders, color, configuration, diameter, and drainage.

Lesion shapes

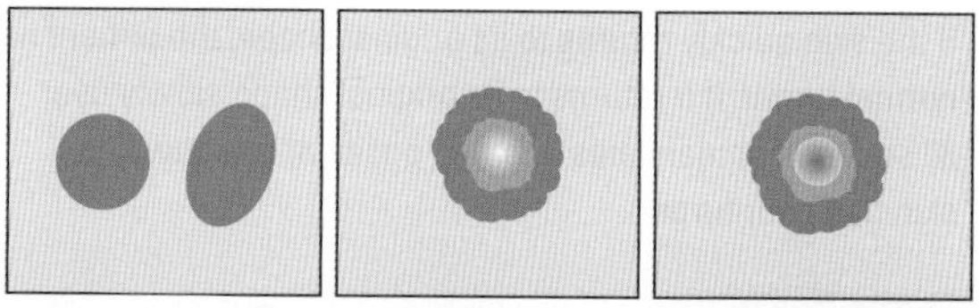

Discoid
Round or oval

Annular
Circular with central clearing

Target (bull's eye)
Annular with central internal activity

Lesion distribution

Generalized—Distributed all over the body
Regionalized—Limited to one area of the body
Localized—Sharply limited to a specific area
Scattered—Dispersed either densely or widely
Exposed areas—Limited to areas exposed to the air or sun
Intertriginous—Limited to areas where skin comes in contact with itself

Lesion configurations

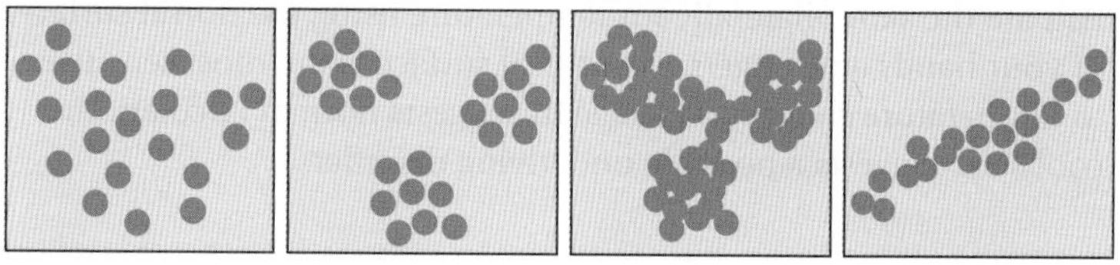

Discrete
Individual lesions are separate and distinct.

Grouped
Lesions are clustered together.

Confluent
Lesions merge so that discrete lesions are not visible or palpable.

Dermatomal
Lesions form a line or an arch and follow a dermatome.

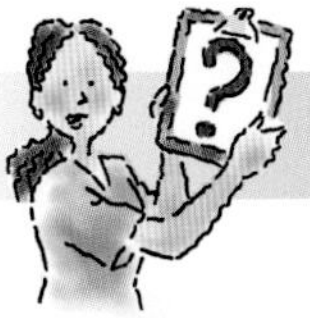

Outside the norm

Types of skin lesions

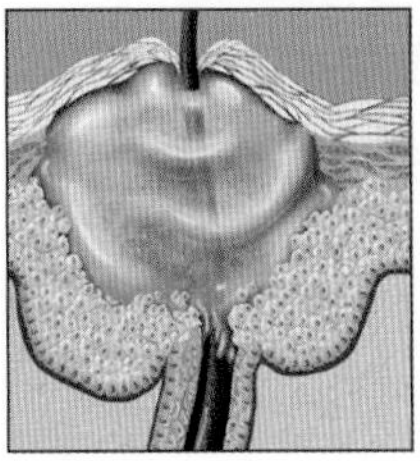

Pustule
A small, pus-filled lesion (called a *follicular pustule* if it contains a hair)

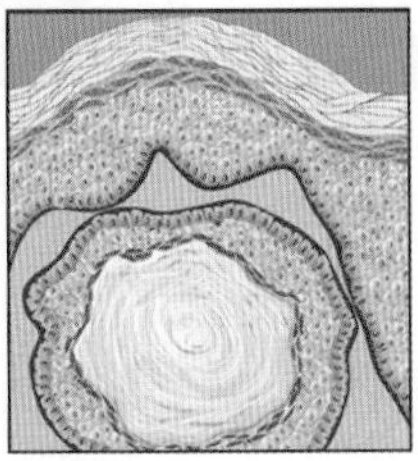

Cyst
A closed sac in or under the skin that contains fluid or semisolid material

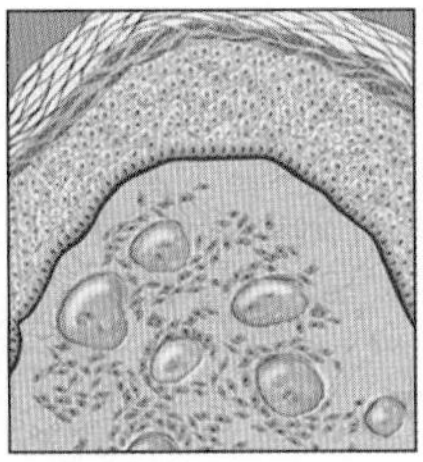

Nodule
A raised lesion detectable by touch that's usually 1 cm or more in diameter

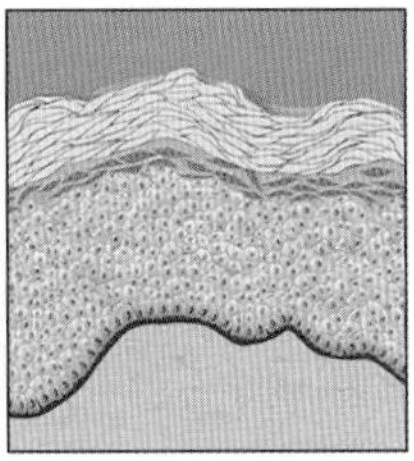

Wheal
A raised, reddish area that's commonly itchy and lasts 24 hours or less

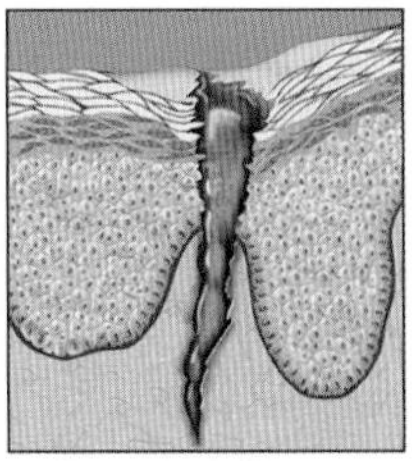

Fissure
A painful, cracklike lesion of the skin that extends at least into the dermis

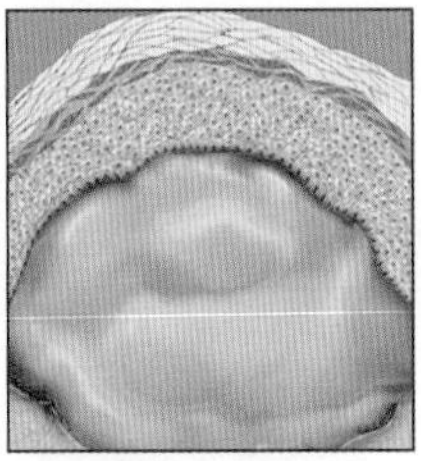

Bulla
A large, fluid-filled blister that's usually 1 cm or more in diameter

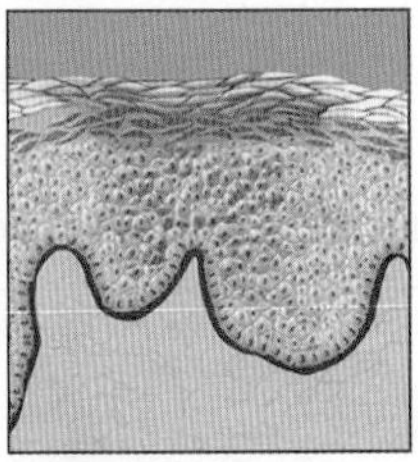

Macule
A small, discolored spot or patch on the skin

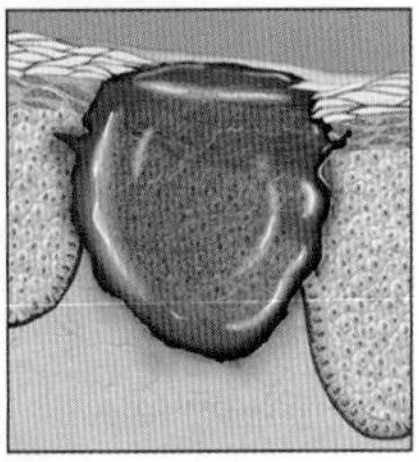

Ulcer
A crater-like lesion of the skin that usually extends at least into the dermis

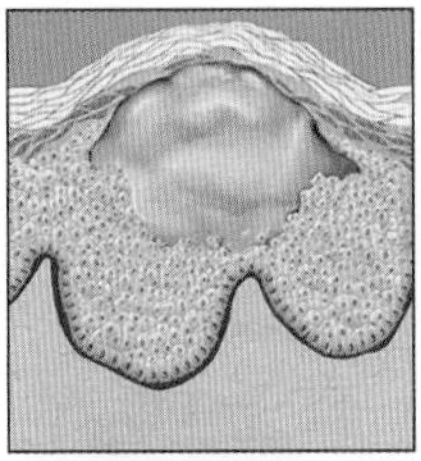

Vesicle
A small, fluid-filled blister that's usually 1 cm or less in diameter

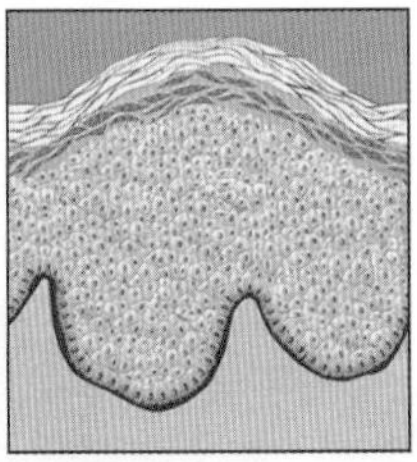

Papule
A solid, raised lesion that's usually less than 1 cm in diameter

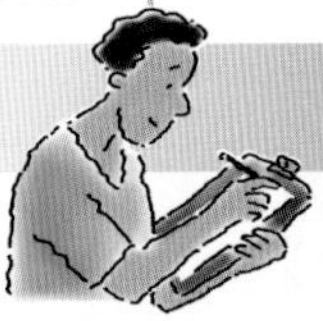

Take note

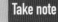

Documenting a skin lesion

4/15/10	0845	At 0820, pt. c/o right shoulder
		blade pain, 4/10 on a 0–10 scale.
		A closed, purulent lesion noted
		in right upper scapular region of
		back, approx. 1.5 cm x 1 cm, with
		3 cm surrounding area of ery-
		thema. T 100.28 F. Call placed to
		Dr. Tomlin's service at 0830.
		Angela Kessler, RN

Benign versus cancerous lesions

Lesions may be benign, such as a benign nevus, or mole. However, changes in an existing growth on the skin or a new growth that ulcerates or doesn't heal could indicate cancer or a precancerous lesion.

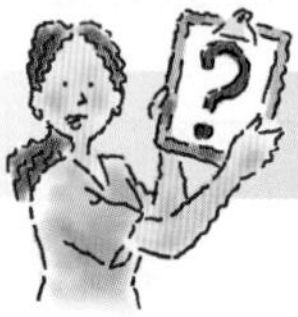

Outside the norm

Types of skin cancer

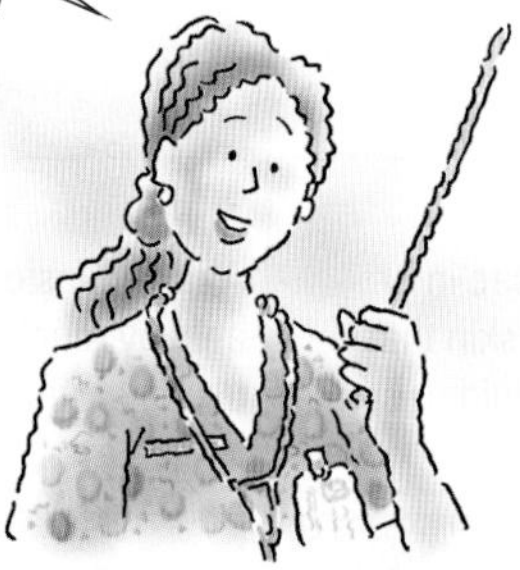
Note the differences between benign and cancerous lesions.

Benign nevus

- Symmetrical, round, or oval shape
- Sharply defined borders
- Uniform, usually tan or brown color
- Less than 6 mm in diameter
- Flat or raised

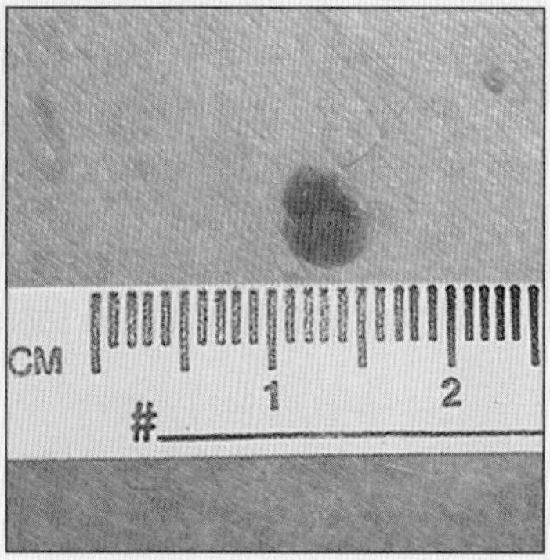
CM
1
2
#

Precancerous actinic keratosis

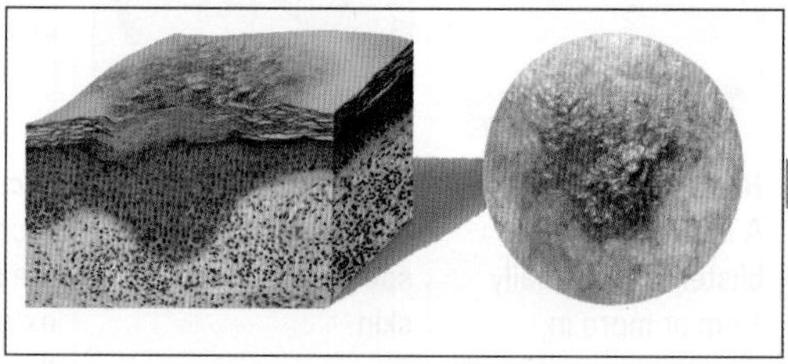

- Abnormal changes in keratinocytes
- Can become squamous cell carcinoma

Dysplastic nevus

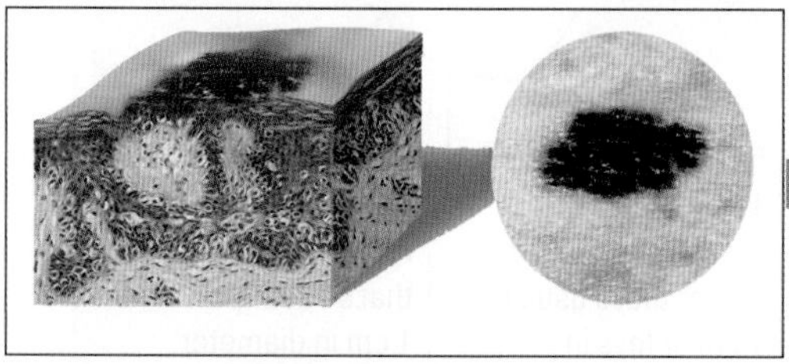

- Abnormal growth of melanocytes in a mole
- Can become malignant melanoma

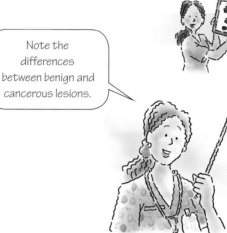

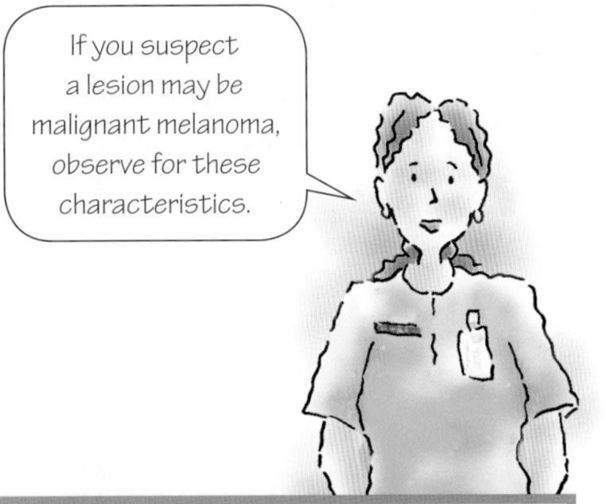
If you suspect a lesion may be malignant melanoma, observe for these characteristics.

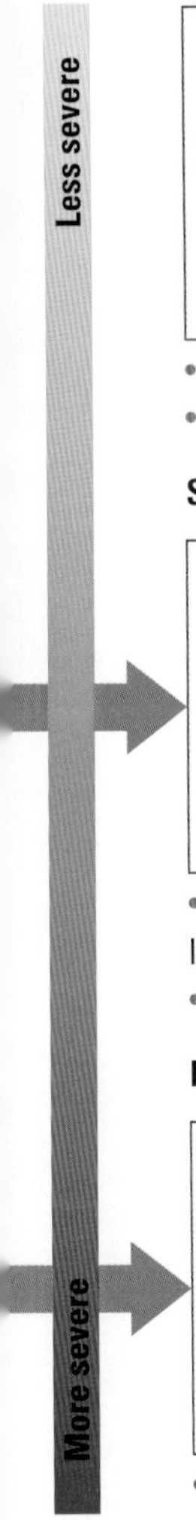
Less severe
More severe

Basal cell carcinoma

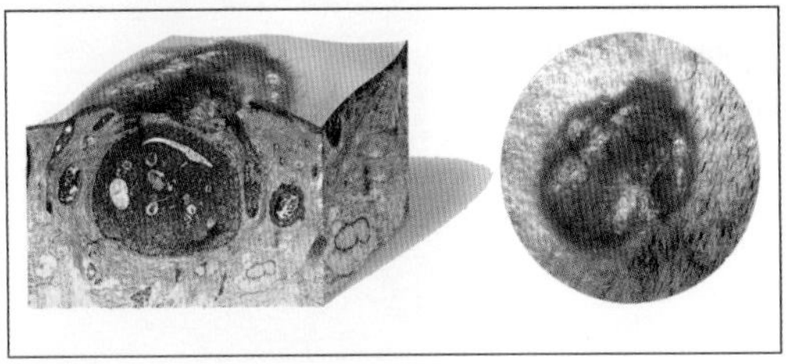

- Most common skin cancer
- Usually spreads only locally

Squamous cell carcinoma

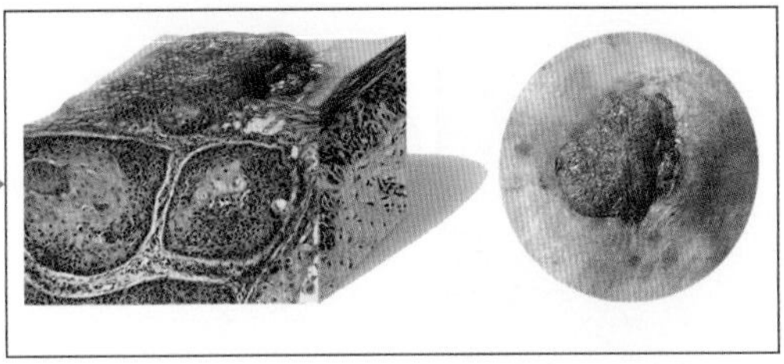

- Begins as a firm, red nodule or scaly, crusted, flat lesion
- Can spread if not treated

Malignant melanoma

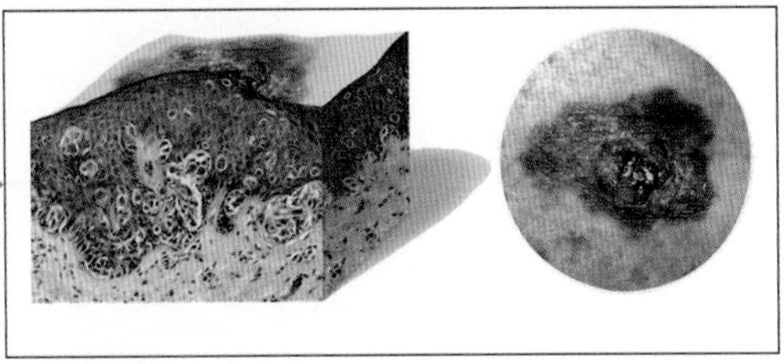

- Can arise on normal skin or from an existing mole
- If not treated promptly, can spread to other areas of skin, lymph nodes, or internal organs

memory board

ABCDEs of malignant melanoma

A = Asymmetrical lesion

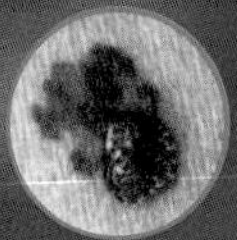

B = Border irregular

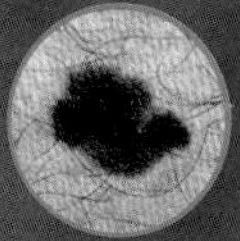

C = Color of lesion varies with shades of tan, brown, or black and, possibly, red, blue, or white

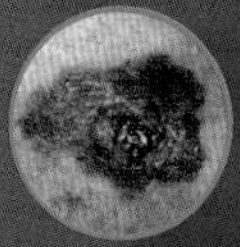

D = Diameter greater than 6 mm

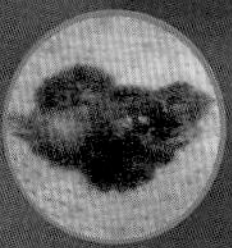

E = Elevated or enlarging lesion

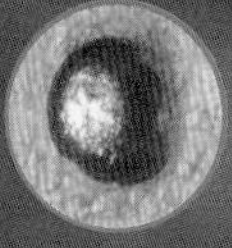

Common skin disorders

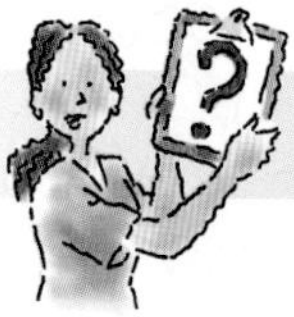
?

Outside the norm

Psoriasis

Psoriasis is a chronic disease of marked epidermal thickening. Plaques are symmetrical and generally appear as red bases topped with silvery scales. The lesions, which may connect with one another, occur most commonly on the scalp, elbows, and knees.

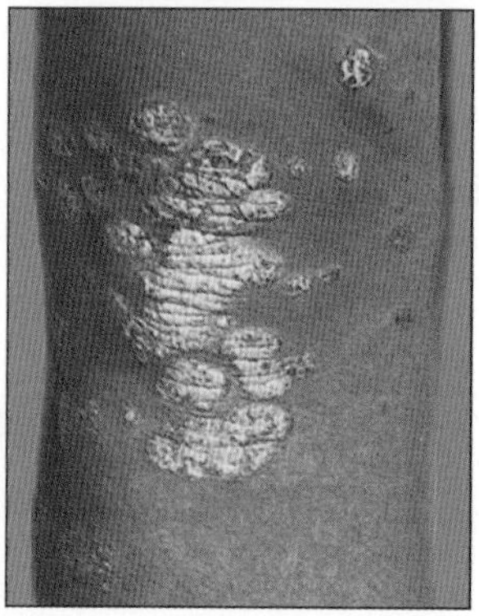

Contact dermatitis

Contact dermatitis is an inflammatory disorder that results from contact with an irritant. Primary lesions include vesicles, large oozing bullae, and red macules that appear at localized areas of redness. These lesions may itch and burn.

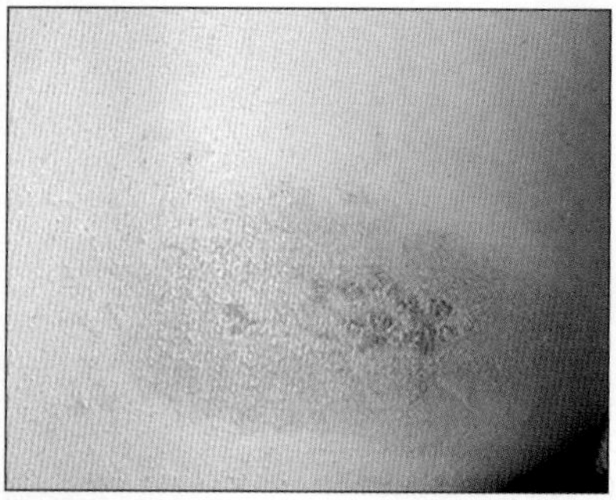

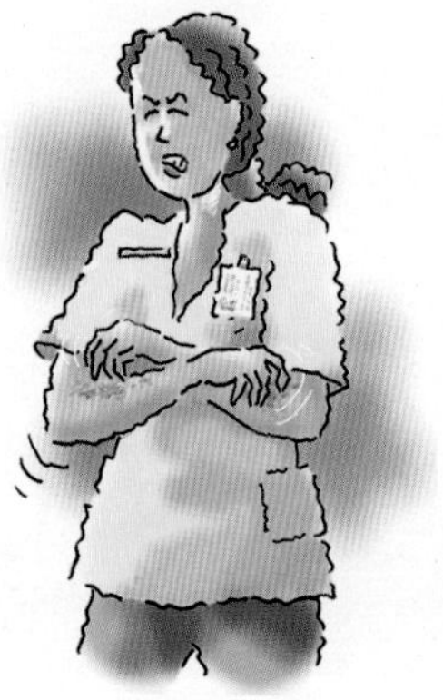

Urticaria (hives)

Occurring as an allergic reaction, urticaria appears suddenly as pink, edematous papules or wheals (round elevations of the skin). Itching is intense. The lesions may become large and contain vesicles.

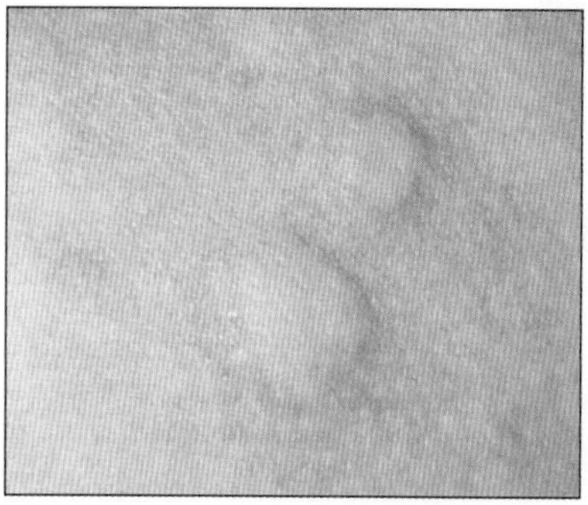

Herpes zoster

Herpes zoster appears as a group of vesicles or crusted lesions along a nerve root. The vesicles are usually unilateral and appear mostly on the trunk. These lesions cause pain but not a rash.

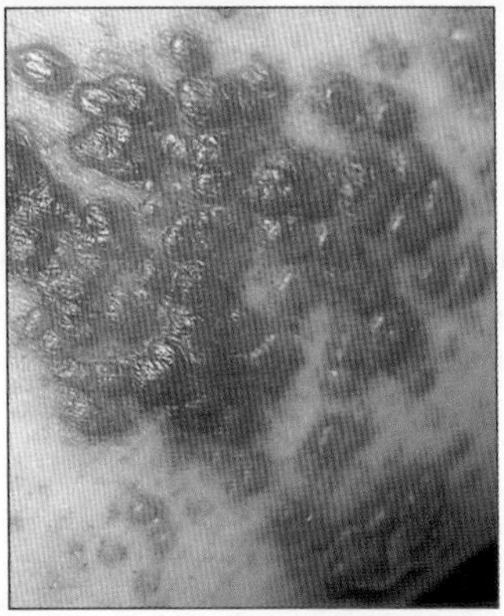

Scabies

Mites, which can be picked up from an infested person, burrow under the skin and cause scabies lesions. The lesions appear in a straight or zigzagging line about 3/8" (1 cm) long with a black dot at the end. Commonly seen between the fingers, at the bend of the elbow and knee, and around the groin, abdomen, or perineal area, scabies lesions itch and may cause a rash.

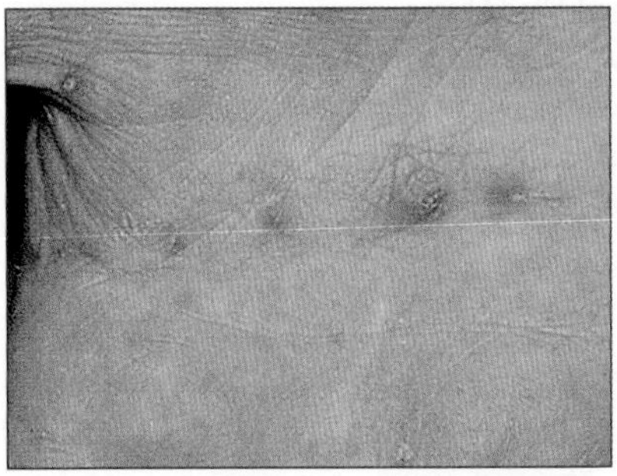

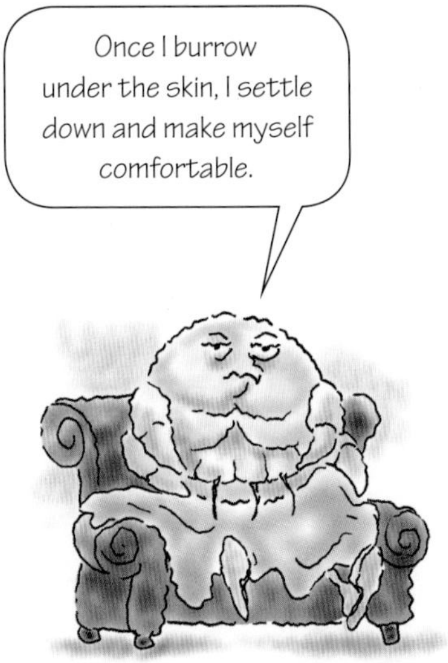
Once I burrow under the skin, I settle down and make myself comfortable.

Tinea corporis (ringworm)

Tinea corporis is characterized by round, red, scaly lesions that are accompanied by intense itching. These lesions have slightly raised, red borders consisting of tiny vesicles. Individual rings may connect to form patches with scalloped edges. They usually appear on exposed areas of the body.

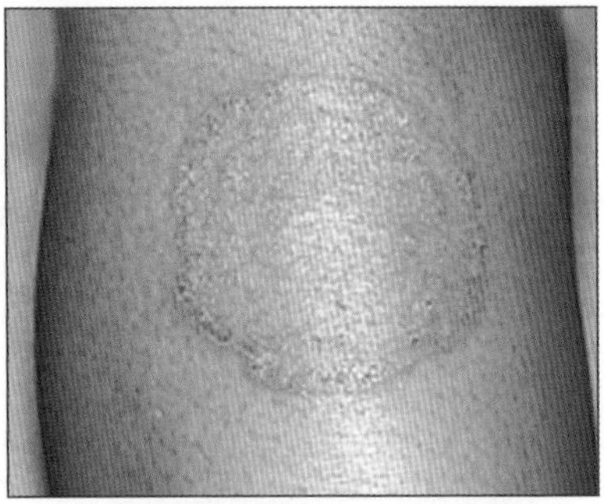

Pressure ulcers

Pressure ulcers are localized areas of skin breakdown that occur as a result of prolonged pressure. Necrotic tissue develops because the vascular supply to the area is diminished.

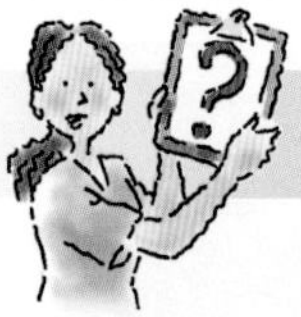

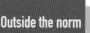

Outside the norm

Staging pressure ulcers

You can use characteristics gained from your assessment to stage a pressure ulcer, as described here. Staging reflects the anatomic depth of exposed tissue. Keep in mind that if the wound contains necrotic tissue, you won't be able to determine the stage until you can see the wound base.

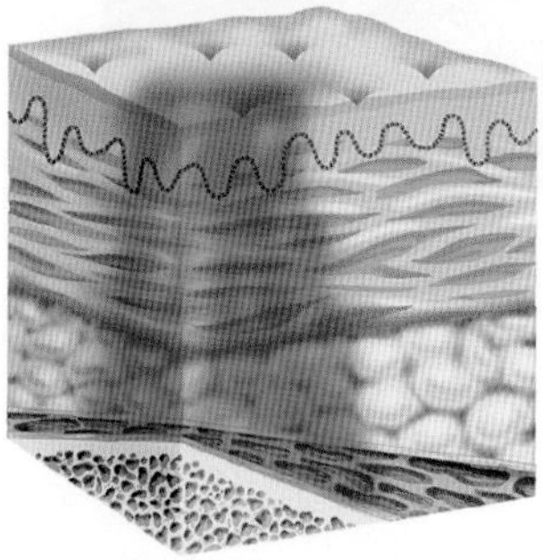

Suspected deep tissue injury

- Maroon or purple intact skin or blood-filled blister
- May be painful; mushy, firm, or boggy; and warmer or cooler than other tissue before discoloration occurs

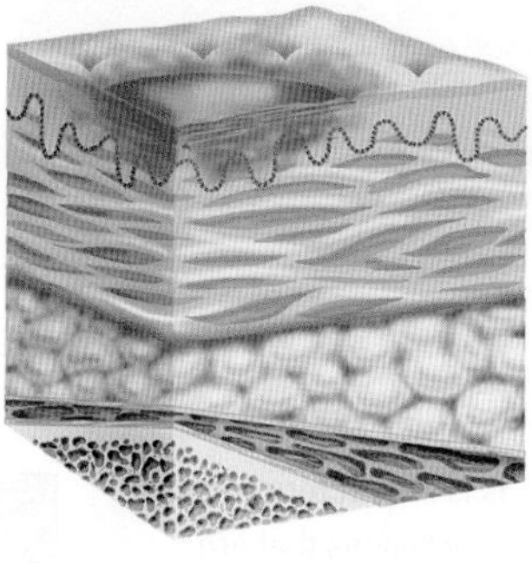

Stage I

- Intact skin that doesn't blanch
- May differ in color from surrounding area in people with darkly pigmented skin
- Usually over a bony prominence
- May be painful, firm or soft, and warmer or cooler than surrounding tissue

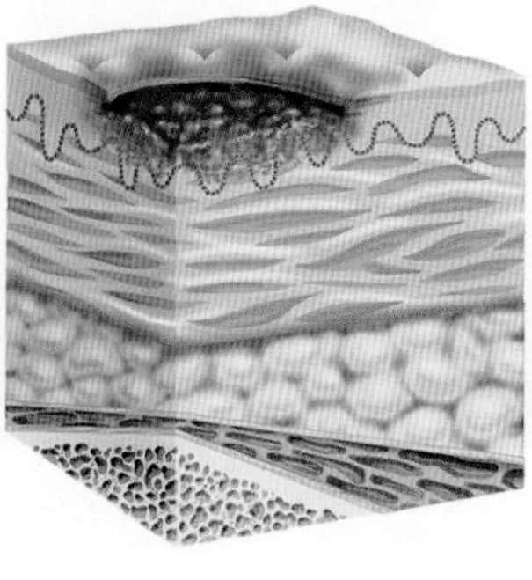

Stage II

- Superficial partial-thickness wound
- Presents as a shallow, open ulcer without slough and with a red and pink wound bed

Note: This stage shouldn't be used to describe perineal dermatitis, maceration, tape burns, skin tears, or excoriation.

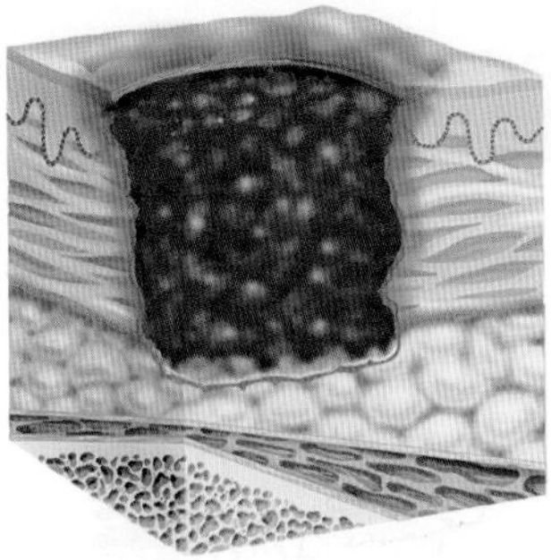

Stage III
- Involves full-thickness wound with tissue loss and possibly visible subcutaneous tissue but no exposed muscle, tendon, or bone
- May have slough but not enough to hide the depth of tissue loss
- May be accompanied by undermining and tunneling

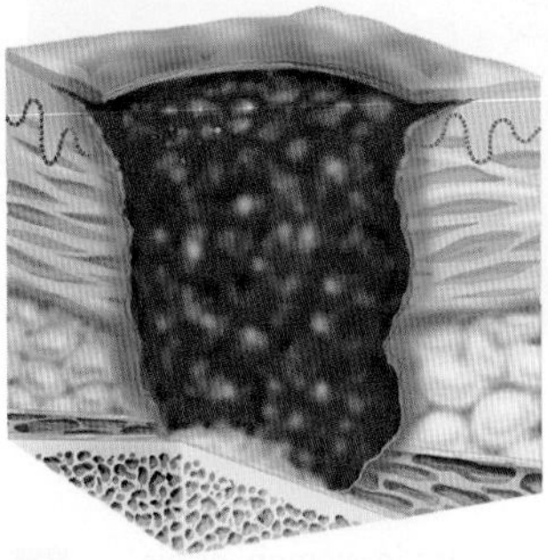

Stage IV
- Involves full-thickness skin loss, with exposed muscle, bone, and tendon
- May be accompanied by eschar, slough, undermining, and tunneling

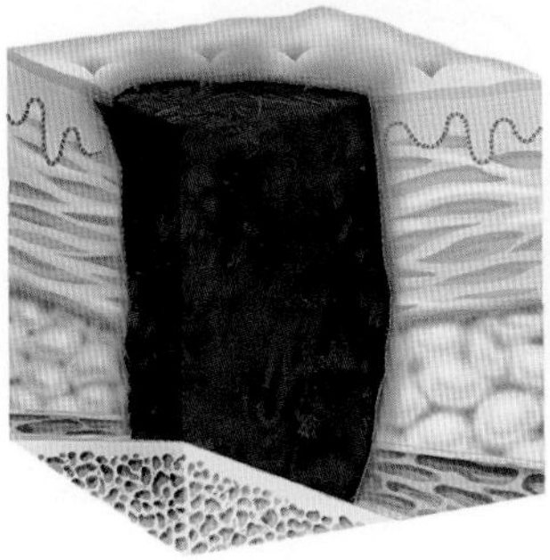

Unstageable
- Involves full-thickness tissue loss, with base of ulcer covered by slough and yellow, tan, gray, green, or brown eschar
- Can't be staged until enough slough and eschar are removed to expose the wound base

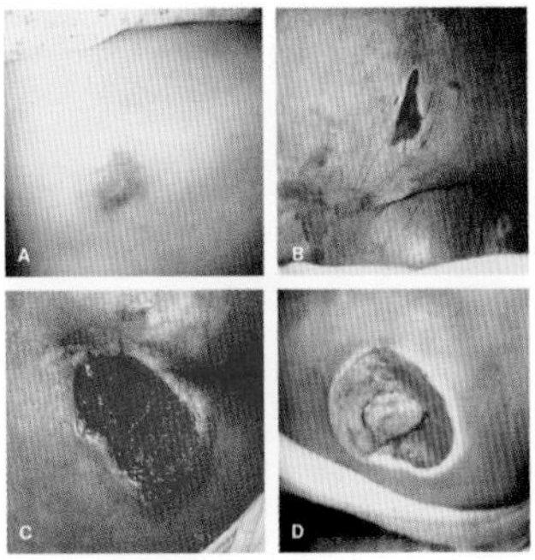
A
B
C
D

Hair abnormalities

Typically stemming from other problems, hair abnormalities can cause patients emotional distress. Among the most common hair abnormalities are alopecia and hirsutism.

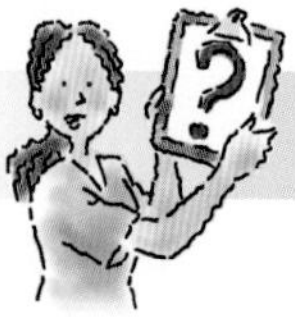

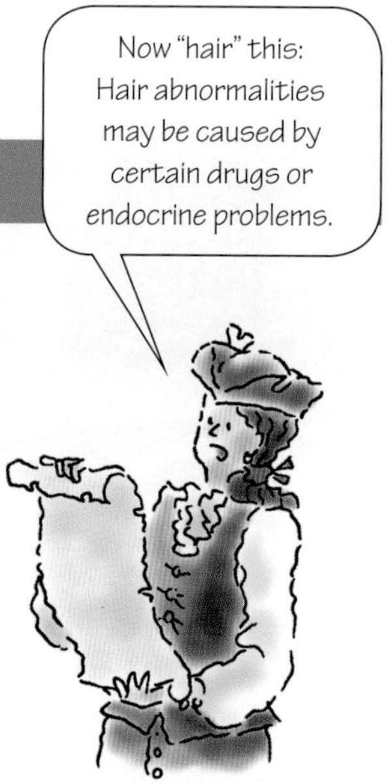
Now "hair" this: Hair abnormalities may be caused by certain drugs or endocrine problems.

Outside the norm

Alopecia

Alopecia occurs more commonly and extensively in men than in women. Diffuse hair loss, though commonly a normal part of aging, may occur as a result of pyogenic infections, chemical trauma, ingestion of certain drugs, and endocrinopathy and other disorders. Tinea capitis, trauma, and full-thickness burns can cause patchy hair loss.

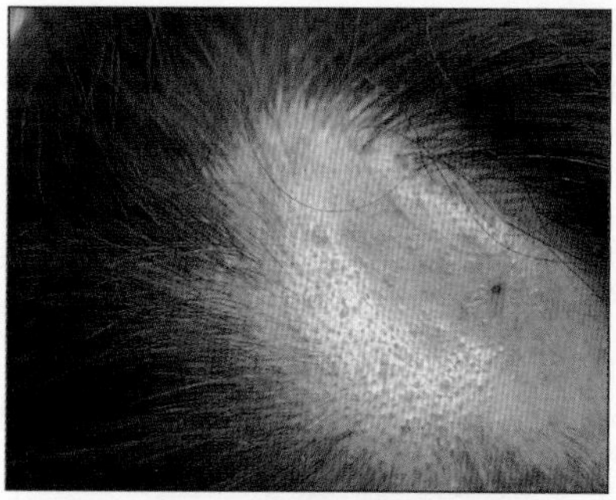

Hirsutism

Excessive hairiness in women, or hirsutism, can develop on the body and face, affecting the patient's self-image. Localized hirsutism may occur on pigmented nevi. Generalized hirsutism can result from certain drug therapy or from such endocrine problems as Cushing syndrome, polycystic ovary syndrome, and acromegaly.

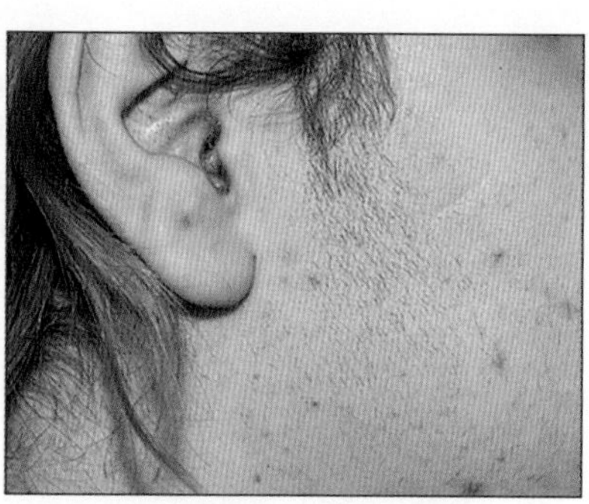

Nail abnormalities

Although many nail abnormalities are harmless, some point to serious underlying problems. Nail abnormalities include clubbed fingers, splinter hemorrhages of the nail bed, and Muehrcke lines.

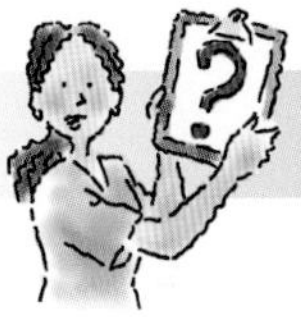

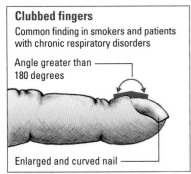

Outside the norm

Clubbed fingers

Clubbed fingers can result from chronic tissue hypoxia. Normally, the angle between the fingernail and the point where the nail enters the skin is about 160 degrees. Clubbing occurs when that angle increases to 180 degrees or more.

Normal fingers

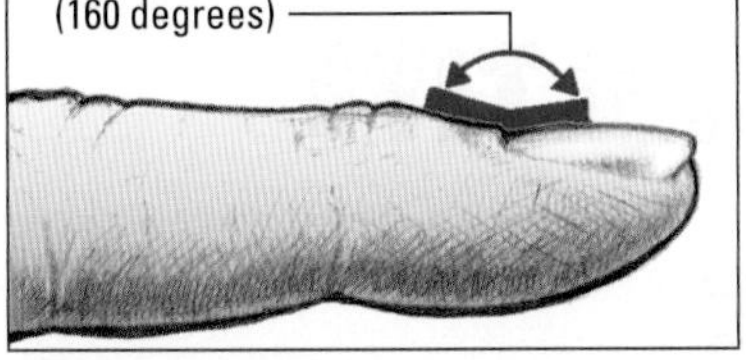
Normal angle
(160 degrees)

Clubbed fingers

Common finding in smokers and patients with chronic respiratory disorders

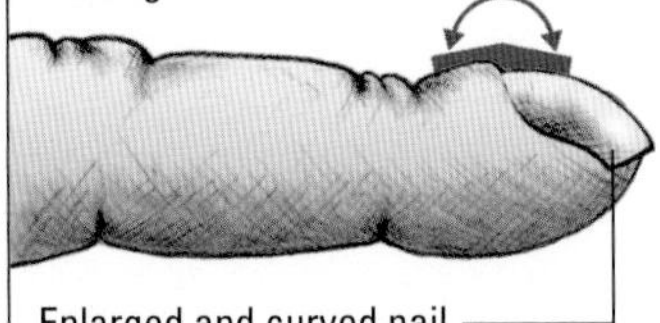
Angle greater than
180 degrees
Enlarged and curved nail

Splinter hemorrhages

Splinter hemorrhages are reddish brown narrow streaks under the nails. They run in the same direction as nail growth and are caused by minor trauma. They can also occur in patients with bacterial endocarditis.

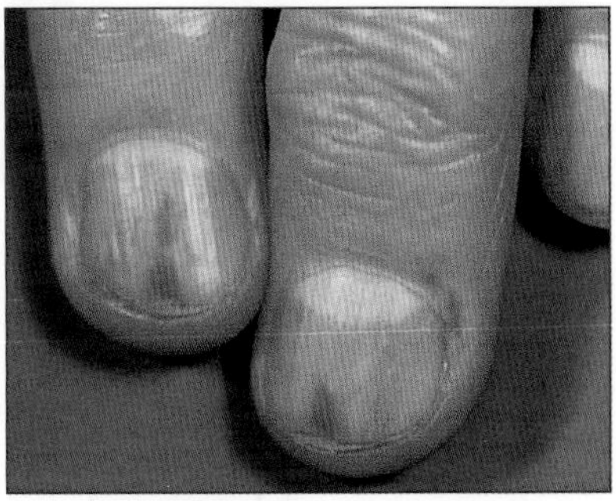

Muehrcke lines

Muehrcke lines or leukonychia striata are longitudinal white lines that can indicate trauma but may also be associated with metabolic stress, which impairs the body from using protein.

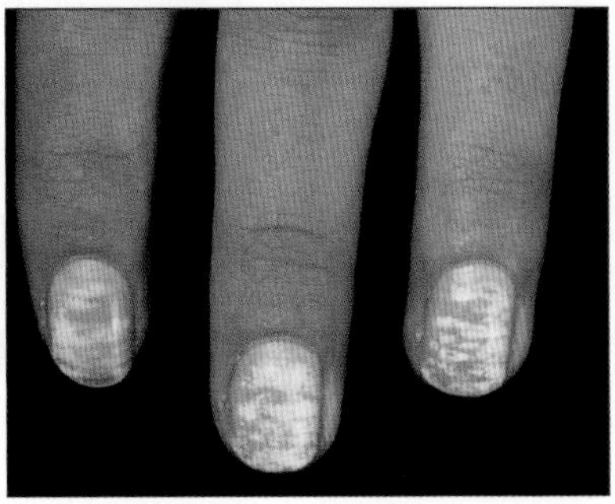

Q&A

Able to label?

Identify the skin structures indicated on this illustration.

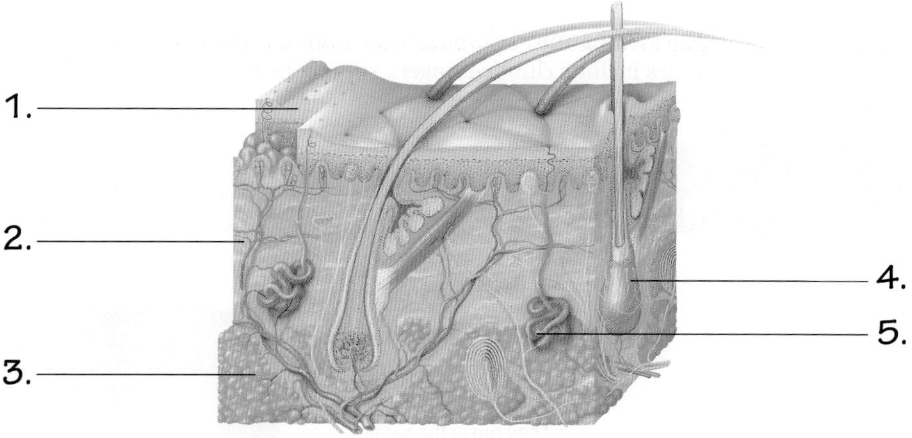
1.
2.
3.
4.
5.

Rebus riddle

Sound out each group of pictures and symbols to reveal terms that complete this assessment consideration.

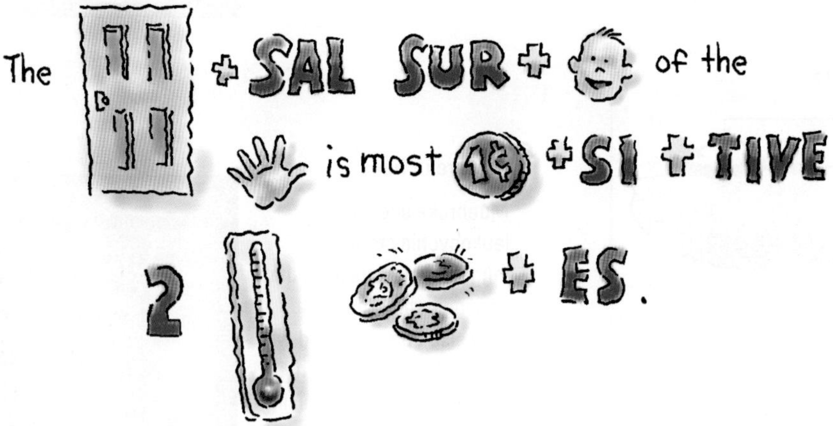
The
+ SAL SUR +
of the
is most
+ SI + TIVE
2
+ ES.

Test your knowledge!

Match the term in the left column with its definition in the right column. Each letter can only be used once.

____Jaundice	A. Paleness, absence of color
____Erythema	B. Yellowish appearance of the skin
____Cyanosis	C. Redness of the skin
____Pallor	D. Grayish blue tone

1. Which of the following lesion characteristics indicates the need for further assessment?
   A. Round shape with distinct borders
   B. Bleeds easily
   C. Light brown in color
   D. Nonpalpable

2. Assessment of the older adult reveals significant tenting of the skin over his forearm. Which of the following explains this finding?
   A. Loss of adipose tissue and elasticity
   B. Parchment-like skin
   C. Significant flaking and dryness
   D. Skin tags

Answers: Able to label 1. Epidermis, 2. Dermis, 3. Subcutaneous tissue, 4. Hair bulb, 5. Eccrine sweat gland; Rebus riddle The dorsal surface of the hand is most sensitive to temperature changes; Matching B, C, D, A; Multiple choice 1. B 2. A

Selected References

Agency for Healthcare Research and Quality (US). (2013). *Making healthcare safer II: An updated critical analysis of the evidence for patient safety practices (Evidence Reports/Technology Assessments, No. 211)*. Rockville, MD: Agency for Healthcare Research and Quality.

Bale, T. (2010). Disorders of the scalp. *Practice Nurse, 40*. Retrieved from http://web.a.ebscohost.com/detaiol/detail?sid=80dd2523-cded-48

Bardsley, A. (July 3, 2013). Prevention and management of incontinence-associated dermatitis. *Nursing Standard, 27*, 41–46.

Pontius, D. (2014). Demystifying pediculosis: School nurses taking the lead. *Pediatric Nursing, 40*, 226–235.

Sullivan, N. (2013). *Preventing in-facility pressure ulcers (Agency for Healthcare Research and Quality (US) 2013 March (Evidence Reports/Technical Assessments, No. 211))*. Rockville, MD: Agency for Healthcare Research and Quality.

Voegeli, D. (2013). Moisture-associated skin damage: An overview for community nurses. *British Journal of Community Nursing, 18(1)*, 6–12.

Watkins, J. (2014). Diagnosing rashes, part 7: Purpuric rashes. *Practice Nursing, 25*, 22–28.

Watkins, J. (2015). Looking at the diagnosis and treatment of head lice. *British Journal of School Nursing, 10*, 90–92.

Winnicki, M., & Shear, N. (2011). A systematic approach to systemic contact dermatitis and symmetric drug-related intertriginous and flexural exanthema (SDRIFE). *American Journal of Clinical Dermatology, 12*, 171–180.

Chapter 3

Eyes and ears

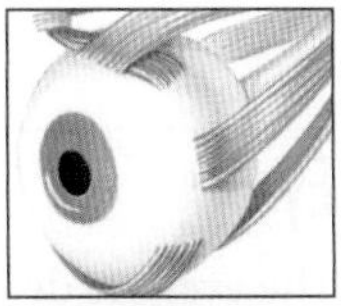

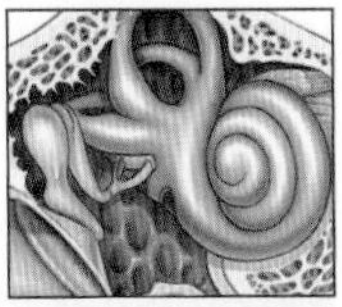

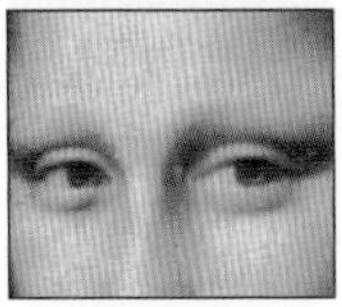

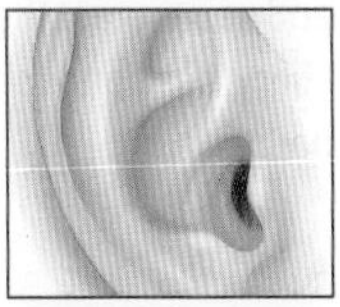

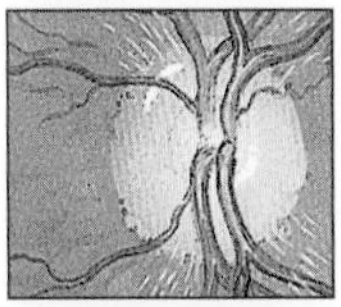

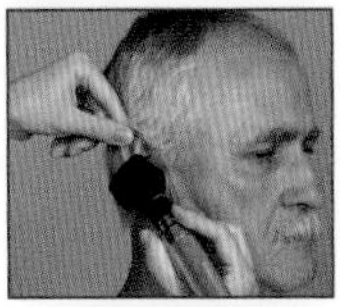

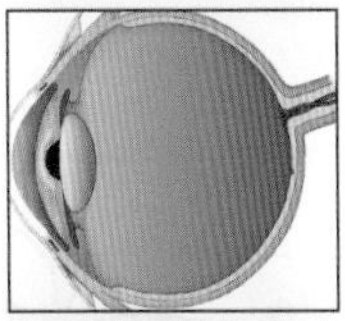

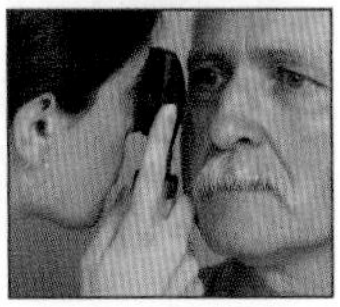

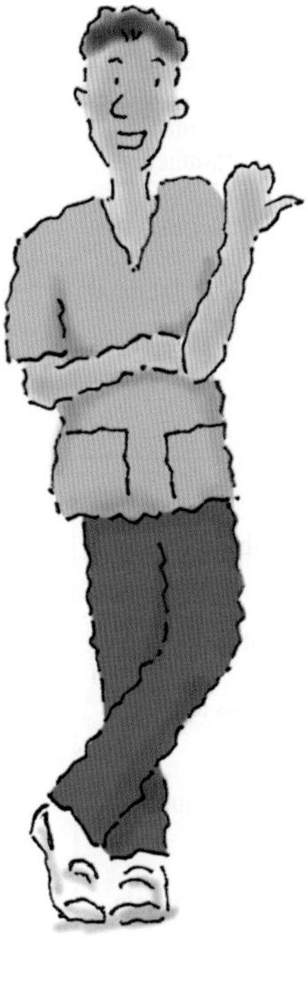

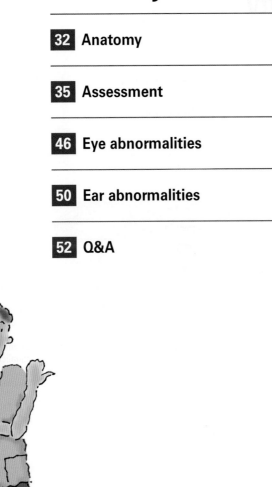

Anatomy

Eye

The eyes are delicate sensory organs equipped with many extraocular and intraocular structures. Some structures are easily visible, whereas others can only be viewed with special instruments, such as an ophthalmoscope.

Extraocular structures

The bony orbits protect the eyes from trauma. The eyelids (or palpebrae), lashes, lacrimal gland, punctum, canaliculi, and sac protect the eyes from injury, dust, and foreign bodies.

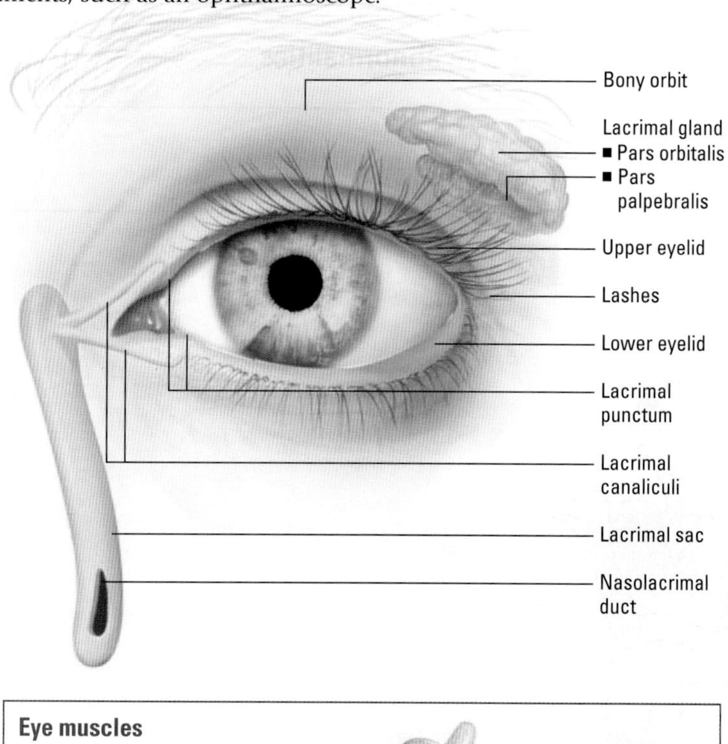
Bony orbit
Lacrimal gland
■ Pars orbitalis
■ Pars palpebralis
Upper eyelid
Lashes
Lower eyelid
Lacrimal punctum
Lacrimal canaliculi
Lacrimal sac
Nasolacrimal duct

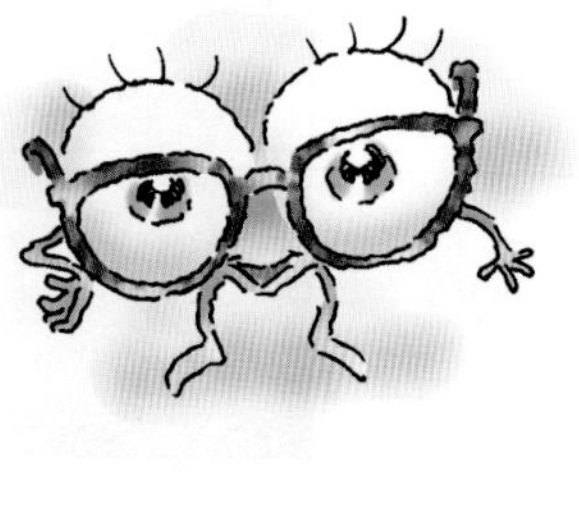

Eye muscles

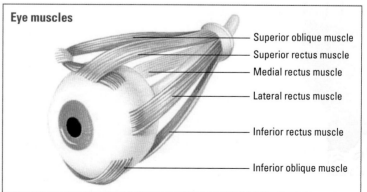

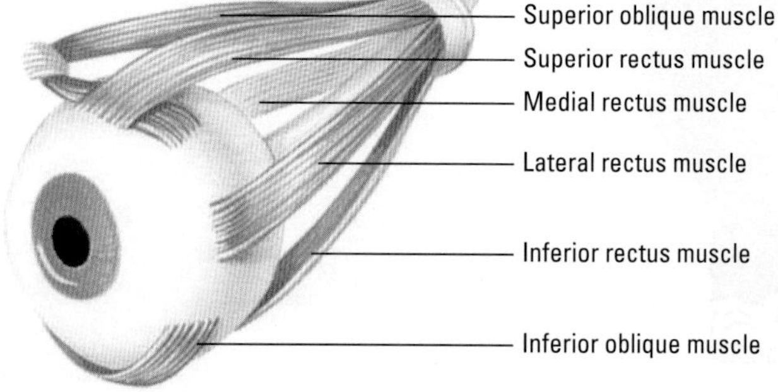
Superior oblique muscle
Superior rectus muscle
Medial rectus muscle
Lateral rectus muscle
Inferior rectus muscle
Inferior oblique muscle

Intraocular structures

The intraocular structures of the eye are directly involved in vision. The eye has three layers of tissue:

- The outermost layer includes the transparent cornea and the sclera, which maintain the form and size of the eyeball.
- The middle layer includes the choroid, ciliary body, and iris. Pupil size is controlled by involuntary muscles in this region.
- The innermost layer is the retina, which receives visual stimuli and sends them to the brain.

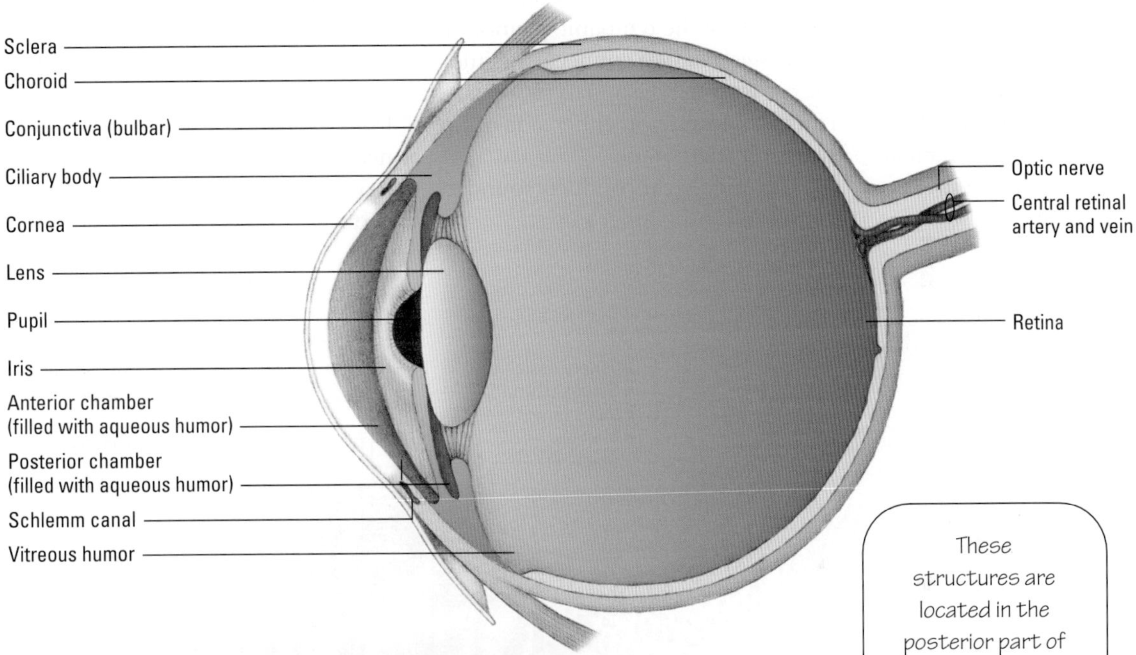
Sclera
Choroid
Conjunctiva (bulbar)
Ciliary body
Cornea
Lens
Pupil
Iris
Anterior chamber (filled with aqueous humor)
Posterior chamber (filled with aqueous humor)
Schlemm canal
Vitreous humor
Optic nerve
Central retinal artery and vein
Retina

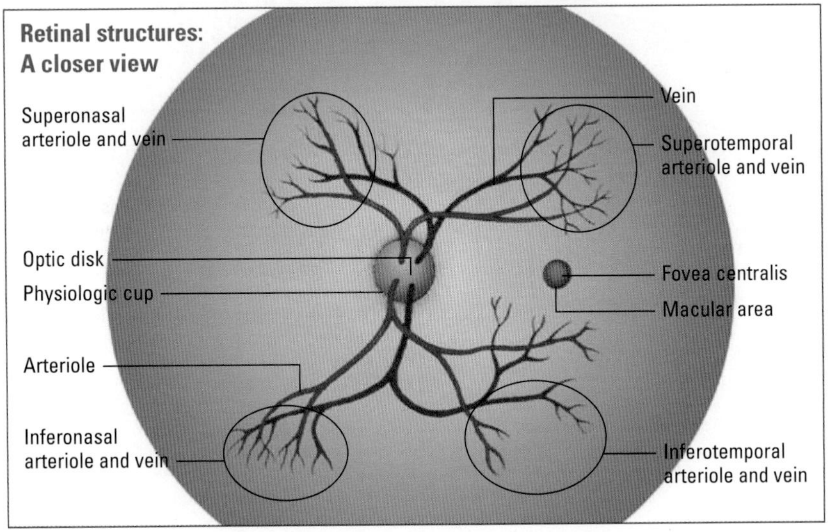
Retinal structures: A closer view
Superonasal arteriole and vein
Vein
Superotemporal arteriole and vein
Optic disk
Physiologic cup
Fovea centralis
Macular area
Arteriole
Inferonasal arteriole and vein
Inferotemporal arteriole and vein

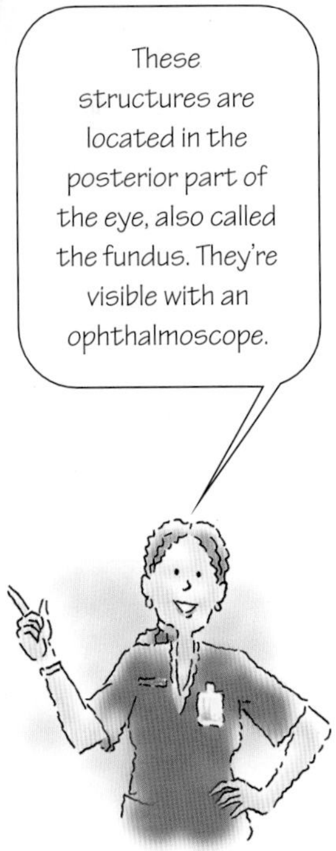
These structures are located in the posterior part of the eye, also called the fundus. They're visible with an ophthalmoscope.

Ear

External ear

The flexible external ear consists mainly of elastic cartilage. It contains the ear flap, also known as the *auricle* or *pinna*, and the auditory canal.

This part of the ear collects and transmits sound to the middle ear.

Middle ear

The *tympanic membrane* separates the external and middle ear. The center, or umbo, is attached to the tip of the long process of the *malleus* on the other side of the tympanic membrane. The *eustachian tube* connects the middle ear with the nasopharynx, equalizing air pressure on either side of the tympanic membrane.

The middle ear conducts sound vibrations to the inner ear.

Inner ear

The *inner ear* consists of closed, fluid-filled spaces within the temporal bone. It contains the bony labyrinth, which includes three connected structures: the *vestibule*, the *semicircular canals*, and the *cochlea*.

The inner ear receives vibrations from the middle ear that stimulate nerve impulses. These impulses travel to the brain, and the cerebral cortex interprets the sound.

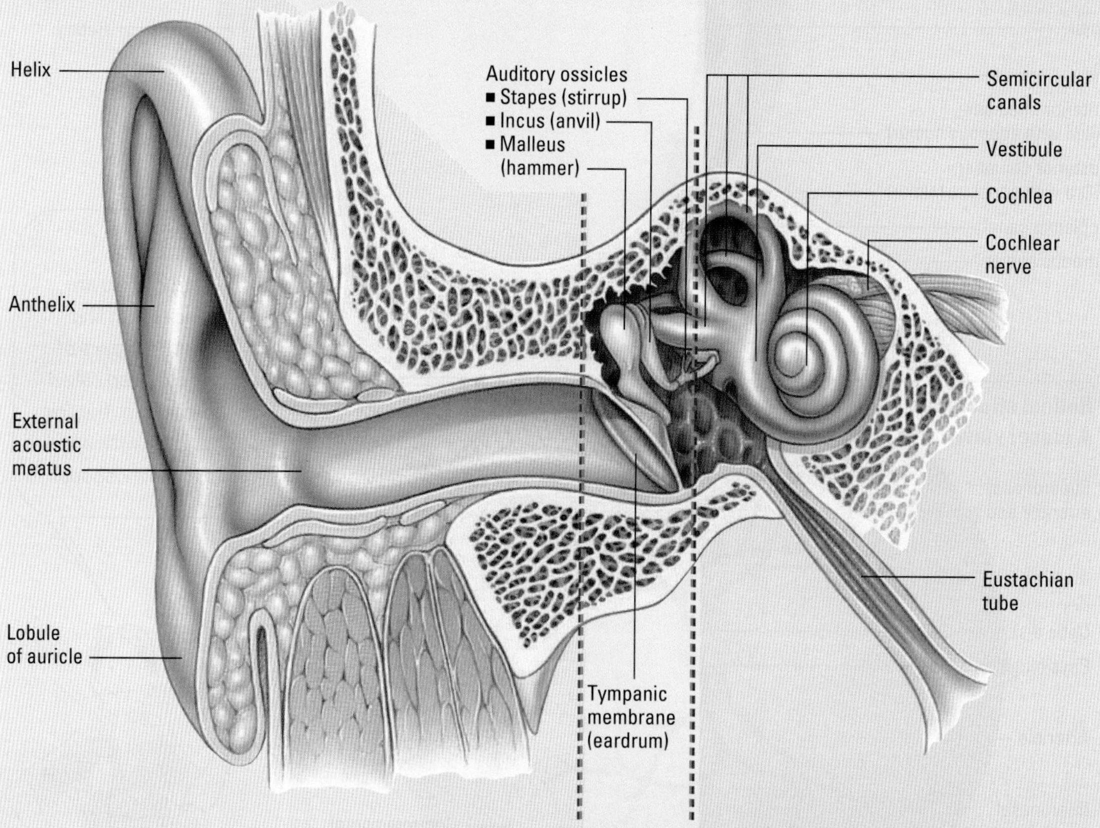
Helix
Anthelix
External acoustic meatus
Lobule of auricle
Auditory ossicles
■ Stapes (stirrup)
■ Incus (anvil)
■ Malleus (hammer)
Tympanic membrane (eardrum)
Semicircular canals
Vestibule
Cochlea
Cochlear nerve
Eustachian tube

Assessment

Eyes

Distance vision

To measure distance vision:

1. Have the patient sit or stand 20′ (6.1 m) from the chart.
2. Cover the left eye with an opaque object.
3. Ask the patient to read the letters on one line of the chart and then to move downward to increasingly smaller lines until he or she can no longer discern all of the letters.
4. Have the patient repeat the test covering the right eye.
5. Have the patient read the smallest line he or she can read with both eyes uncovered to test the binocular vision.
6. If the patient wears corrective lenses, have the patient repeat the test wearing them.
7. Record the vision with and without correction.

Snellen charts

The Snellen alphabet chart and the Snellen E chart are used to test distance vision and measure visual acuity.

Snellen alphabet chart

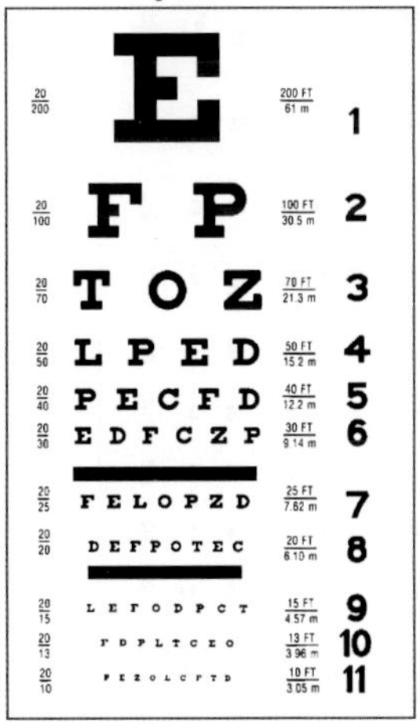
20/200 E 200 FT 61 m 1
20/100 F P 100 FT 30.5 m 2
20/70 T O Z 70 FT 21.3 m 3
20/50 L P E D 50 FT 15.2 m 4
20/40 P E C F D 40 FT 12.2 m 5
20/30 E D F C Z P 30 FT 9.14 m 6
20/25 F E L O P Z D 25 FT 7.62 m 7
20/20 D E F P O T E C 20 FT 6.10 m 8
20/15 L E F O D P C T 15 FT 4.57 m 9
20/13 F D P L T C E O 13 FT 3.96 m 10
20/10 P E Z O L C F T D 10 FT 3.05 m 11

Snellen E chart

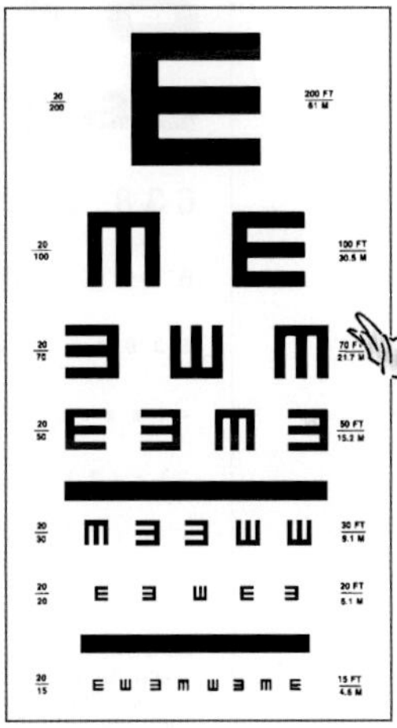

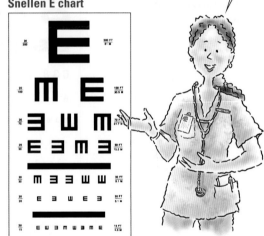

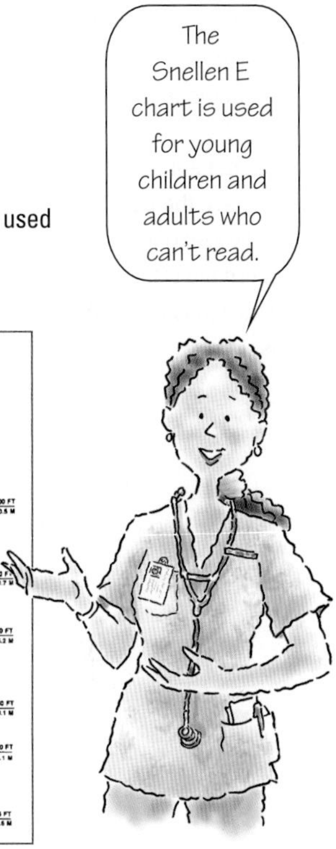
The Snellen E chart is used for young children and adults who can't read.

Recording results

Visual acuity is recorded as a fraction. The top number (20) is the distance between the patient and the chart. The line for which two or fewer letters are missed is recorded as the visual acuity (20/20 is normal). The first number indicates the number of feet from the chart that the patient is standing; the bottom number is the distance at which a normal-sighted person can read the same line.

Age differences

20/20 In adults and children age 6 and older, normal vision is measured as 20/20.

20/30 For children age 5, normal vision is 20/30.

20/40 For children age 4, normal vision is 20/40.

20/50 For children age 3 and younger, normal vision is 20/50.

Near vision

To measure near vision:

1. Cover one of the patient's eyes with an opaque object.
2. Hold the Rosenbaum card 14" (35.6 cm) from the eyes.
3. Have the patient read the line with the smallest letters he or she can distinguish.
4. Repeat the test with the other eye.
5. If the patient wears corrective lenses, have the patient repeat the test while wearing them.
6. Record the visual accommodation with and without corrective lenses.

Rosenbaum card

The Rosenbaum card is used to evaluate near vision. This small, handheld card has a series of numbers, E's, X's, and O's in graduated sizes. Visual acuity is indicated on the right side of the chart in either distance equivalents or Jaeger equivalents.

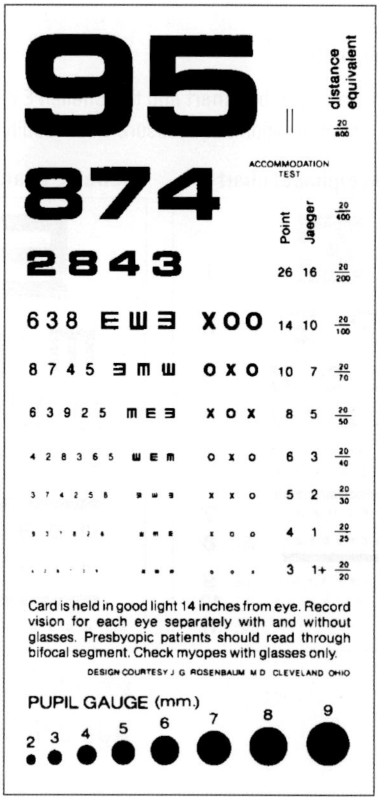
95
distance equivalent
20/800
ACCOMMODATION TEST
874
Point Jaeger
20/400
2843 26 16 20/200
638 XOO 14 10 20/100
8745 OXO 10 7 20/70
63925 XOX 8 5 20/50
6 3 20/40
5 2 20/30
4 1 20/25
3 1+ 20/20
Card is held in good light 14 inches from eye. Record vision for each eye separately with and without glasses. Presbyopic patients should read through bifocal segment. Check myopes with glasses only.
DESIGN COURTESY J G ROSENBAUM M D CLEVELAND OHIO
PUPIL GAUGE (mm.)
2 3 4 5 6 7 8 9

Confrontation

Test peripheral vision using confrontation. Confrontation can help identify such abnormalities as homonymous hemianopsia and bitemporal hemianopsia. Here's how to test confrontation:

- Sit or stand directly across from the patient and have the patient focus the gaze on your eyes.
- Place your hands on either side of the patient's head at the level of the ears so that they're about 28 apart.
- Tell the patient to focus the gaze on you as you gradually bring your wiggling fingers into his or her visual field.
- Instruct the patient to tell you as soon as he or she can see your wiggling fingers; the patient should see them at the same time you do.
- Repeat the procedure while holding your hands at the superior and inferior positions.

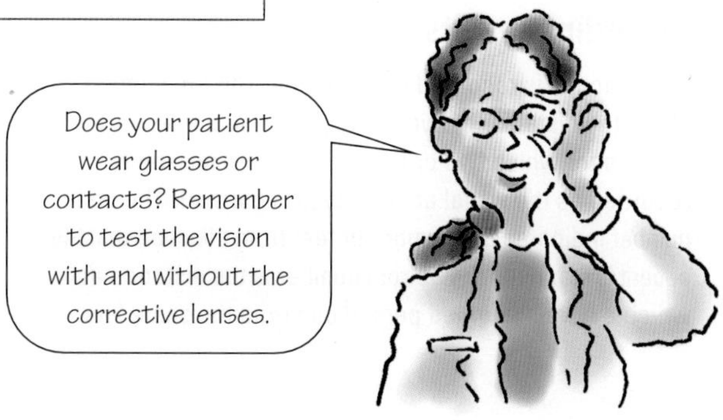
Does your patient wear glasses or contacts? Remember to test the vision with and without the corrective lenses.

Inspecting the eyes

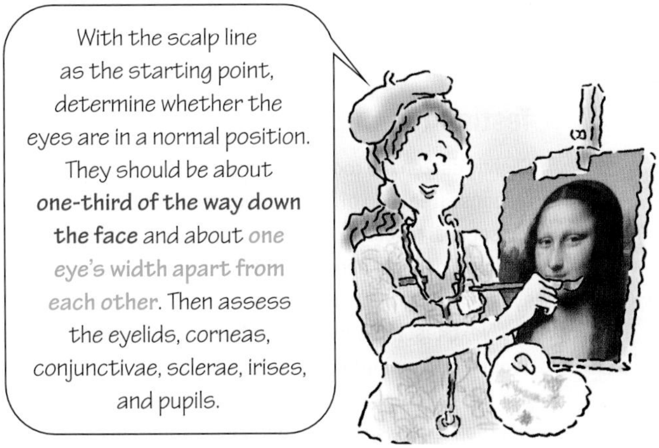
With the scalp line as the starting point, determine whether the eyes are in a normal position. They should be about **one-third of the way down the face** and about **one eye's width apart from each other**. Then assess the eyelids, corneas, conjunctivae, sclerae, irises, and pupils.

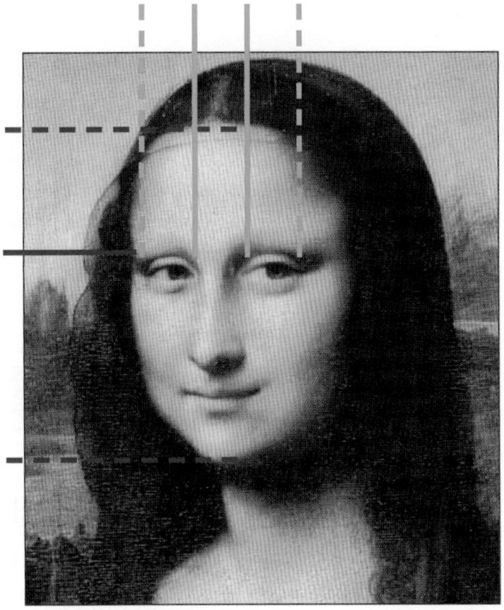

Eyelids

Each upper eyelid should cover the top quarter of the iris so the eyes look alike. Look for redness, edema, inflammation, or lesions on the lids.

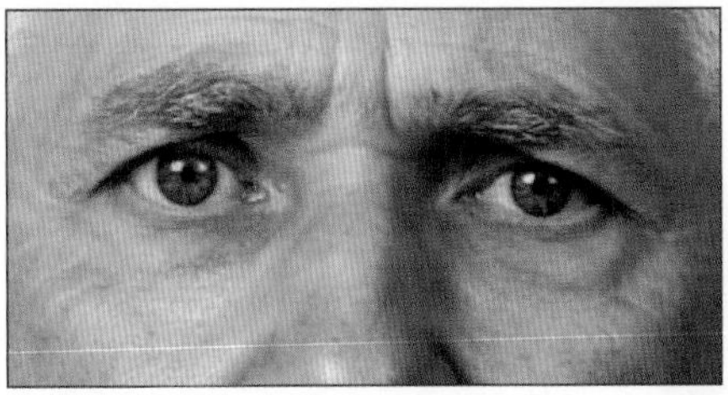

Corneas

The corneas should be clear and without lesions and should appear convex.

Examining the corneas

Examine the corneas by shining a penlight first from both sides and then from straight ahead. Test corneal sensitivity by lightly touching the cornea with a wisp of cotton.

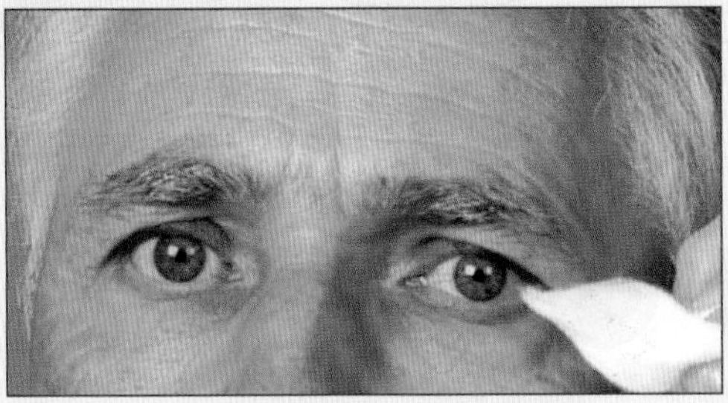

Age differences

Pediatrics

- Eyes set too narrow or too wide may indicate a systemic disorder.
- Dark circles under eyes may indicate chronic allergies.

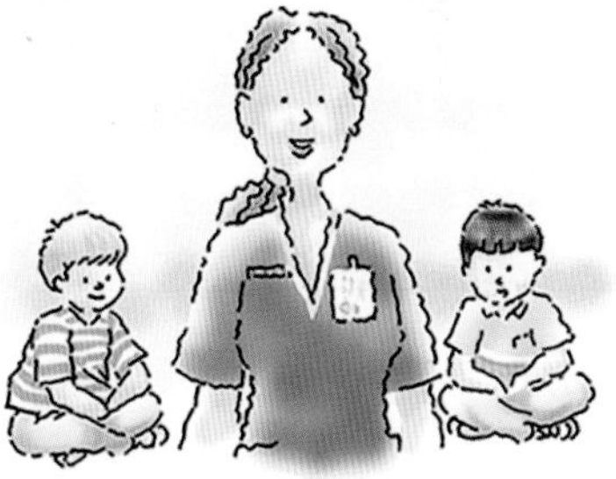

Geriatrics

- Eyes may have a sunken appearance due to loss of periorbital fat.

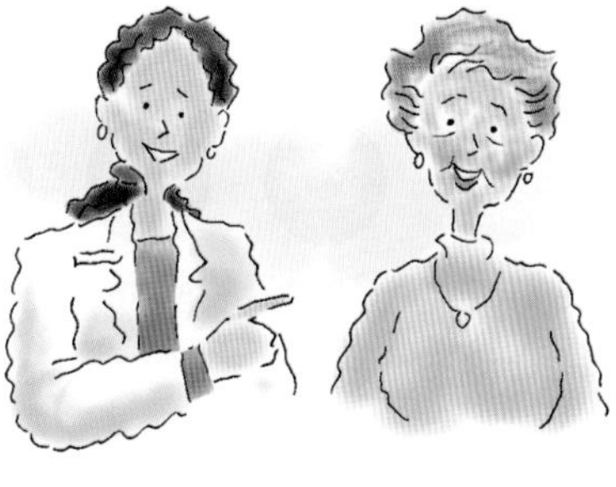

Irises

The irises should appear flat and should be the same size, color, and shape.

Conjunctivae and sclerae

The conjunctivae should be clear and shiny. Note excessive redness or exudate. The sclerae should be white or buff.

Skill check

Inspecting the conjunctiva and sclera

To inspect the bulbar conjunctiva, ask the patient to look up and gently pull the lower eyelid down. Then have the patient look down and lift the upper lid to examine the palpebral conjunctiva.

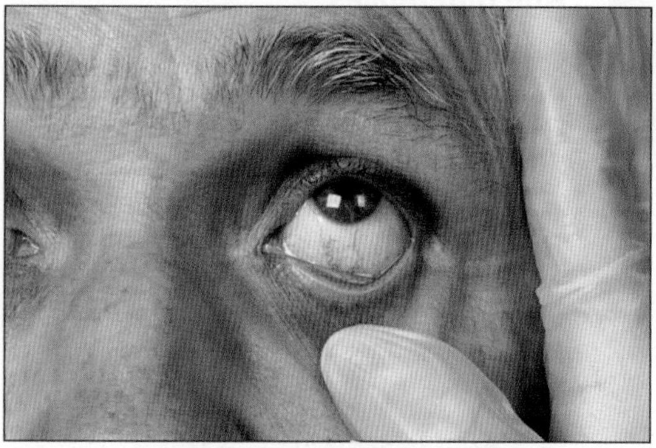

Pupils

Each pupil should be equal in size, round, and about one-fourth the size of the iris in normal room light.

Testing the pupils

Slightly darken the room. Then test the pupils for direct response (reaction of the pupil you're testing) and consensual response (reaction of the opposite pupil) by holding a penlight about 20" (51 cm) from the patient's eyes, directing the light at the eye from the side.

Next, test accommodation by placing your finger about 4" (10 cm) from the bridge of the patient's nose. Ask the patient to look at a fixed object in the distance and then to look at your finger. The patient's eyes should converge and pupils should constrict.

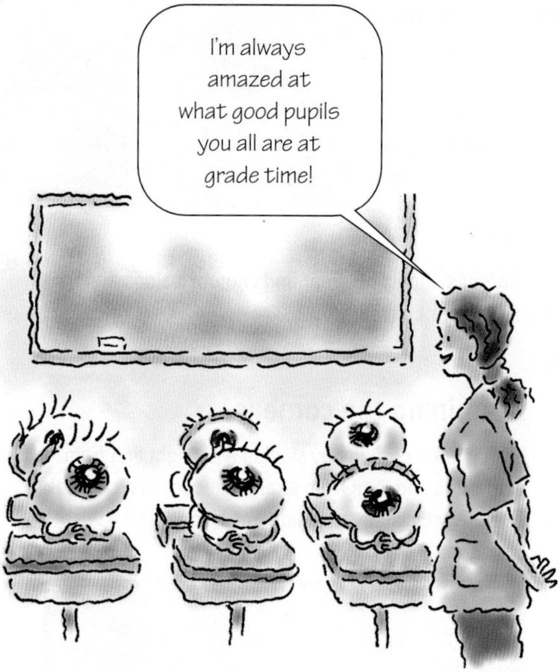
I'm always amazed at what good pupils you all are at grade time!

Grading pupil size

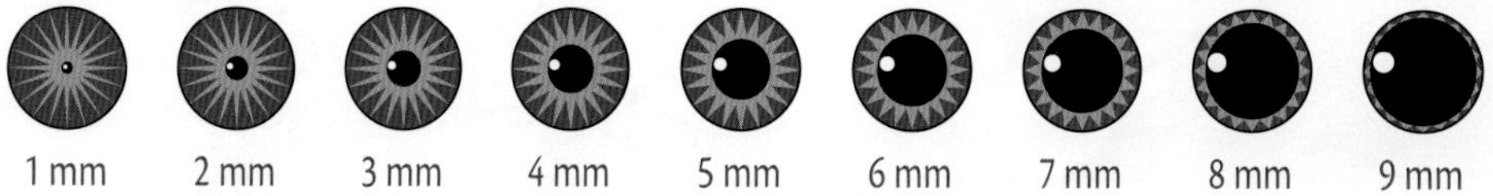
1 mm
2 mm
3 mm
4 mm
5 mm
6 mm
7 mm
8 mm
9 mm

Assessing eye muscle function

Corneal light reflex

Ask the patient to look straight ahead; then shine a penlight on the bridge of the patient's nose from 12" to 15" (30.5 to 38 cm) away. The light should fall at the same spot on each cornea. If it doesn't, the eyes aren't being held in the same plane by the extraocular muscles. The patient likely lacks muscle coordination, a condition called *strabismus*.

Cardinal positions of gaze

Cardinal positions of gaze evaluate the oculomotor, trigeminal, and abducens cranial nerves and the extraocular muscles.

1. Ask the patient to remain still while you hold a pencil or other small object directly in front of his or her nose at a distance of about 18" (45 cm).
2. Ask the patient to follow the object with the eyes, without moving the head.
3. Move the object to each of the six cardinal positions shown, returning to the midpoint after each movement.

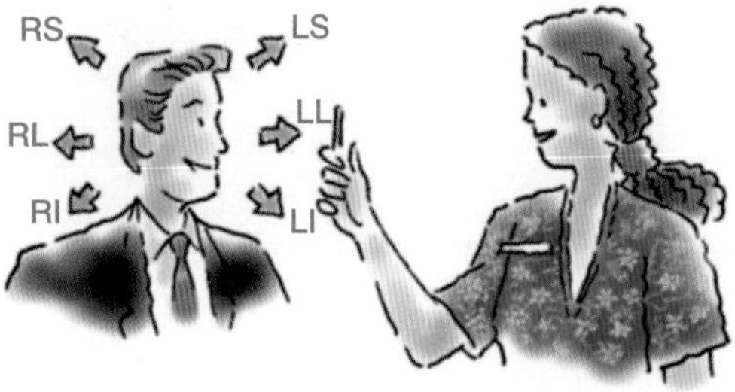
RS
LS
RL
LL
RI
LI

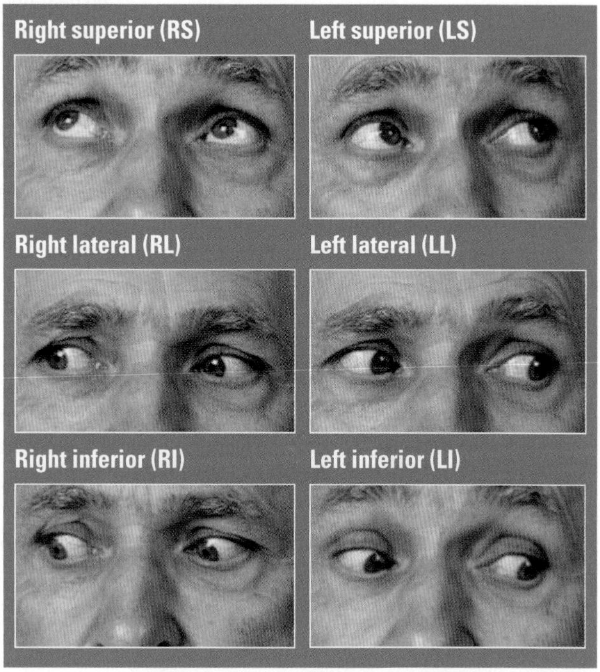
Right superior (RS)
Left superior (LS)
Right lateral (RL)
Left lateral (LL)
Right inferior (RI)
Left inferior (LI)

4. Note abnormal findings, such as nystagmus (involuntary, rhythmic oscillation of the eyeballs) or amblyopia (failure of one eye to follow an object).

Skill check

Examining intraocular structures

Before beginning your examination, ask the patient to remove his or her contact lenses or eyeglasses. Then darken the room to dilate the patient's pupils and make your examination easier. Ask the patient to focus on a point behind you.

Positioning suggestions:

- Make sure the patient is comfortably positioned.
- Position yourself to the side of the patient.

Use the right eye-to-right eye, left eye-to-left eye approach when examining the patient to keep from bumping noses as you move in toward the patient.

Set the lens disc at zero diopter, hold the *ophthalmoscope* about 4" (10 cm) from the patient's eye, and direct the light through the pupil to elicit the red reflex. The red reflex is reflection of the retina, which should appear as pinkish red in color. Check the red reflex for depth of color.

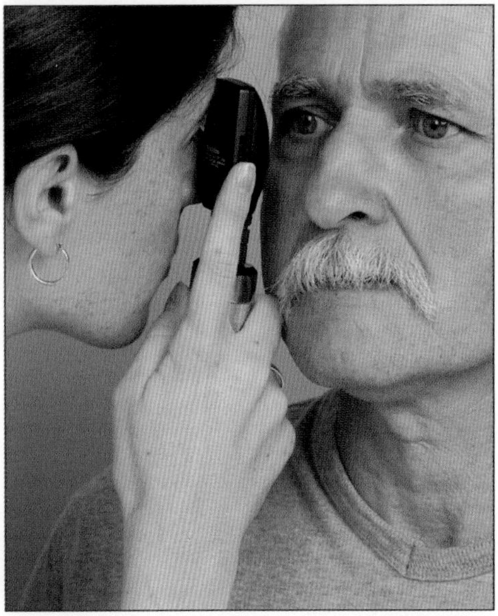

Adjust the lens disc so you can focus on the anterior chamber and lens. Look for clouding, foreign matter, or opacities.

The ophthalmoscope

The ophthalmoscope allows you to directly observe the eye's internal structures. Use the green, positive numbers on the ophthalmoscope's lens disc to focus on near objects such as the patient's cornea and lens. Use the red, minus numbers to focus on distant objects such as the retina.

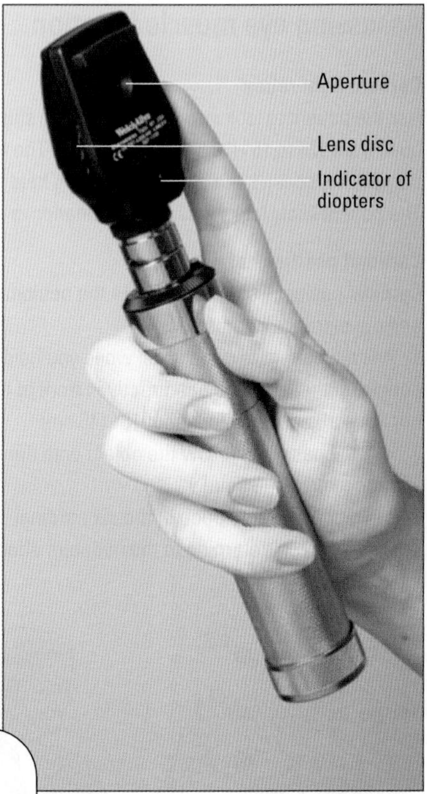
Aperture
Lens disc
Indicator of diopters

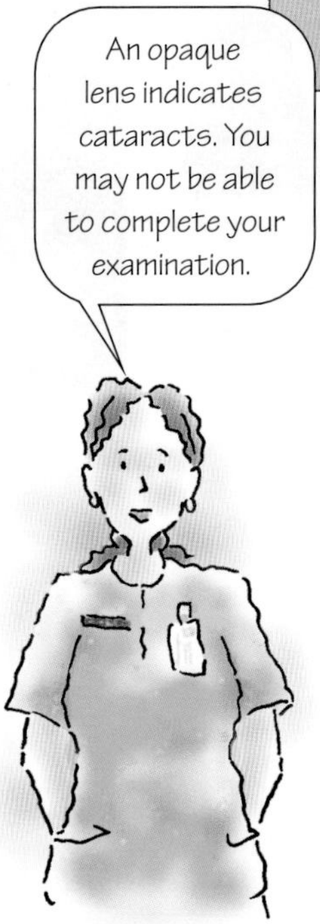
An opaque lens indicates cataracts. You may not be able to complete your examination.

Retinal structures

To examine the retina, start with the lens disc turned to zero. Rotate the lens disc to adjust for your refractive correction and the patient's refractive error. The first retinal structures you'll see are the blood vessels. Rotate the lens disc into the negative numbers to bring the blood vessels into focus.

Follow one of the vessels along its path toward the nose until you reach the optic disk. Examine arteriovenous crossings for localized constrictions in the retinal vessels, which might be a sign of hypertension.

The fundus

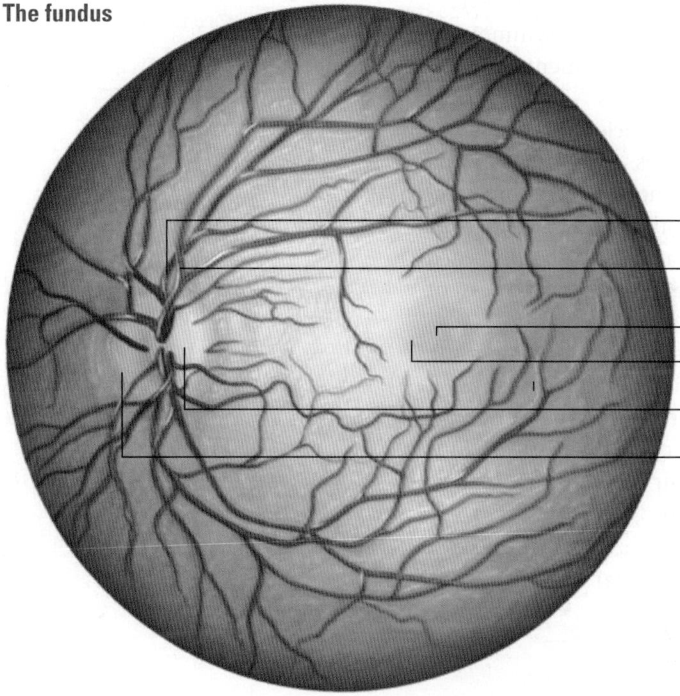
Artery
Vein
Fovea
Macula
Optic disc
Physiologic cup

Optic disk

The optic disk is located toward the nasal side of the retina. The optic disk is a creamy pink to yellow-orange structure with clear borders and a round-to-oval shape; the physiologic cup is a small depression that occupies about one-third of the disk's diameter. Arteries and veins run together in pairs. Arteries are smaller and are bright red in color; veins are larger and are darker red. The artery/vein pairs travel in four directions and narrow as you move away from the optic disc.

Retina

Completely scan the retina by following four blood vessels from the optic disk to different peripheral areas. The retina should have a uniform color and be free from scars and pigmentation.

Macula

Move the light laterally from the optic disk to locate the macula, the part of the eye most sensitive to light. It appears as a darker structure, free from blood vessels.

Fovea

The fovea is a tiny area located in the center of the macula. The fovea contains only cones and is responsible for sharp central vision.

Ears

External observation

Observe the ears for position and symmetry. The top of the ear should line up with the outer corner of the eye, and the ears should look symmetrical, with an angle of attachment of no more than 10 degrees.

Inspect the auricle for lesions, drainage, nodules, or redness. Pull the helix back and note if it's tender, which may indicate otitis externa. Inspect and palpate the mastoid area behind each auricle, noting tenderness, redness, or warmth.

Finally, inspect the opening of the ear canal, noting discharge, redness, odor, or the presence of nodules or cysts. Patients normally have varying amounts of hair and cerumen (earwax) in the ear canal.

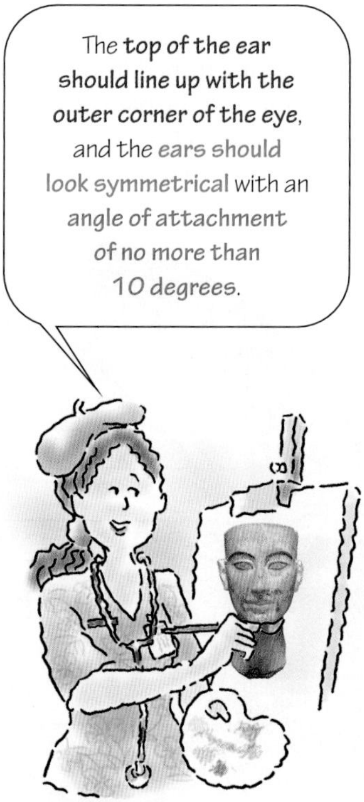
The top of the ear should line up with the outer corner of the eye, and the ears should look symmetrical with an angle of attachment of no more than 10 degrees.

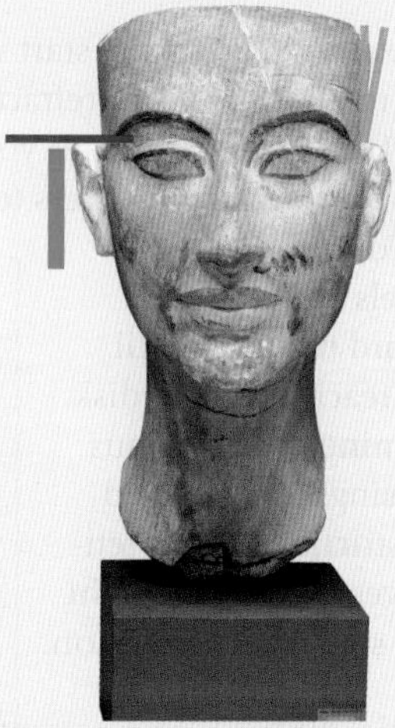

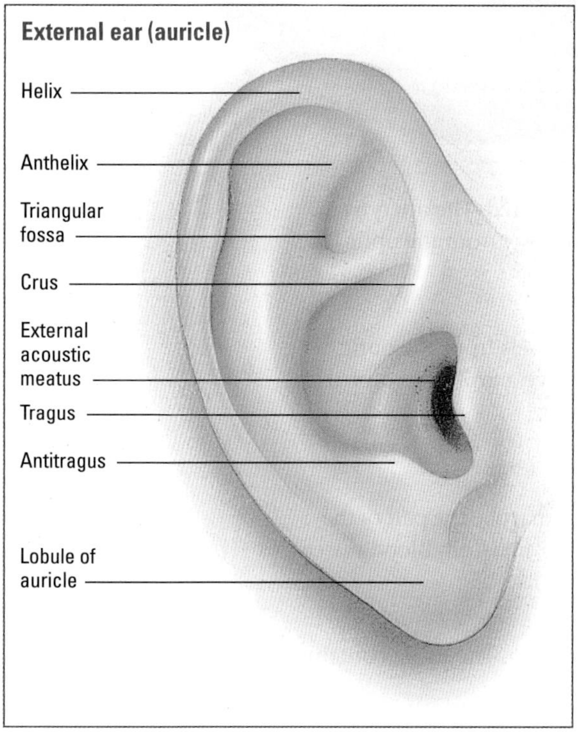
External ear (auricle)
Helix
Anthelix
Triangular fossa
Crus
External acoustic meatus
Tragus
Antitragus
Lobule of auricle

Genes and the cerumen scene

The presence of cerumen in the ear canal doesn't indicate poor hygiene. In fact, the appearance and type of cerumen are genetically determined. There are two types of cerumen:

- Dry cerumen—gray and flaky; mostly found in Asians and Native Americans (including Eskimos)
- Wet cerumen—dark brown and moist; commonly found in Blacks and Whites

Skill check

Otoscopic examination

1

Positioning the patient

Ask the patient to sit with back straight and head tilted away from you and toward the opposite shoulder. Straighten the ear canal by grasping the auricle and pulling it up and back for adults and down and back for children.

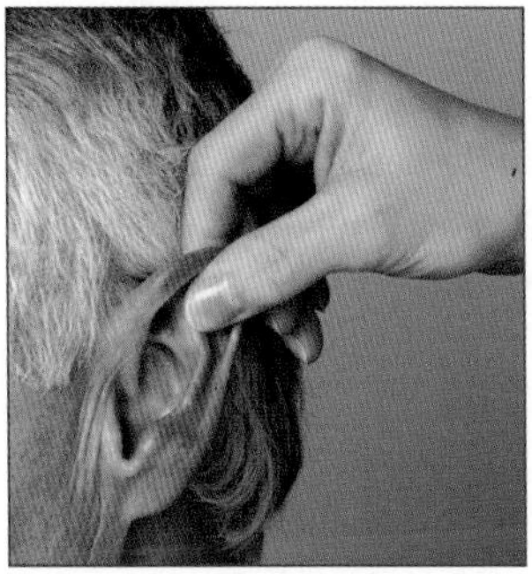

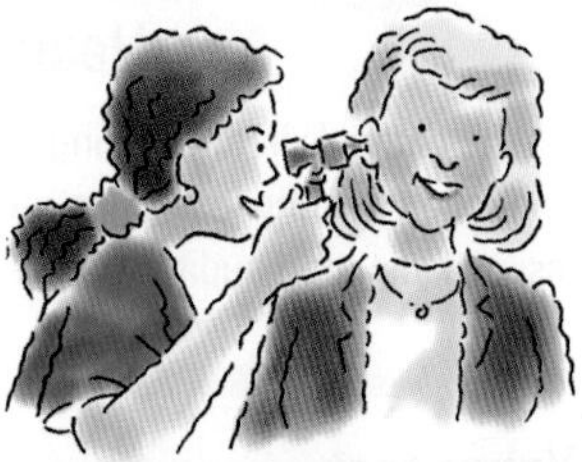

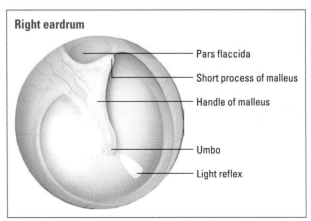

2

Positioning the scope

Hold the otoscope handle between your thumb and fingers and brace your hand firmly against the patient's head. Doing so keeps you from hitting the canal with the speculum.

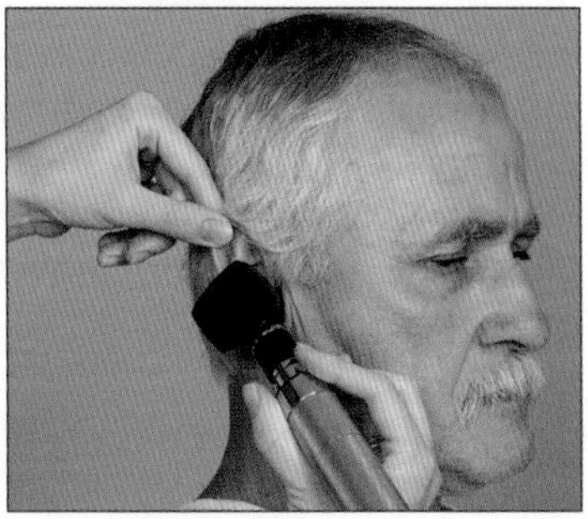

3

Inserting the speculum

Insert the speculum one-third its length gently down and forward into the ear canal. Be careful not to touch either side of the inner portion of the ear canal wall because this area is covered by a thin epithelial layer that's sensitive to pressure.

4

Viewing the structures

Once the otoscope is positioned properly, you should see the tympanic membrane, pars flaccida, and the bony structures, as shown. The tympanic membrane should be pearl gray, glistening, and transparent. Inspect the membrane for bulging, retraction, bleeding, lesions, and perforations.

The light reflex in the right ear should be between 4 and 6 o'clock; in the left ear, it should be between 6 and 8 o'clock. Finally, look for the bony landmarks. The malleus will appear as a dense, white streak at 12 o'clock. The umbo is the inferior portion of the malleus.

Right eardrum

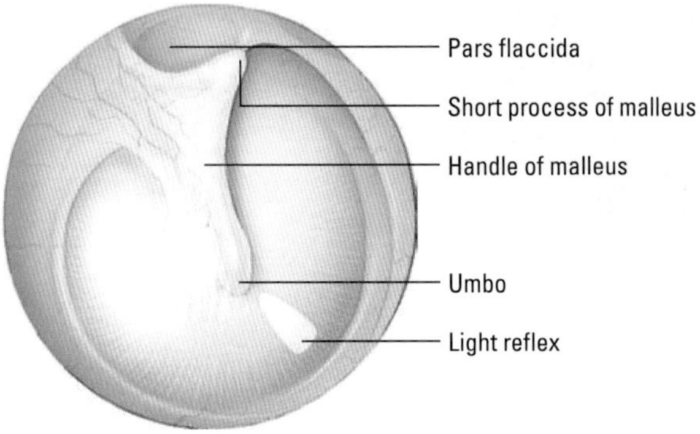
Pars flaccida
Short process of malleus
Handle of malleus
Umbo
Light reflex

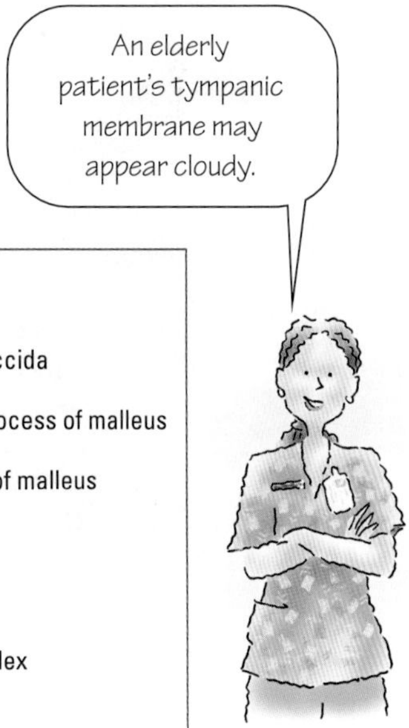
An elderly patient's tympanic membrane may appear cloudy.

Skill check

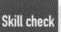

Hearing acuity tests

Test the patient's hearing using the Weber test and the Rinne test. These tests assess conduction hearing loss, impaired sound transmission to the inner ear, sensorineural hearing loss, and impaired auditory nerve conduction or inner ear function.

Weber test

In the Weber test, a tuning fork is used to evaluate bone conduction. The tuning fork should be tuned to the frequency of normal human speech, 512 cycles/second. To perform the Weber test:

- Strike the tuning fork lightly against your hand.
- Place the vibrating fork on the patient's forehead at the midline or on the top of the patient's head.

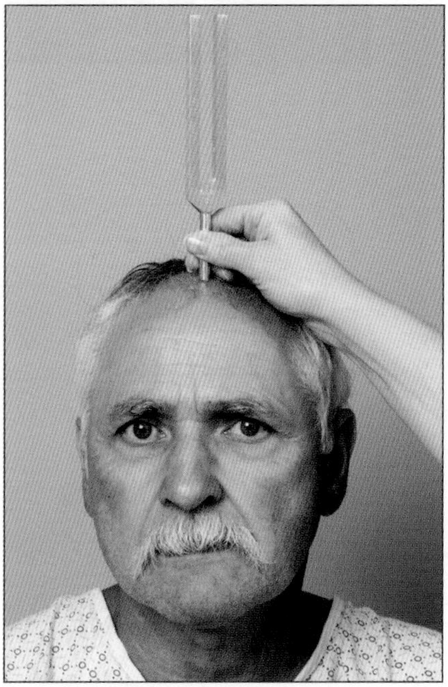

Results	Description
Normal	Patient hears tone equally well in both ears.
Right or left lateralization	Patient hears tone better in one ear.
Conductive hearing loss	Patient hears tone only in the impaired ear.
Sensorineural hearing loss	Patient hears tone only in the unaffected ear.

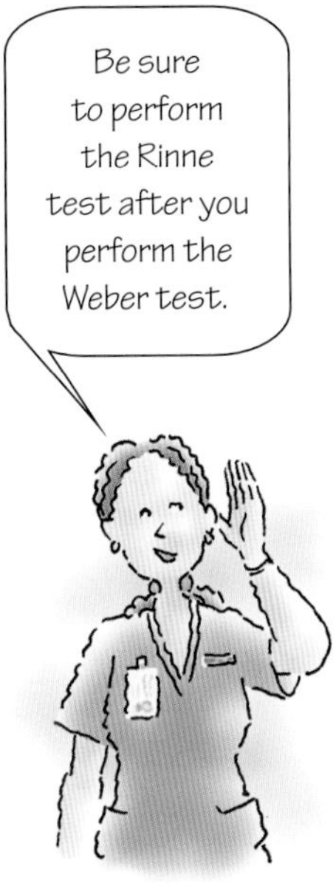
Be sure to perform the Rinne test after you perform the Weber test.

Rinne test

The Rinne test is used to compare air conduction (AC) of sound with bone conduction (BC) of sound. To perform this test:

- Strike the tuning fork against your hand.
- Place the vibrating fork over the patient's mastoid process.

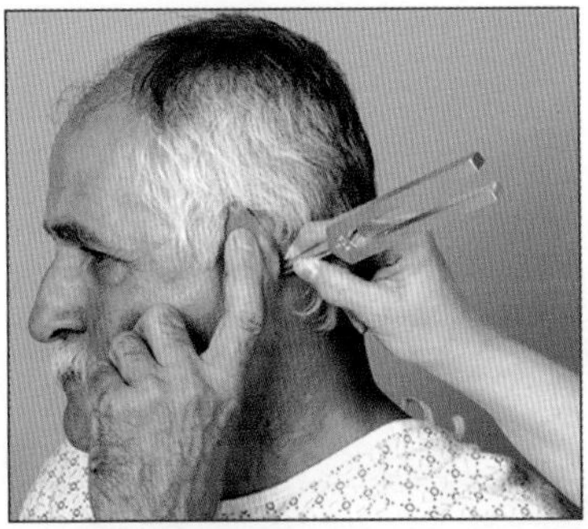

- Ask the patient to tell you when the tone stops; note this time in seconds.
- Move the still-vibrating tuning fork to the ear's opening without touching the ear.

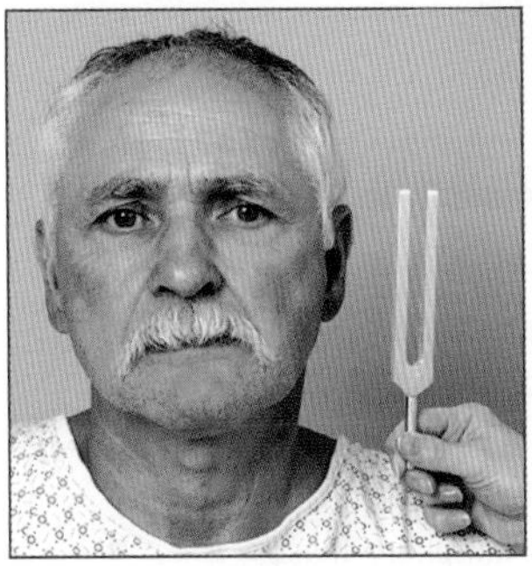

- Ask the patient to tell you when the tone stops; note this time in seconds.

Results	Description
Normal hearing	Patient hears AC tone twice as long as he or she hears BC tone (AC > BC).
Conductive hearing loss	Patient hears BC tone as long as or longer than he or she hears AC tone (BC > AC).
Sensorineural hearing loss	Patient hears AC tone longer than he or she hears BC tone (AC > BC).

Age differences

Pediatrics

- Look for symmetry and position of the ears in relation to location of the eyes as congenital abnormalities can result in abnormal positioning.
- For older children and adolescents, the ear should be pulled down and back, as in adults.
- Indicators of hearing problems in children may be indicated by language delays or frequent ear infections.

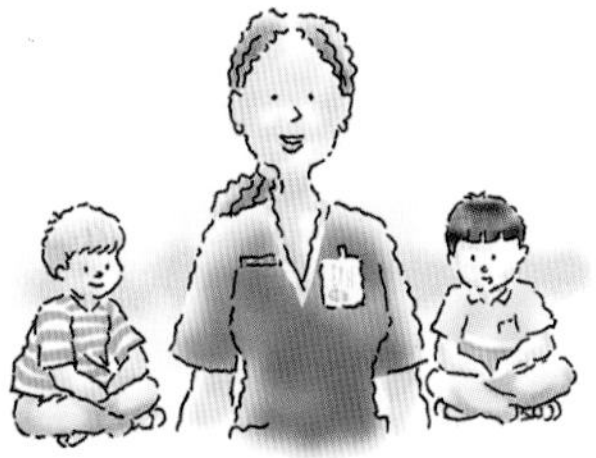

Geriatrics

- An elderly patient's tympanic membrane may appear cloudy.
- An increase in the amount of hair within the ear can create an accumulation of cerumen and cause mild hearing loss.
- Hearing loss is common with age. Loss of higher tones typically occurs first.

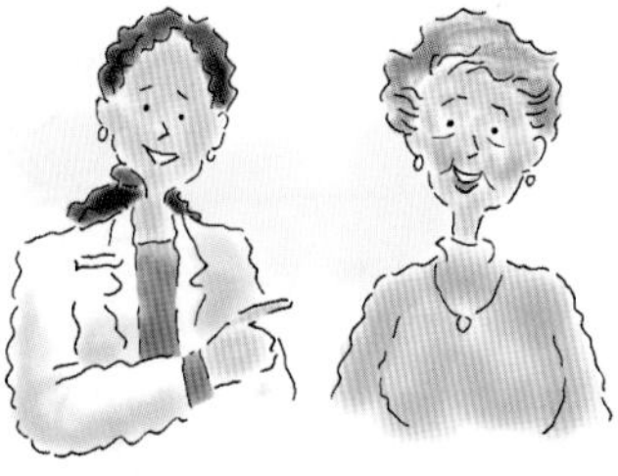

Eye abnormalities

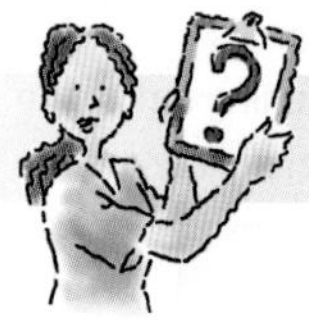

Outside the norm

Conjunctivitis

This condition is characterized by hyperemia of the conjunctiva with predominate redness in the eye periphery. It usually begins in one eye and rapidly spreads by contamination to the other eye. The patient experiences mild discomfort rather than severe pain. Vision isn't affected except for some blurring because of watery or mucopurulent eye discharge.

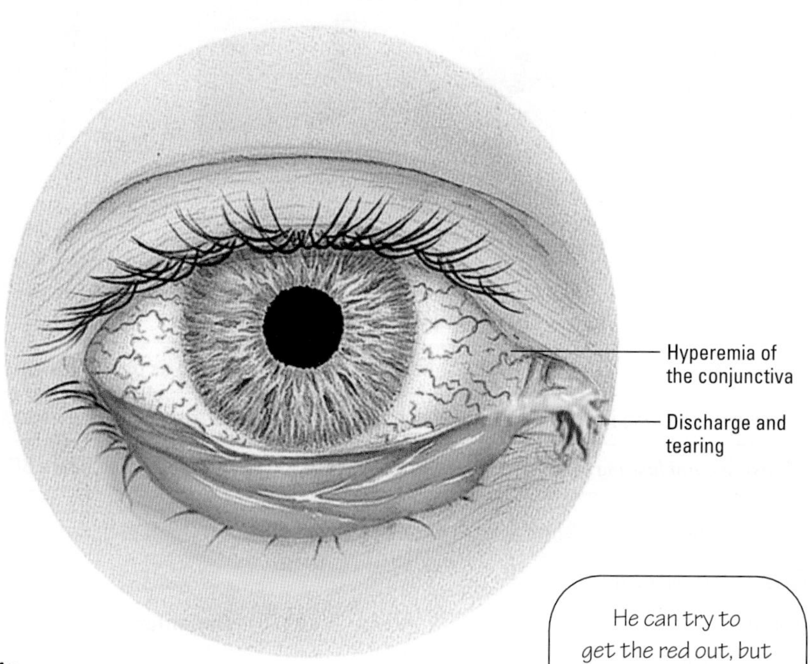
Hyperemia of the conjunctiva
Discharge and tearing

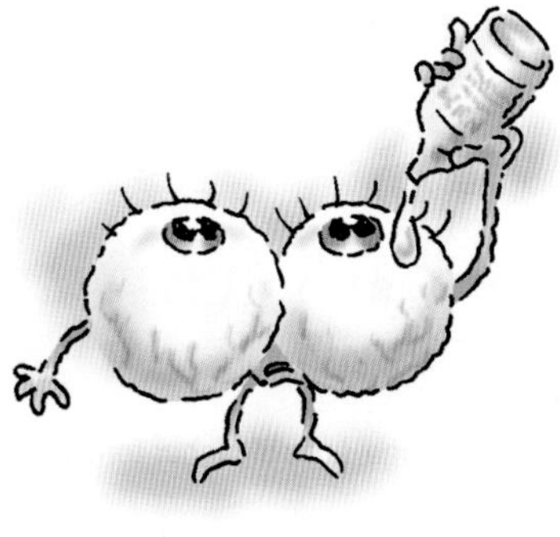

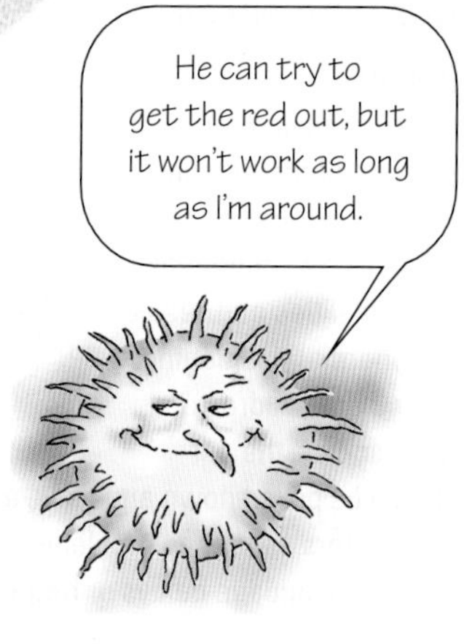
He can try to get the red out, but it won't work as long as I'm around.

Acute angle-closure glaucoma

Acute angle-closure glaucoma is characterized by a rapid onset of unilateral inflammation, severe eye pain and pressure, and photophobia. It also causes decreased vision, moderate pupil dilation, nonreactive pupillary response, and clouding of the cornea but no eye discharge. Ophthalmoscopic examination reveals changes in the retinal vessels and enlargement of the physiologic cup.

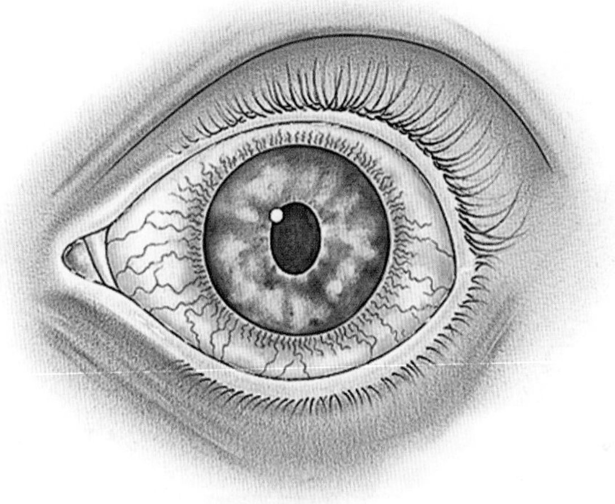

Disk changes associated with glaucoma

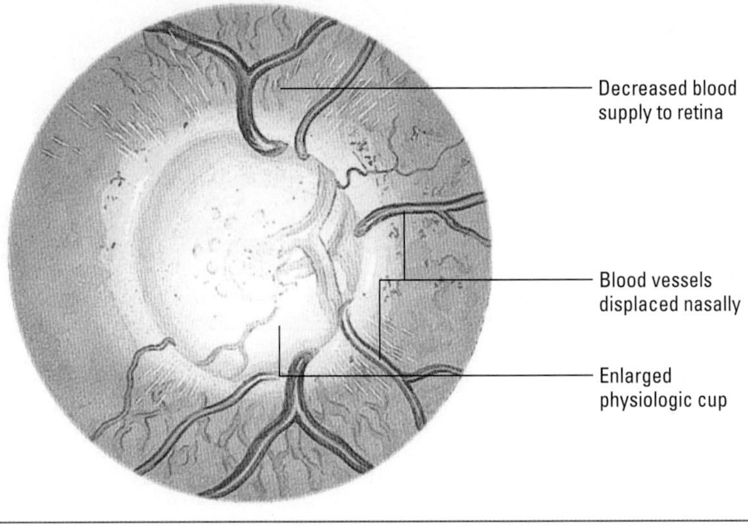
Decreased blood supply to retina
Blood vessels displaced nasally
Enlarged physiologic cup

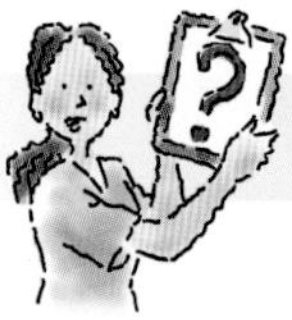

Outside the norm

Periorbital edema

Swelling around the eyes, or periorbital edema, may result from allergies, local inflammation, fluid-retaining disorders, or crying.

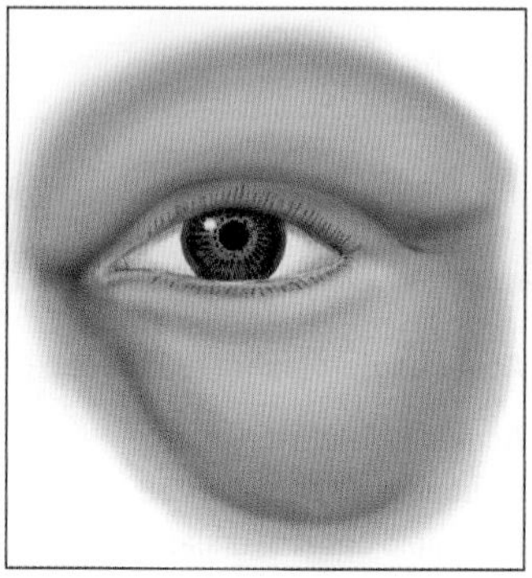

Ptosis

Ptosis, or a drooping upper eyelid, may be caused by an interruption in sympathetic innervation to the eyelid, muscle weakness, or damage to the oculomotor nerve.

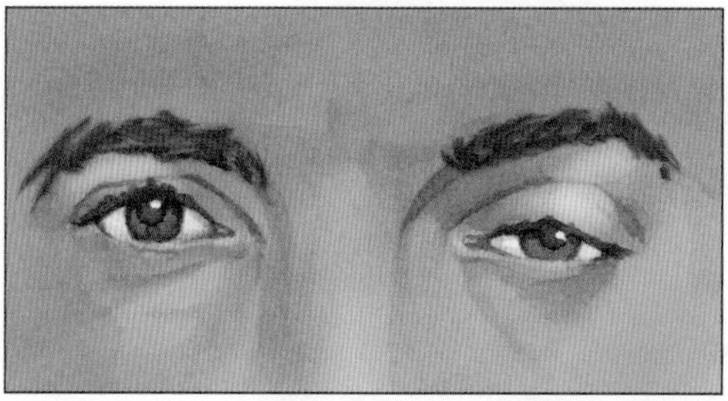

Cataract

A common cause of vision loss, a cataract is a clouding of the lens or lens capsule of the eye that can result from trauma, diabetes, and some medications.

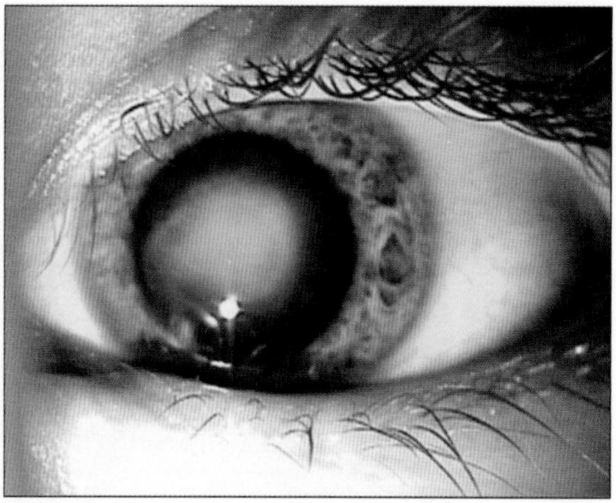

Macular degeneration

Macular degeneration—atrophy or deterioration of the macular disk—is a cause of severe irreversible loss of central vision in people older than age 50. Dry macular degeneration, in which tissue deterioration isn't accompanied by bleeding, is the most common form.

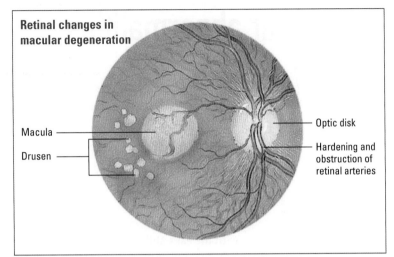

Retinal changes in macular degeneration

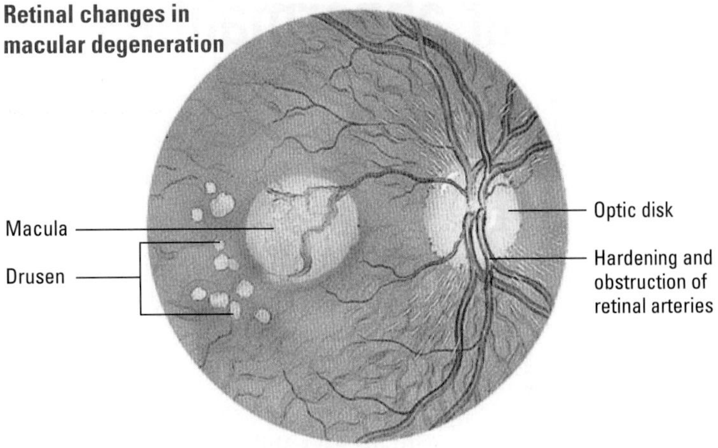
Macula
Drusen
Optic disk
Hardening and obstruction of retinal arteries

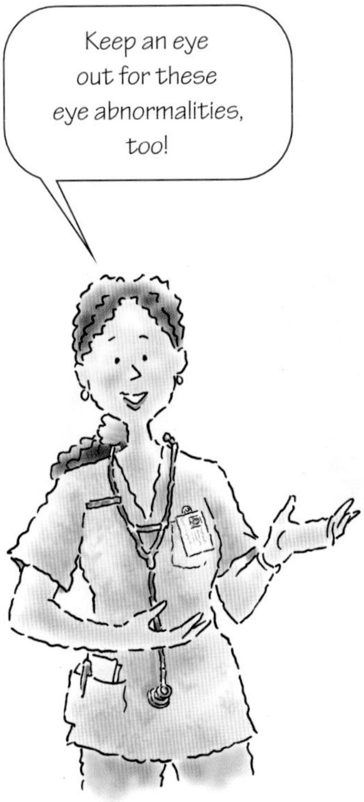
Keep an eye out for these eye abnormalities, too!

Decreased visual acuity

Decreased visual acuity—the inability to see clearly—commonly occurs with refractive errors. In nearsightedness, or *myopia,* vision at a distance is blurry. In farsightedness, or hyperopia, vision in close view is blurry.

Diplopia

Diplopia, or double *vision,* occurs when the extraocular muscles are misaligned.

Discharge

Discharge may occur in one or both eyes and may be scant or copious. The discharge may be purulent, frothy, mucoid, cheesy, serous, or clear or may have a stringy, white appearance. Eye discharge commonly results from inflammatory and infectious eye disorders such as conjunctivitis.

Pain

Eye pain may signal an emergency and requires immediate attention. Diseases causing eye pain include acute angle-closure glaucoma and blepharitis. Corneal damage caused by a foreign body or abrasions as well as trauma to the eye can also cause eye pain.

Vision loss

Disorders of any structure of the eye can result in vision loss. Types of vision loss include central vision loss, peripheral vision loss, or a blind spot in the middle of an area of normal vision (scotoma).

Visual halos

Increased intraocular pressure, which occurs in glaucoma, causes the patient to see halos and rainbows around bright lights.

Ear abnormalities

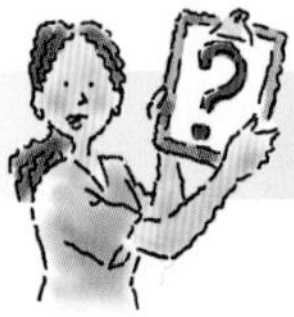

Outside the norm

Earache

Earaches usually result from disorders of the external and middle ear and are associated with infection, hearing loss, and otorrhea.

Hearing loss

Several factors can interfere with the ear's ability to conduct sound waves. Cerumen, a foreign body, or a polyp may obstruct the ear canal. Otitis media may thicken the fluid in the middle ear, which interferes with the vibrations that transmit sound. Otosclerosis, a hardening of the bones in the middle ear, also interferes with the transmission of sound vibrations. Trauma can disrupt the middle ear's bony chain.

Otitis media

Otitis media, inflammation of the middle ear, results from disruption of eustachian tube patency. It can be suppurative or secretory, acute (as shown at right) or chronic.

Acute otitis media
- Infected fluid in middle ear
- Rapid onset and short duration

Otoscopic view

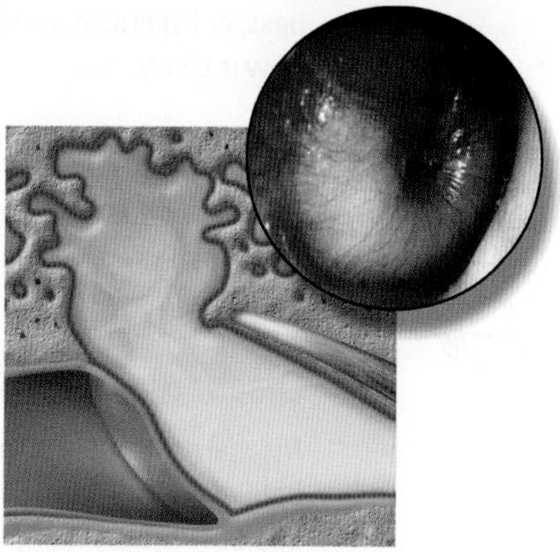

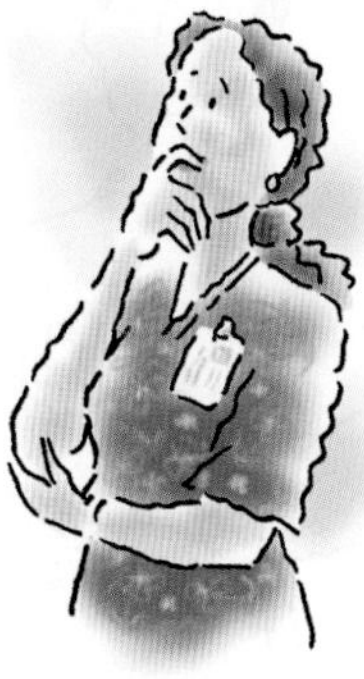

Complications of otitis media

Otitis media with effusion
- Characterized by fluid in middle ear that may not cause symptoms
- May be acute, subacute, or chronic

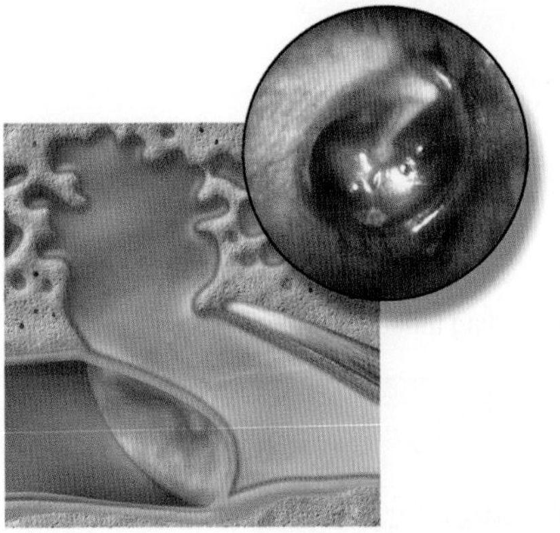

Cholesteatoma
- Abnormal skin growth or epithelial cyst in middle ear that usually results from repeated ear infections

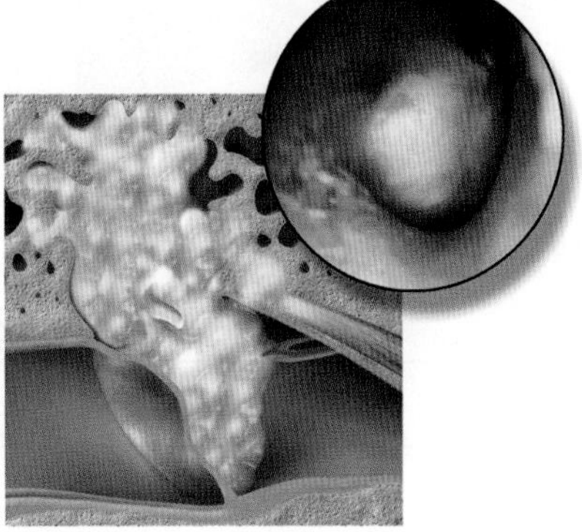

Perforation
- Hole in tympanic membrane caused by chronic negative middle ear pressure, inflammation, or trauma

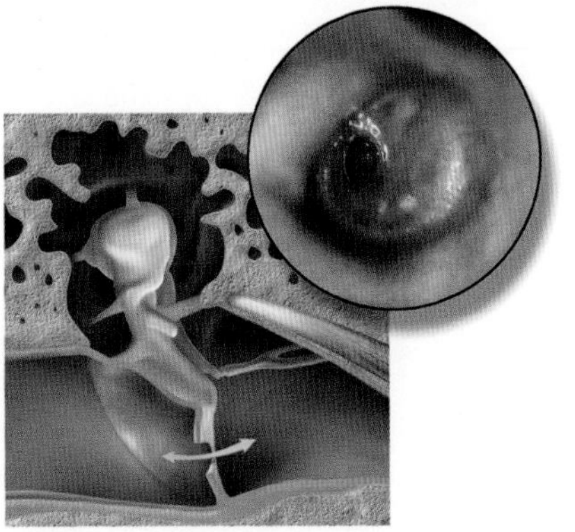

Q&A

Able to label?

Identify the intraocular structures indicated on this illustration.

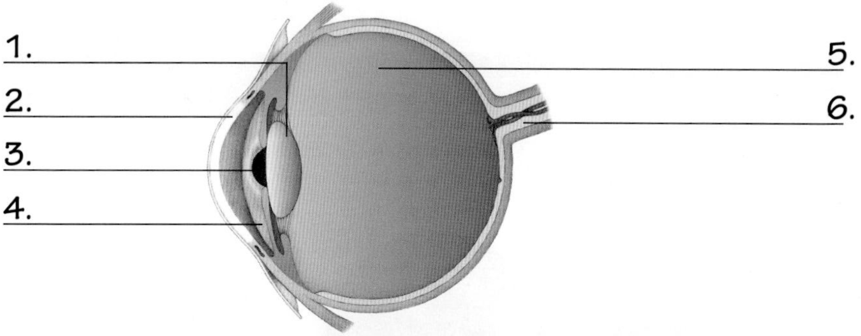
1.
2.
3.
4.
5.
6.

Show and tell

Describe the steps for performing the Rinne test, including those shown below.

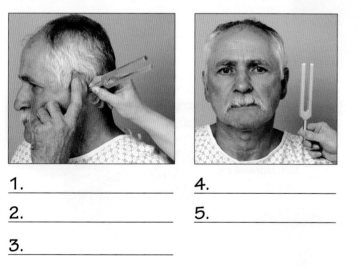

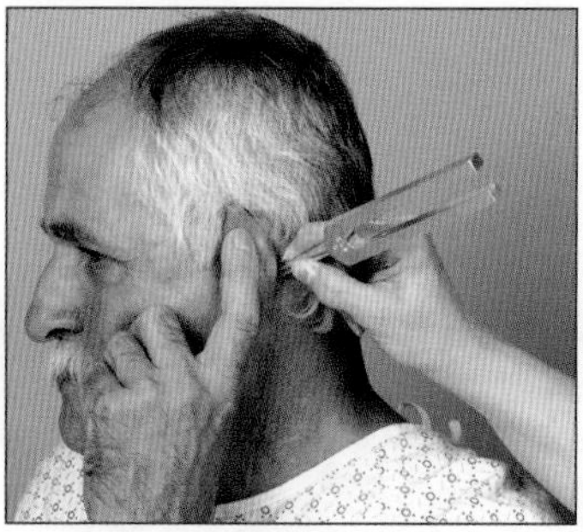

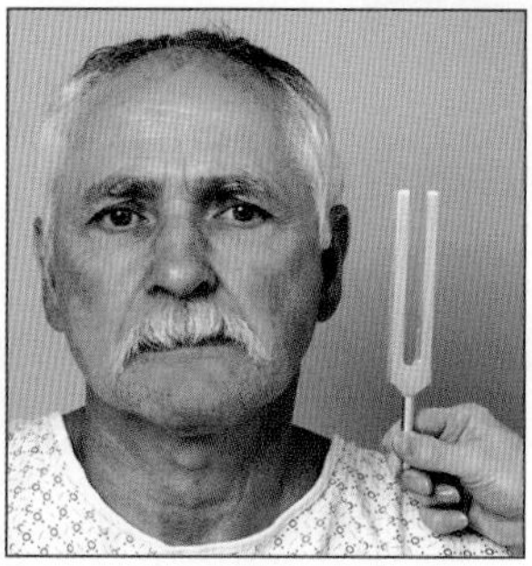

1. ______________________

2. ______________________

3. ______________________

4. ______________________

5. ______________________

Test your knowledge!

1. Which of the following is a normal finding when viewing the tympanic membrane with the otoscope?
   A. A glistening pearly-gray transparent surface
   B. A pink surface with a small opening in the lower quadrant and appearance of small air bubbles
   C. A reddened bulging surface
   D. A dull gray surface

2. A patient asks what her Snellen eye test results mean. Her acuity for both eyes together is 20/30. Which of the following is the nurse's best response?
   A. "You see at 30 feet what the normal-sighted person sees at 20 feet."
   B. "You see at 20 feet what the normal-sighted person sees at 30 feet."
   C. "You see at 10 feet what the normal-sighted person sees at 50 feet."
   D. You see at 50 feet what the normal-sighted person sees at 10 feet."

3. What part of the eye exam should occur first?
   A. Extraocular movements
   B. Internal structures
   C. Visual fields
   D. Visual acuity

4. When inspecting the internal ear with an otoscope, the nurse should pull the ear _____ and back for adults and older children and _____ and back for infants and small children.

Answers: Able to label? 1. Lens, 2. Cornea, 3. Pupil, 4. Iris, 5. Vitreous humor, 6. Optic nerve; Show and tell 1. Strike the tuning fork against your hand. 2. Place the vibrating fork over the patient's mastoid process. 3. Ask the patient to tell you when the tone stops; note this time in seconds. 4. Move the still-vibrating tuning fork to the ear's opening without touching the ear. 5. Ask the patient to tell you when the tone stops; note this time in seconds.
Test your Knowledge! 1. A 2. B 3. D 4. up, down

Selected References

Christoff, A. (2015). Examining pediatric eyes. *Ophthalmology Times, March; Supplement 1-10*. ISSN: 0193-032X

McCullagh, M. C., & Frank, K. (2013). Addressing hearing loss in primary care. *Journal of Advanced Nursing, 69*(4), 896–904.

Chapter 4

Nose, mouth, throat, and neck

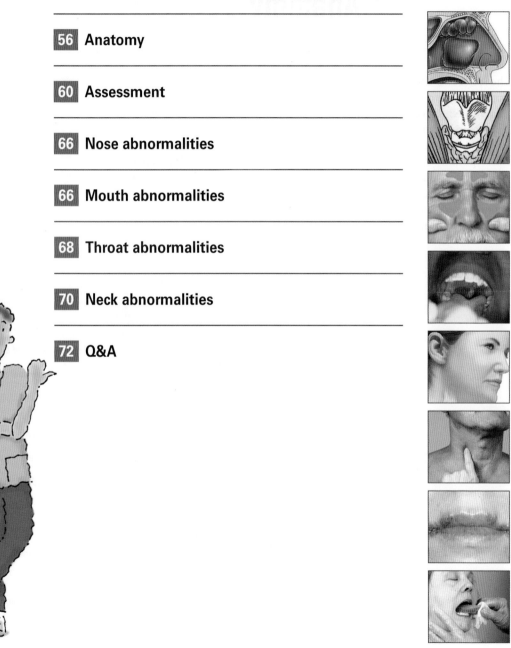

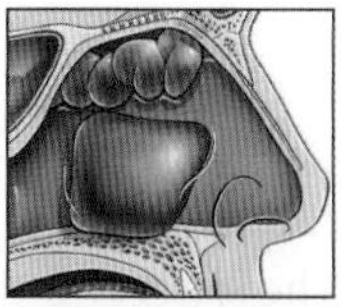

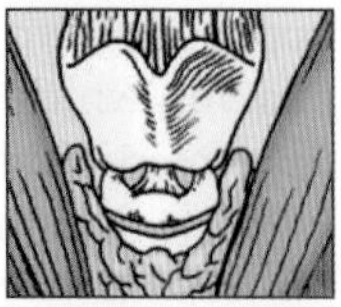

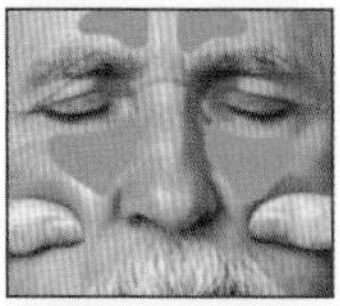

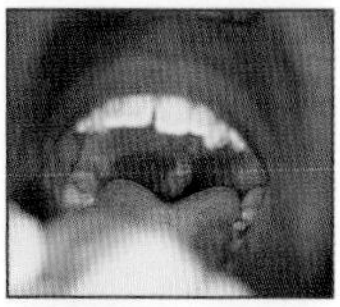

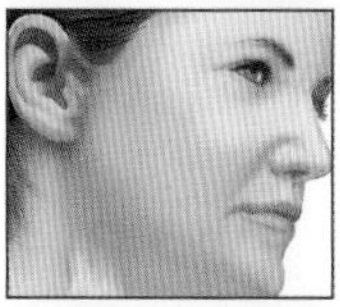

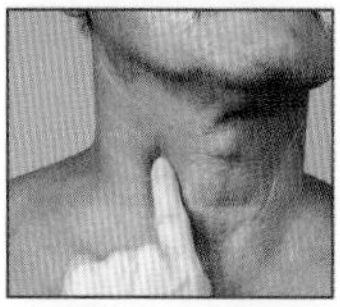

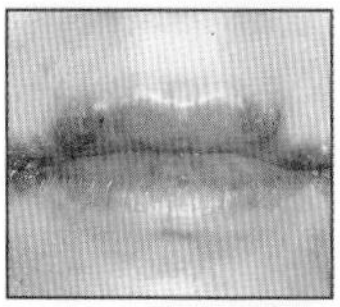

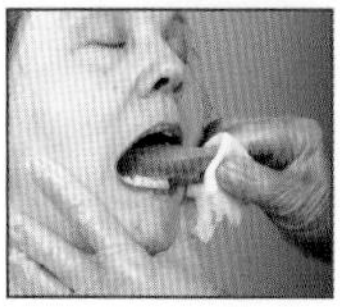

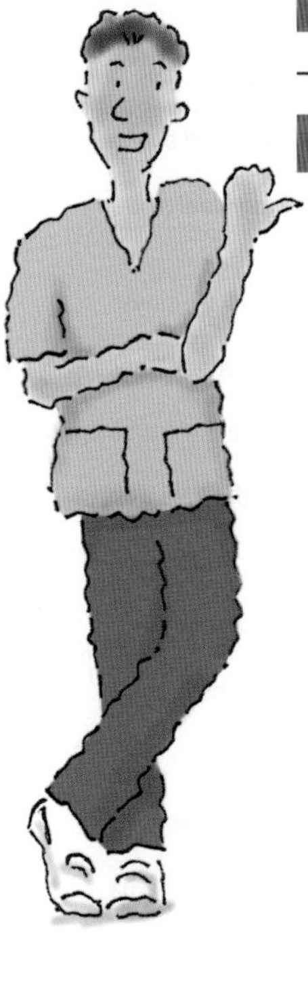

Anatomy

Nose

The lower two-thirds of the external nose consists of flexible cartilage, and the upper one-third is rigid bone. Posteriorly, the internal nose merges with the pharynx, which is divided into the *nasopharynx, oropharynx,* and *laryngopharynx*. Anteriorly, it merges with the external nose.

More than just the sensory organ of smell, the nose also plays a key role in the respiratory system by filtering, warming, and humidifying inhaled air.

The internal and external nose are divided vertically by the nasal septum. Kiesselbach area, the most common site of nosebleeds, is located in the anterior portion of the septum. Air entering the nose passes through the vestibule, which is lined with coarse hair that helps filter dust.

Nasopharyngeal structures

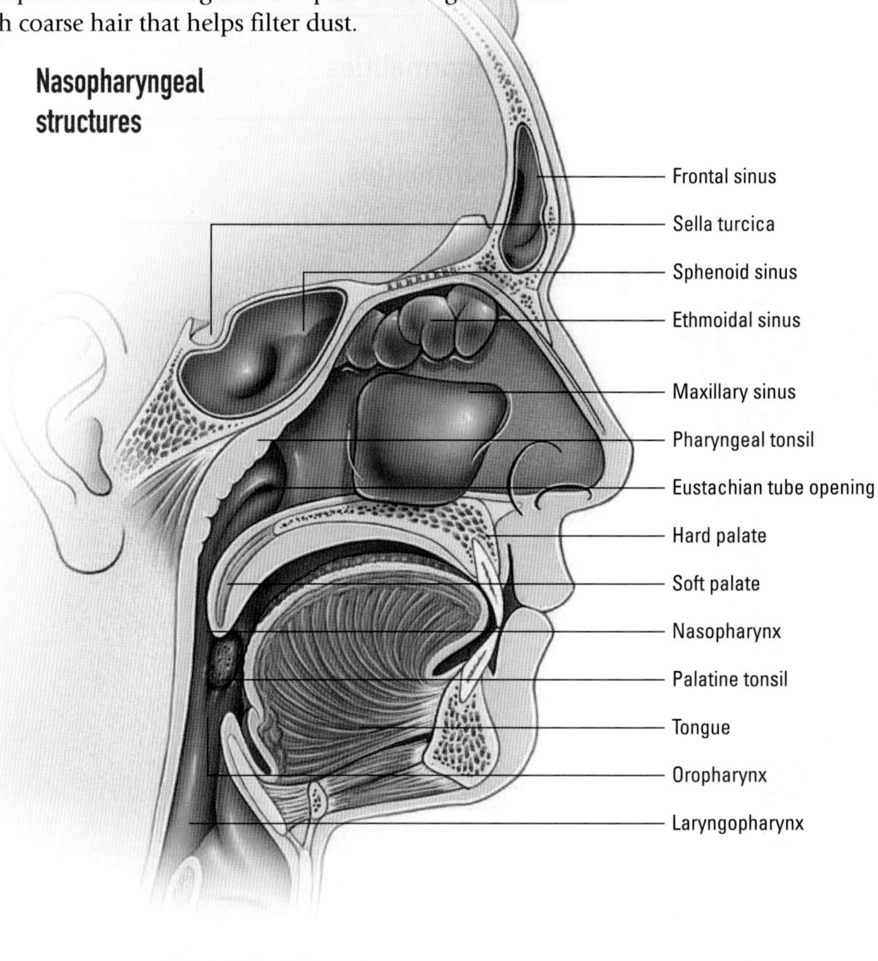
Frontal sinus
Sella turcica
Sphenoid sinus
Ethmoidal sinus
Maxillary sinus
Pharyngeal tonsil
Eustachian tube opening
Hard palate
Soft palate
Nasopharynx
Palatine tonsil
Tongue
Oropharynx
Laryngopharynx

Sinuses

Four pairs of paranasal sinuses open into the internal nose:

- Maxillary sinuses, located on the cheeks below the eyes
- Frontal sinuses, located above the eyebrows
- Ethmoidal and sphenoidal sinuses, located behind the eyes and nose in the head

The sinuses serve as resonators for sound production and provide mucus. You'll be able to assess the maxillary and frontal sinuses, but the ethmoidal and sphenoidal sinuses aren't readily accessible.

Paranasal sinuses

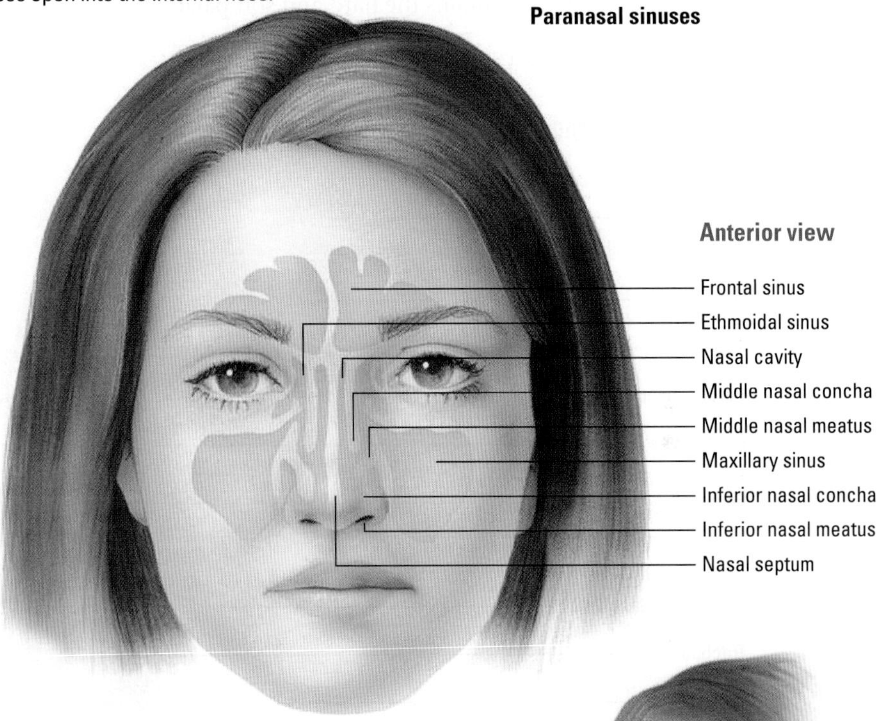
Anterior view
Frontal sinus
Ethmoidal sinus
Nasal cavity
Middle nasal concha
Middle nasal meatus
Maxillary sinus
Inferior nasal concha
Inferior nasal meatus
Nasal septum

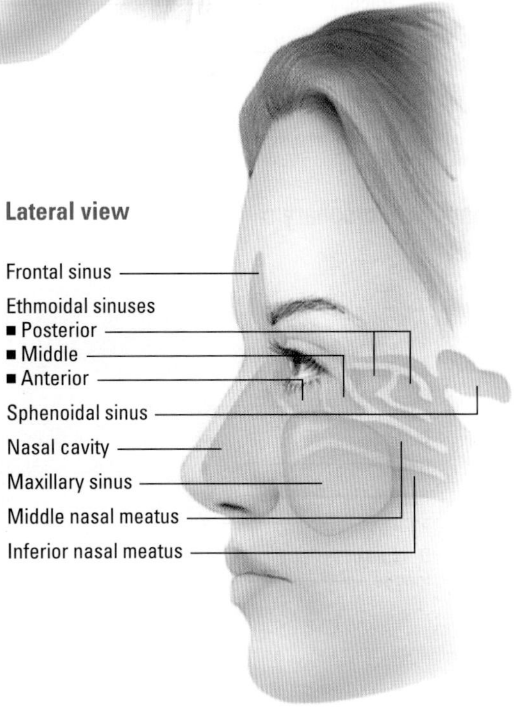
Lateral view
Frontal sinus
Ethmoidal sinuses
■ Posterior
■ Middle
■ Anterior
Sphenoidal sinus
Nasal cavity
Maxillary sinus
Middle nasal meatus
Inferior nasal meatus

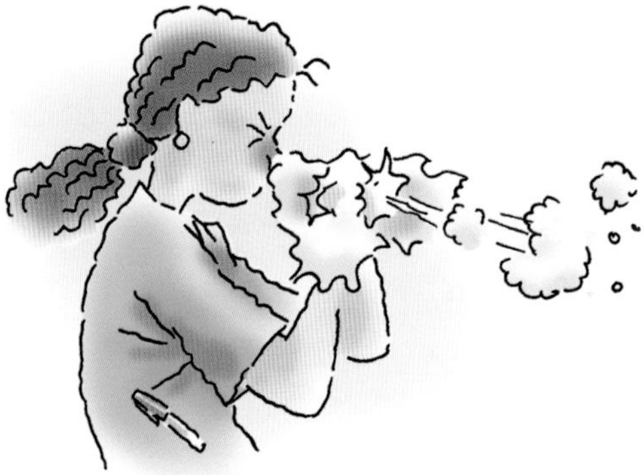

Mouth and throat

The mouth is bounded by the lips, cheeks, palate, and tongue and contains the teeth. The throat, or pharynx, contains the hard and soft palates, the uvula, and the tonsils.

Structures of the mouth and throat

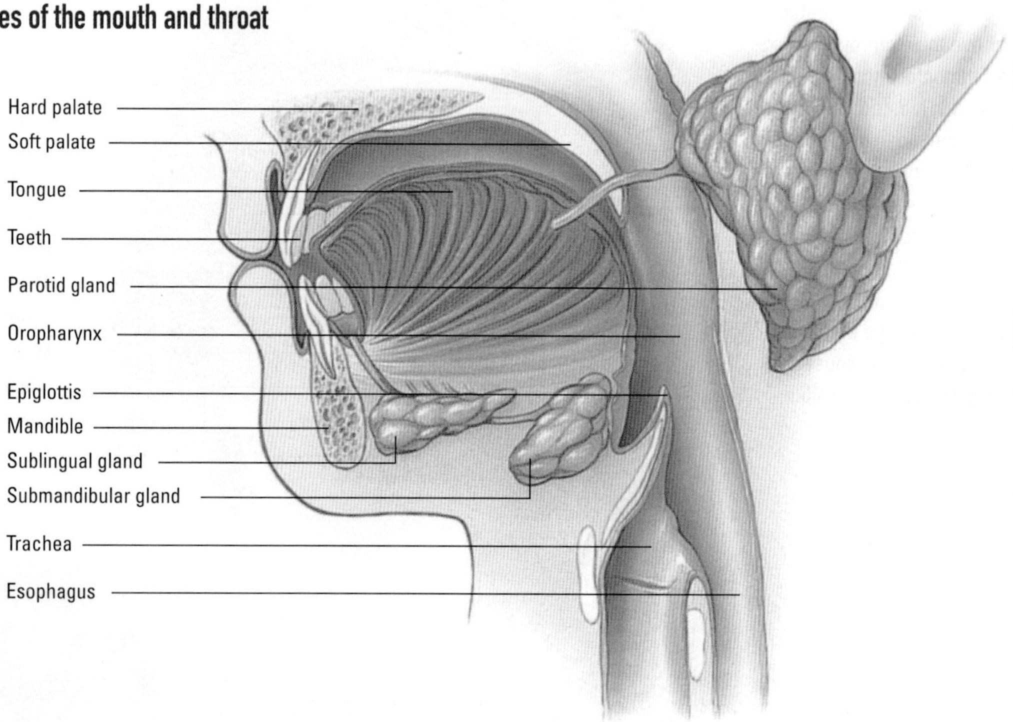
Hard palate
Soft palate
Tongue
Teeth
Parotid gland
Oropharynx
Epiglottis
Mandible
Sublingual gland
Submandibular gland
Trachea
Esophagus

Mouth and oropharynx

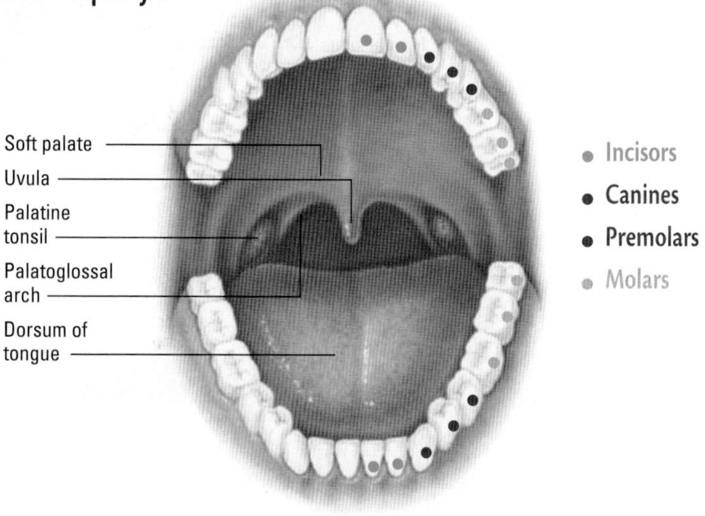
Soft palate
Uvula
Palatine tonsil
Palatoglossal arch
Dorsum of tongue
Incisors
Canines
Premolars
Molars

Neck

The neck is formed by the cervical vertebrae, the major neck and shoulder muscles, and their ligaments. Other important structures of the neck include the trachea, thyroid gland, and chains of lymph nodes.

The thyroid gland lies in the anterior neck, just below the larynx. Its two cone-shaped lobes are located on either side of the trachea and are connected by an isthmus below the cricoid cartilage, which gives the gland its butterfly shape.

Structures of the neck

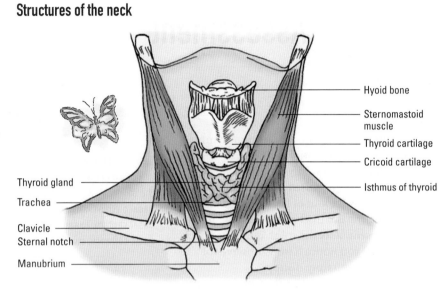

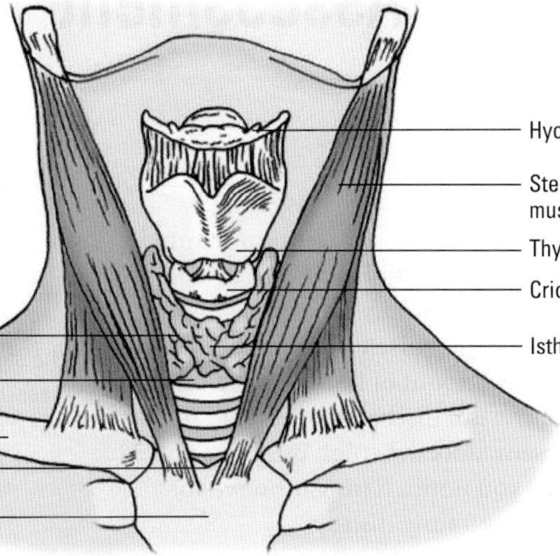
Hyoid bone
Sternomastoid muscle
Thyroid cartilage
Cricoid cartilage
Isthmus of thyroid
Thyroid gland
Trachea
Clavicle
Sternal notch
Manubrium

Lymph node locations

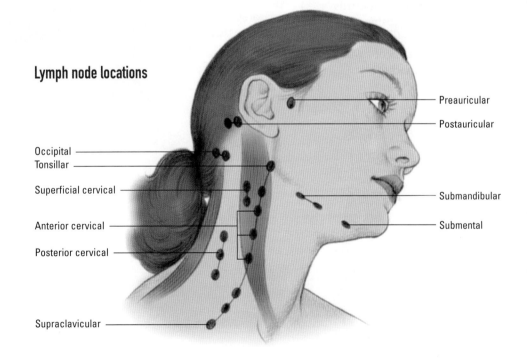

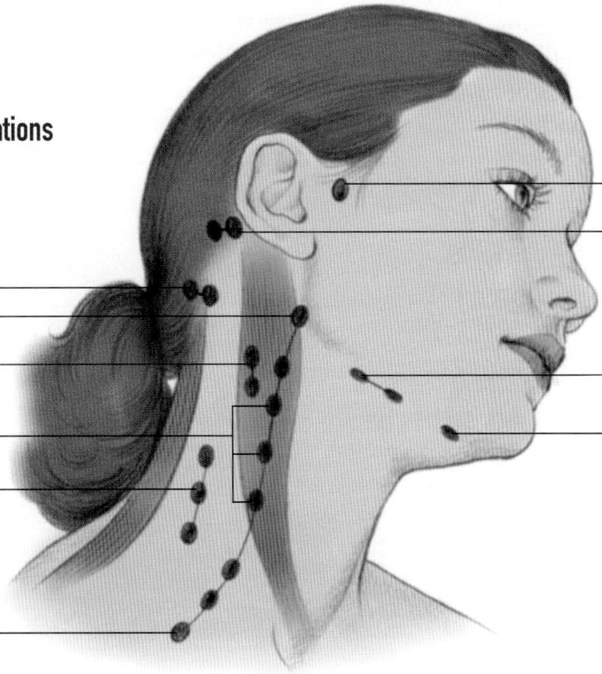
Preauricular
Postauricular
Occipital
Tonsillar
Superficial cervical
Anterior cervical
Posterior cervical
Supraclavicular
Submandibular
Submental

Assessment

Nose and sinuses

Inspecting the nose

Observe the patient's nose for position, symmetry, and color. Note variations, such as discoloration, swelling, or deformity. Variations in size and shape are largely caused by differences in cartilage and in the amount of fibroadipose tissue.

Observe for nasal discharge or flaring. If discharge is present, note the color, quantity, and consistency. If you notice flaring, observe for other signs of respiratory distress.

Then inspect the nasal cavity. Check patency by occluding one nostril and asking the patient to breathe in through the other nostril. Repeat on the other side. Examine the nostrils by direct inspection using a nasal speculum, a penlight or small flashlight, or an otoscope with a short, wide-tip attachment.

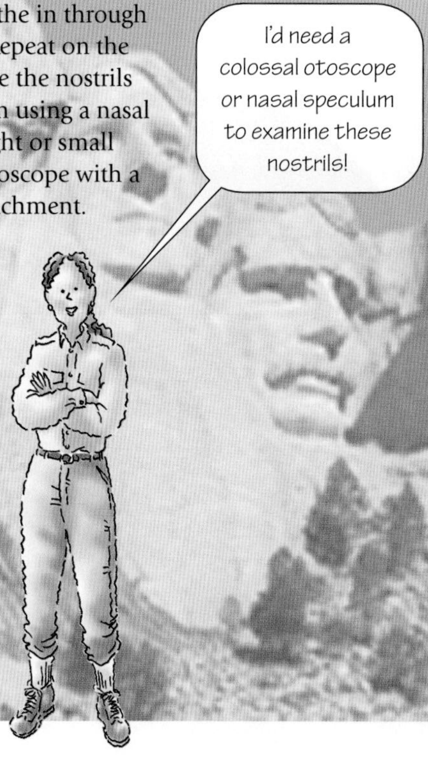
I'd need a colossal otoscope or nasal speculum to examine these nostrils!

Skill check

Inspecting the nasal cavity

To inspect the nose, ask the patient to tilt the head back slightly, and then push up the tip of the nose and gently insert the otoscope. Use the light from the otoscope to illuminate the nasal cavities. Check for severe deviation or perforation of the nasal septum. Examine the vestibule and turbinates for redness, softness, swelling, and discharge.

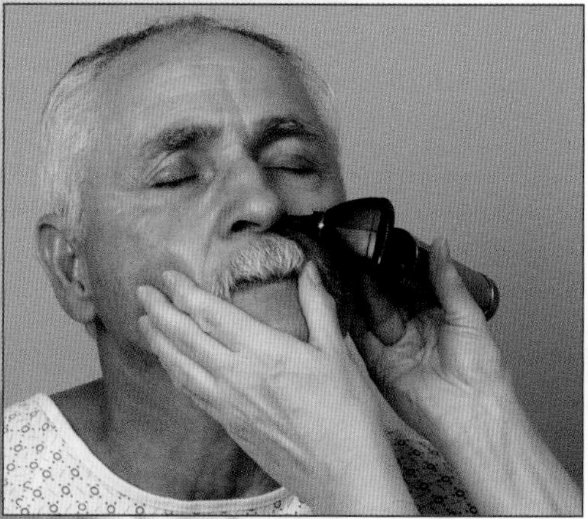

Inspecting the nostrils

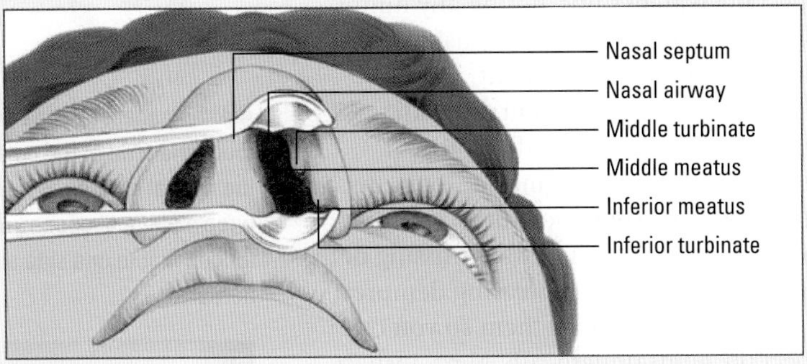
Nasal septum
Nasal airway
Middle turbinate
Middle meatus
Inferior meatus
Inferior turbinate

Have the patient sit in front of you with the head tilted back. Put on gloves and insert the tip of the closed nasal speculum into one nostril to the point where the blade widens. Slowly open the speculum as wide as possible without causing discomfort, as shown. Shine the flashlight in the nostril to illuminate the area.

Observe the color and patency of the nostril, and check for exudate. The mucosa should be moist, pink to light red, and free from lesions and polyps. After inspecting one nostril, close the speculum, remove it, and inspect the other nostril.

Palpating the nose

Palpate the patient's nose with your thumb and forefinger, assessing for pain, tenderness, swelling, and deformity.

Examining the sinuses

Begin by checking for swelling around the eyes, especially over the sinus area. Then palpate the sinuses, checking for tenderness.

If the patient complains of tenderness during sinus palpation, transilluminate the sinuses to see if they're filled with fluid or pus. Transillumination can also help reveal tumors and obstructions.

To perform transillumination, darken the room and have the patient close the eyes. Place a penlight under the eyebrow and direct the light upward to illuminate the frontal sinuses. Place the penlight on the patient's cheekbone just below the eye and ask the patient to open the mouth. A red glow inside the oral cavity indicates normal maxillary sinuses.

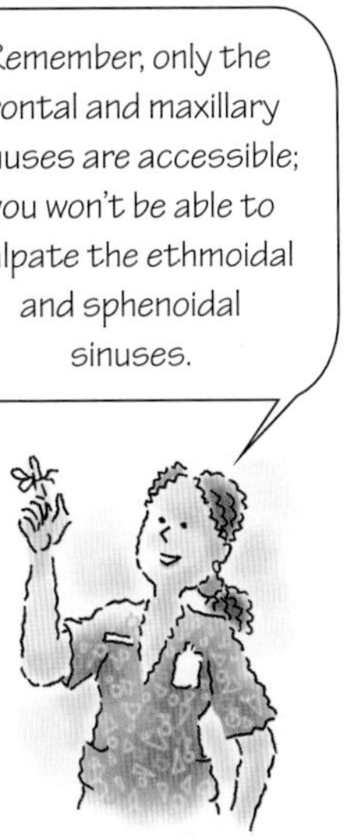
Remember, only the frontal and maxillary sinuses are accessible; you won't be able to palpate the ethmoidal and sphenoidal sinuses.

Skill check

Palpating the maxillary sinuses

To palpate the maxillary sinuses, gently press your thumbs on each side of the nose just below the cheekbones.

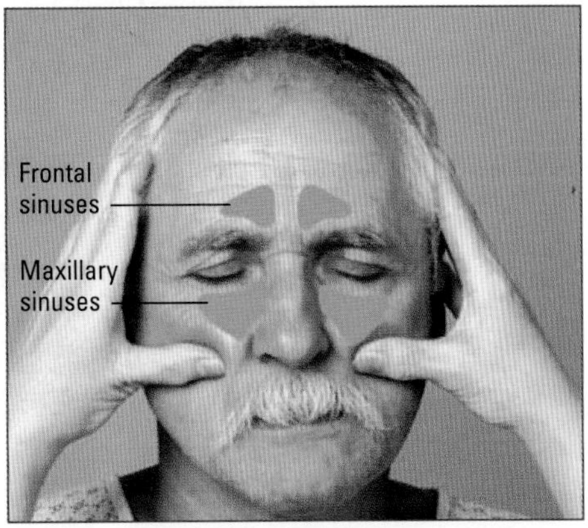
Frontal sinuses
Maxillary sinuses

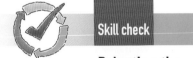

Mouth and throat

Inspect the patient's lips, noting any lumps or surface abnormalities. Then, using a tongue blade and a bright light, inspect the mouth. While the patient's mouth is open, place the tongue blade on top of the tongue. Observe the gingivae, or gums. Then inspect the teeth; note their number, condition, and whether any are missing or crowded. If the patient is wearing dentures, ask the patient to remove them so you can inspect the gums underneath. Next, inspect the tongue and oropharynx.

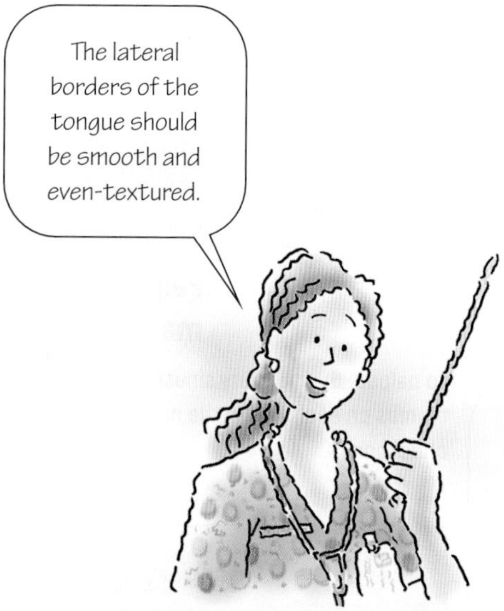
The lateral borders of the tongue should be smooth and even-textured.

Skill check

Inspecting the tongue

Ask the patient to raise the tip of the tongue and use the tongue to touch the area of the palate directly behind the front teeth. Inspect the ventral surface of the tongue and the floor of the mouth. Next, wrap a piece of gauze around the tip of the tongue and move the tongue first to one side and then the other to inspect the lateral borders.

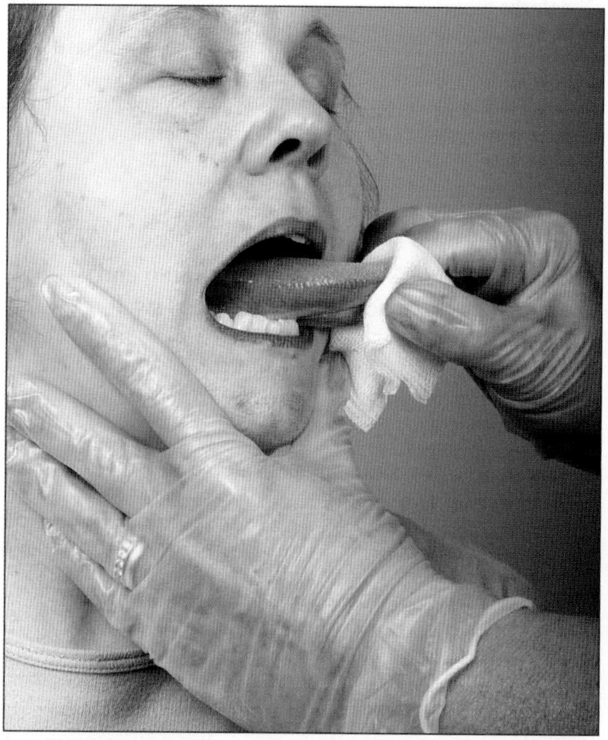

Lips

The lips should be pink, moist, symmetrical, and without lesions. They may have a bluish hue or flecked pigmentation in dark-skinned patients.

Oral mucosa

The oral mucosa should be pink, smooth, moist, and free from lesions and unusual odors. Increased pigmentation may occur in dark-skinned patients.

Gingivae (gums)

The gums should be pink, smooth, and moist, with clearly defined margins at each tooth. They shouldn't be retracted, red, or inflamed.

Inspecting the oropharynx

Inspect the patient's oropharynx by asking the patient to open the mouth while you shine the penlight on the uvula and palate. You may need to insert a tongue blade into the mouth and depress the posterior tongue. Place the tongue blade slightly off center to avoid eliciting the gag reflex. Ask the patient to say "Ahhh." Observe for movement of the soft palate and uvula. Note lumps, lesions, ulcers, or edema of the lips or tongue.

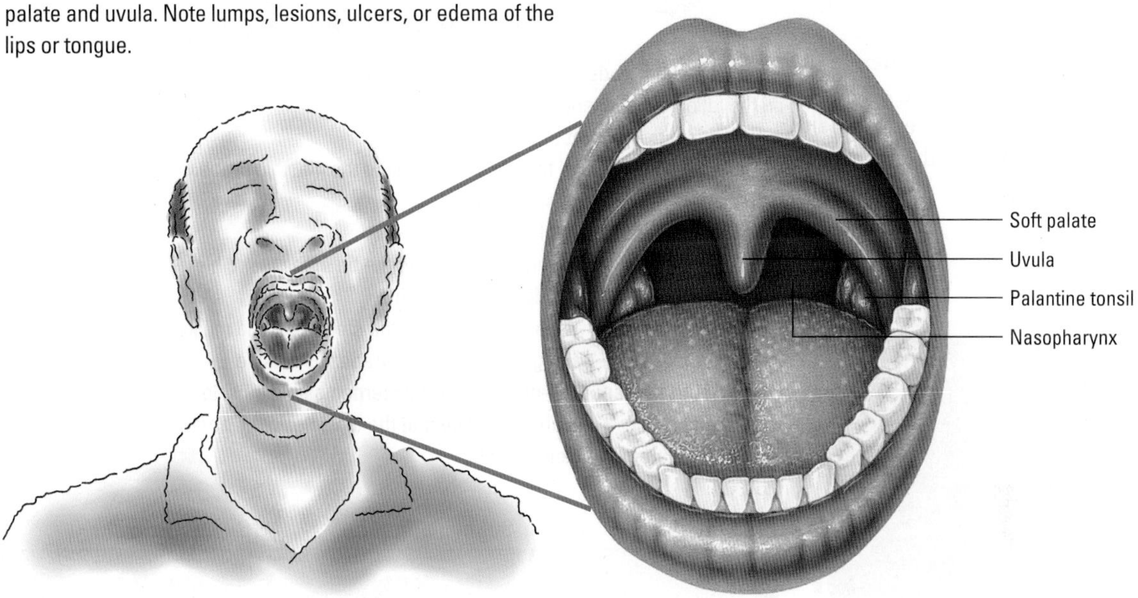

Soft palate
Uvula
Palantine tonsil
Nasopharynx

Finally, assess the patient's gag reflex by gently touching the back of the pharynx with a cotton-tipped applicator or the tongue blade. Doing so should produce a bilateral response.

Tongue

The tongue should be midline, moist, pink, and free from lesions. It should have a smooth posterior surface and slightly rough anterior surface with small fissures. It should move easily in all directions and lie straight to the front at rest.

Oropharynx and uvula

These structures should be pink and moist, without inflammation or exudates.

Tonsils

The tonsils should be pink and without hypertrophy.

Neck

Inspection

Observe the patient's neck. It should be symmetrical, and the skin should be intact. Note any scars. No visible pulsations, masses, swelling, venous distention, or thyroid gland or lymph node enlargement should be present. Ask the patient to gently move the neck through the entire range of motion and then shrug shoulders.

memory board

When assessing the neck, remember to **SPEND** some time evaluating these findings:
Swelling
Pulsations
Enlargement (of thyroid gland or lymph node)
Neck masses
Distention.

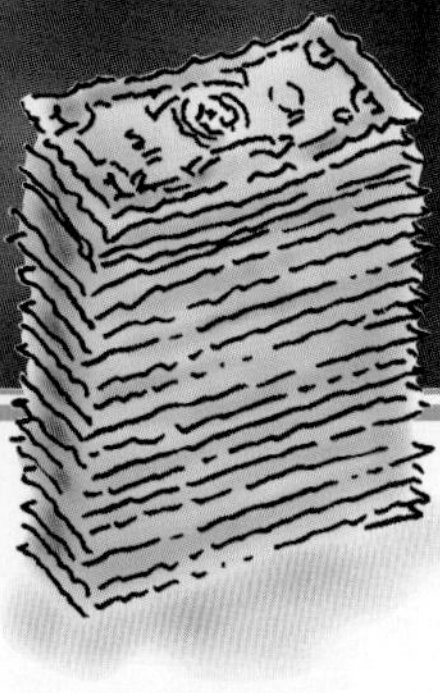

Palpation

Palpate the patient's neck using the finger pads of both hands. Assess the lymph nodes for size, shape, mobility, consistency, temperature, and tenderness, comparing nodes bilaterally.

Skill check

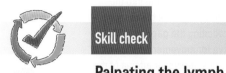

Palpating the lymph nodes

Using the finger pads of both hands, bilaterally palpate the chain of lymph nodes in the following sequence:

- Preauricular—in front of the ear
- Postauricular—behind the ear, superficial to the mastoid process
- Occipital—at the base of the skull
- Tonsillar—at the angle of the mandible
- Submandibular—between the angle and the tip of the mandible
- Submental—behind the tip of the mandible
- Superficial cervical—superficially along the sternomastoid muscle
- Posterior cervical—along the edge of the trapezius muscle
- Deep anterior cervical—deep under the sternomastoid muscle
- Supraclavicular—just above and behind the clavicle, in the angle formed by the clavicle and sternomastoid muscle

Preauricular

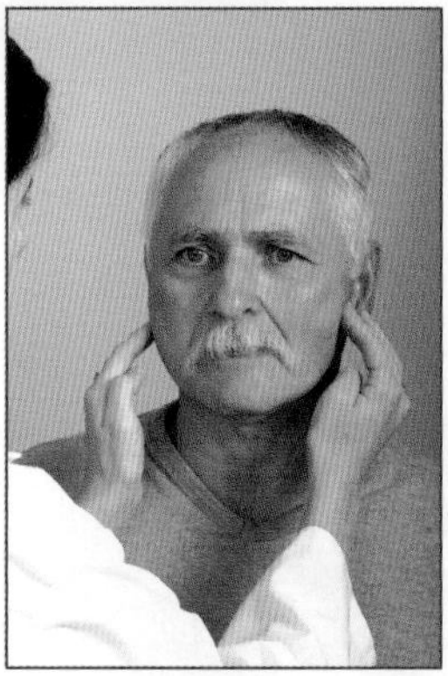

Submandibular

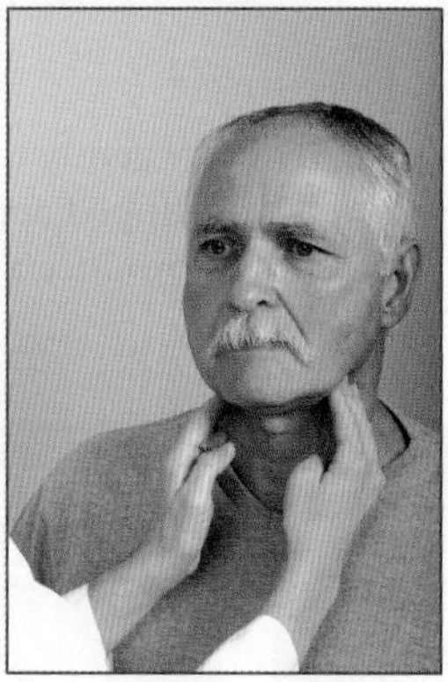

Supraclavicular

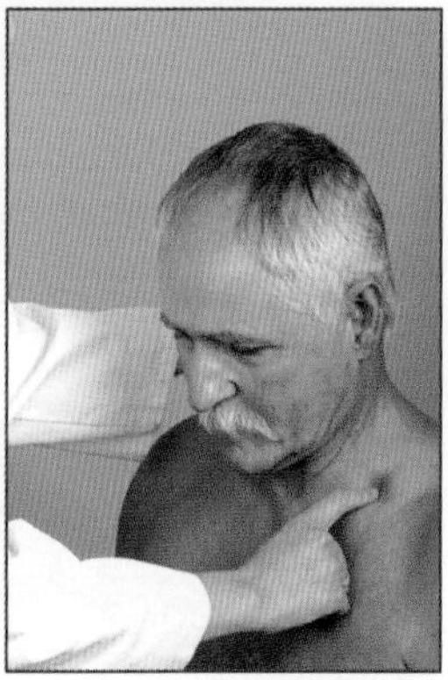

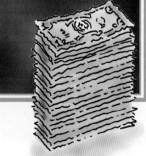

Then palpate the trachea, which is normally located midline in the neck, and the thyroid.

Palpating the trachea

Place your finger along one side of the trachea. Assess the distance between the trachea's outer edge and the sternocleidomastoid muscle. Then assess the distance on the other side, and compare the two distances. They should be the same.

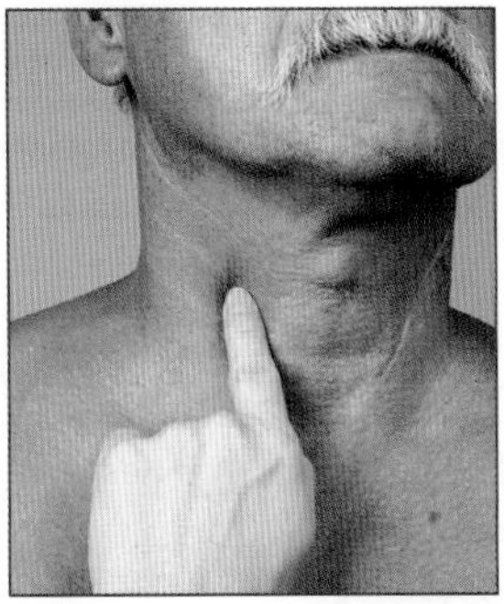

Palpating the thyroid

To palpate the thyroid, stand behind the patient and put your hands gently around the patient's neck, with the fingers of both hands over the lower trachea. Ask the patient to swallow as you feel the thyroid isthmus. The isthmus should rise with swallowing because it lies across the trachea, just below the cricoid cartilage.

Displace the thyroid to the right and then to the left, palpating both lobes for enlargement, nodules, tenderness, or a gritty sensation. Lowering the patient's chin slightly and turning toward the side you're palpating help relax the muscle and may facilitate assessment.

Palpating the thyroid

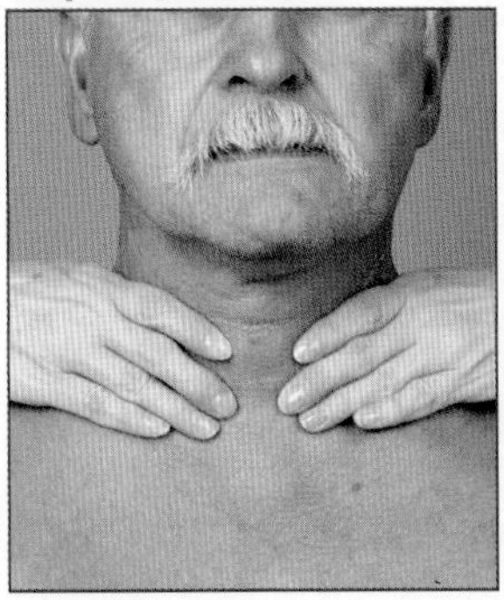

Normal thyroid on swallowing

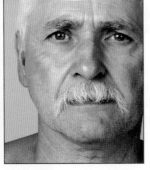

Auscultation

Using light pressure on the bell of the stethoscope, listen over the carotid arteries. Ask the patient to hold the breath while you listen to prevent breath sounds from interfering with the sounds of circulation. Listen for bruits, which signal turbulent blood flow.

If you detect an enlarged thyroid gland during palpation, also auscultate the thyroid area with the bell. Check for a bruit or a soft rushing sound, which indicates a hypermetabolic state.

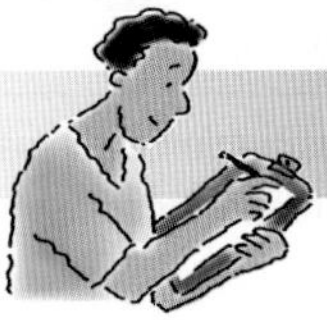

Take note

Documenting a thyroid bruit

4/25/10	0800	Thyroid gland found to be
		enlarged on palpation. Bruit
		heard over the lateral lobes
		of the thyroid gland.
		Lucinda Stevens, RN

Nose abnormalities

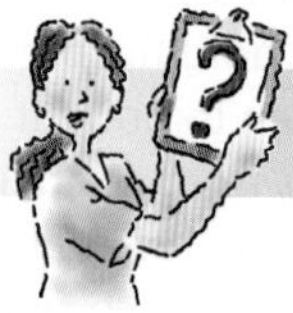

Outside the norm

Symptom synopsis: The nose

Symptom	Key facts	Possible causes
Epistaxis	• Refers to nosebleed	• Coagulation disorders • Trauma • Other hematologic disorders • Renal disorders • Hypertension
Flaring	• Refers to nostril dilation that occurs during inspiration • Normal to some extent during quiet breathing but marked regular flaring is abnormal	• Respiratory distress
Stuffiness and discharge	• Refers to obstruction of the nasal mucous membranes accompanied by secretions	• Common cold • Sinusitis • Trauma • Allergies • Exposure to irritants • Deviated septum

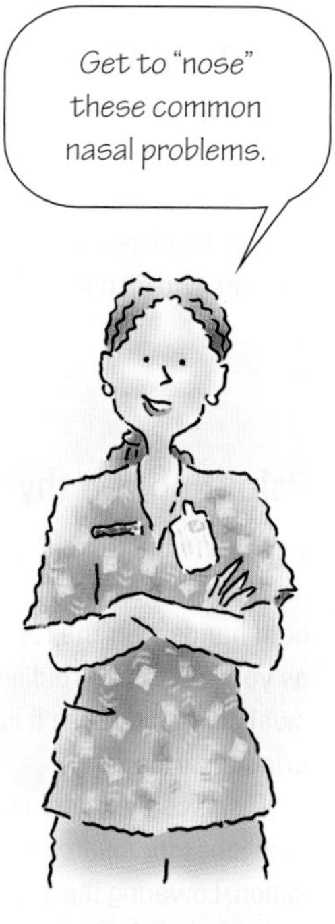
Get to "nose" these common nasal problems.

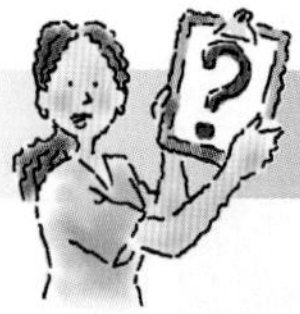

Outside the norm

Mouth abnormalities

Herpes simplex (type 1)

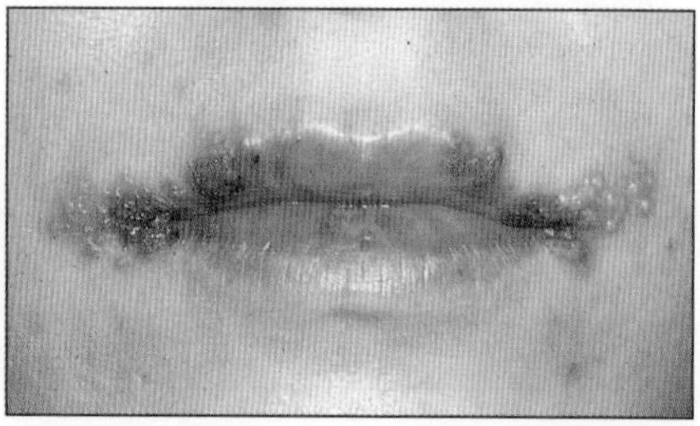

Herpes simplex, a recurrent viral infection, is caused by *human herpesvirus*. It's transmitted by oral and respiratory secretions, affects the mucous membranes, and produces painful cold sores and fever blisters. After a brief period of prodromal tingling and itching, the primary lesions erupt as vesicles on an erythematous base, eventually rupturing and leaving ulcers, followed by a yellow crust. Vesicles may form on any part of the oral mucosa, especially the lips, tongue, chin, and cheek.

Angioedema

Angioedema, commonly associated with urticaria, is usually caused by an allergic reaction. It presents subcutaneously or dermally and produces nonpitted swelling of subcutaneous tissue and deep, large wheals usually on the lips, hands, feet, eyelids, or genitalia. These swellings don't itch but may burn or tingle.

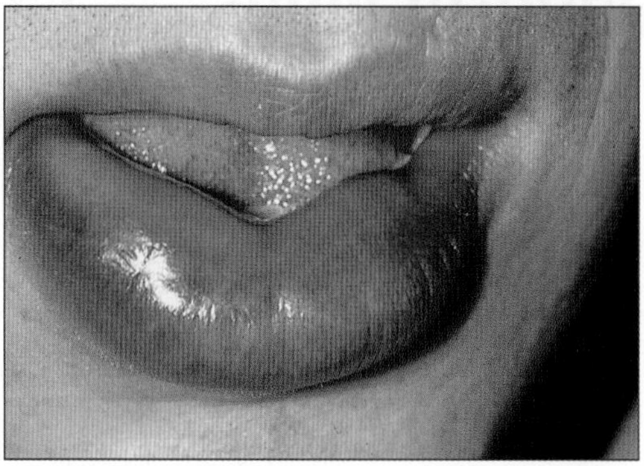

Leukoplakia

Leukoplakia involves painless, white patches that appear on the tongue or the mucous membranes of the mouth. It results from chronic irritation of the membranes due to tobacco use, poor-fitting dentures, use of some medications, or a rough tooth. The white patches are considered precancerous lesions. Biopsy determines whether the lesions are malignant.

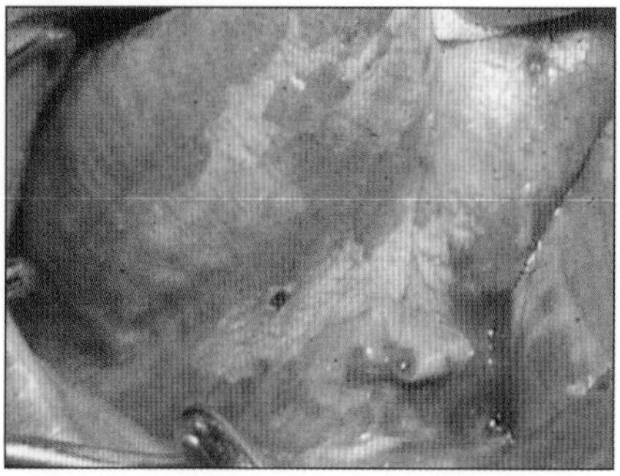

Candidiasis

Candidiasis of the oropharyngeal mucosa causes cream-colored or white patches on the tongue, mouth, or pharynx. Most cases of this infection are caused by *Candida albicans*. Although these fungi are part of the body's normal flora, they can cause infection when changes—such as an elevated blood glucose level in a patient with diabetes, immunosuppression in a patient with human immunodeficiency virus, or use of antibiotics—allow for their sudden proliferation.

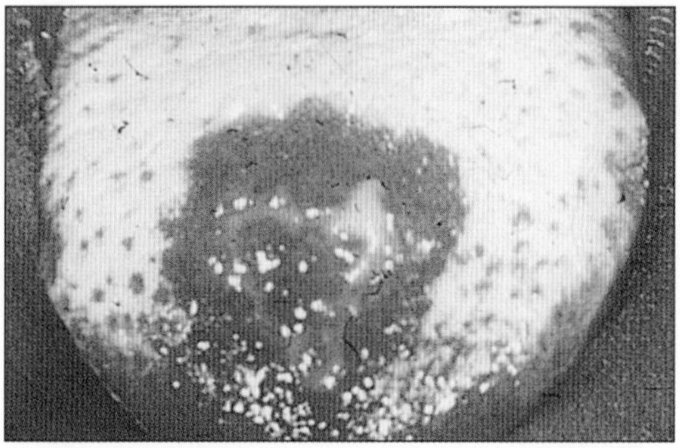

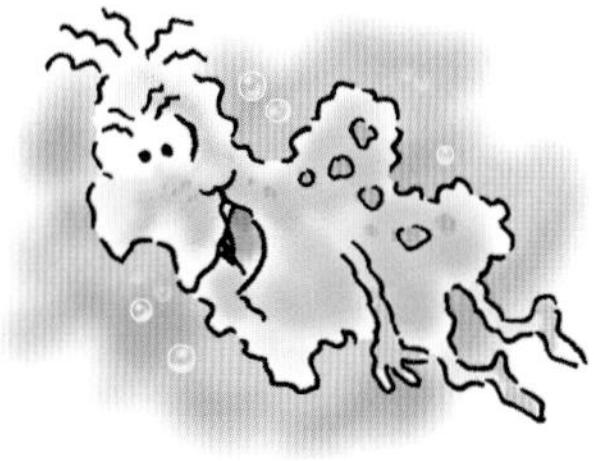

Throat abnormalities

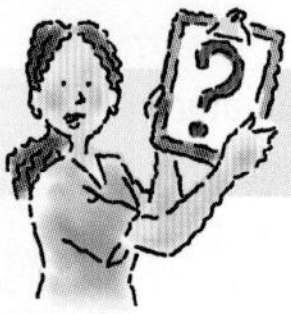

Outside the norm

Symptom synopsis: The throat

Symptom	Key facts	Possible causes
Dysphagia	• Refers to difficulty swallowing	• Esophageal disorders • Oropharyngeal, respiratory, neurologic, or collagen disorders • Certain toxins and treatments
Throat pain	• Commonly known as a *sore throat* • Refers to discomfort in any part of the pharynx • Ranges from a sensation of scratchiness to severe pain	• Infection such as pharyngitis or tonsillitis • Trauma • Allergies • Cancer or a systemic disorder • Surgery • Endotracheal intubation • Mouth breathing • Alcohol consumption • Inhaling smoke or chemicals such as ammonia • Vocal strain

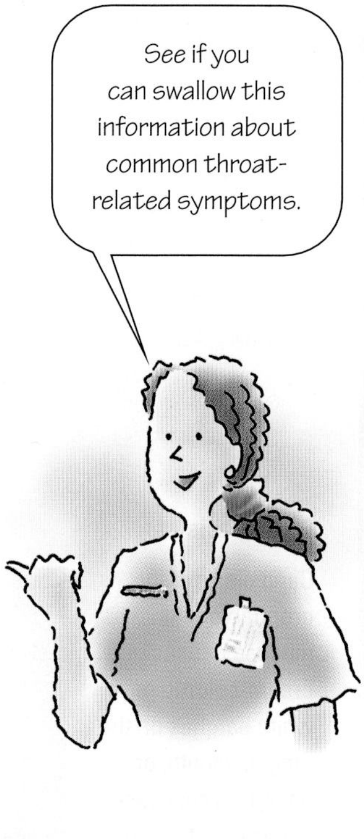
See if you can swallow this information about common throat-related symptoms.

Tonsillitis

Acute tonsillitis commonly begins with a mild to severe sore throat. Tonsillitis may also produce dysphagia, fever, swelling and tenderness of the lymph nodes, and redness in the throat. With exudative tonsillitis, a white exudate appears on the tonsils.

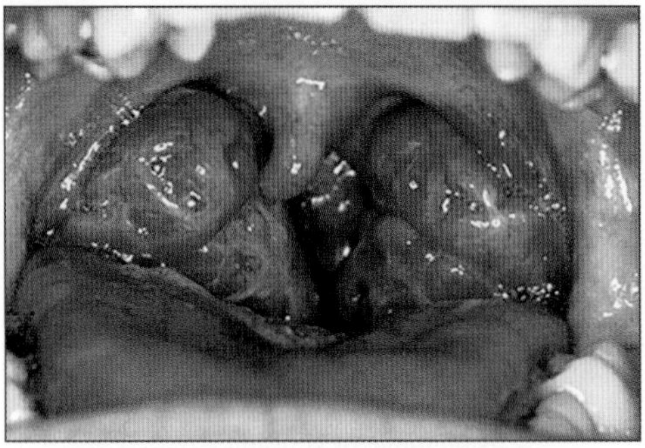

Pharyngitis

Pharyngitis is an acute or chronic inflammation of the pharynx that produces a sore throat and slight difficulty swallowing. It's usually caused by a virus, such as a rhinovirus, coronavirus, or adenovirus. It may also be caused by a bacterial infection, such as from group A beta-hemolytic streptococci.

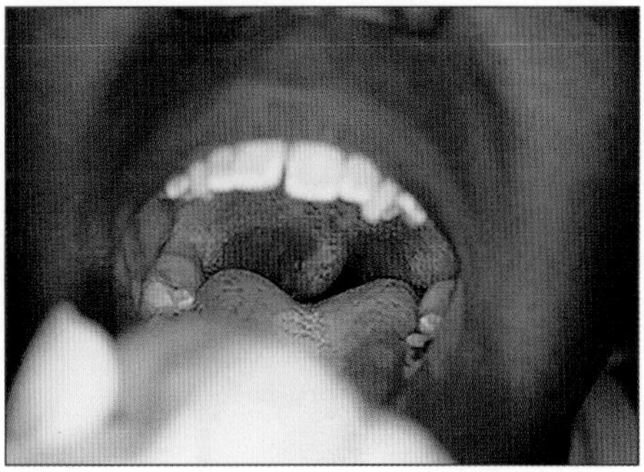

Diphtheria

Diphtheria is an acute, highly contagious, toxin-mediated infection caused by *Corynebacterium diphtheriae*. It causes a sore throat with rasping cough and leads to airway obstruction. The throat appears red with a thick, gray membrane covering the back of the throat.

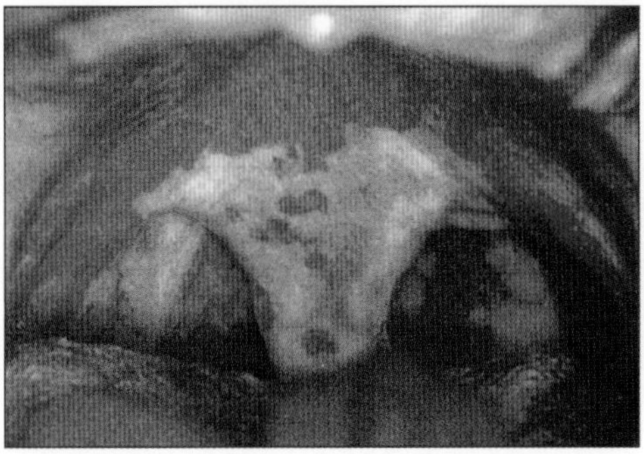

Neck abnormalities

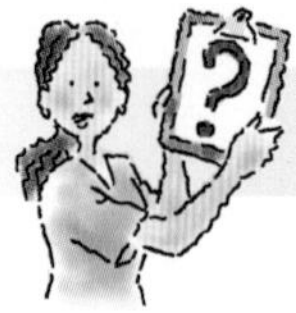

Outside the norm

Simple (nontoxic goiter)

A simple or nontoxic goiter involves thyroid gland enlargement that isn't caused by inflammation or a neoplasm. It's commonly classified as endemic or sporadic. Thyroid enlargement may range from a mildly enlarged gland to massive multinodular goiter.

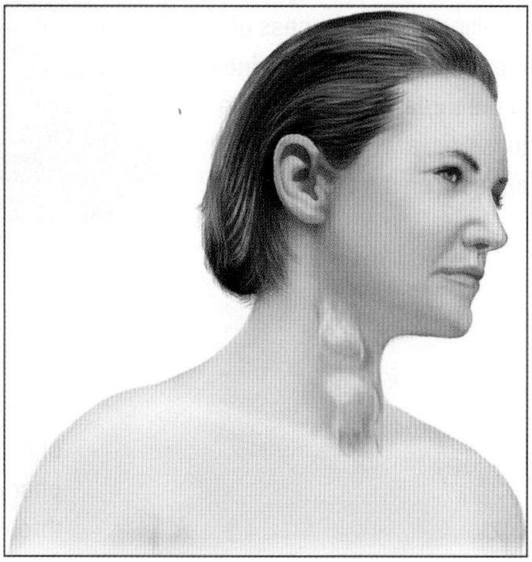

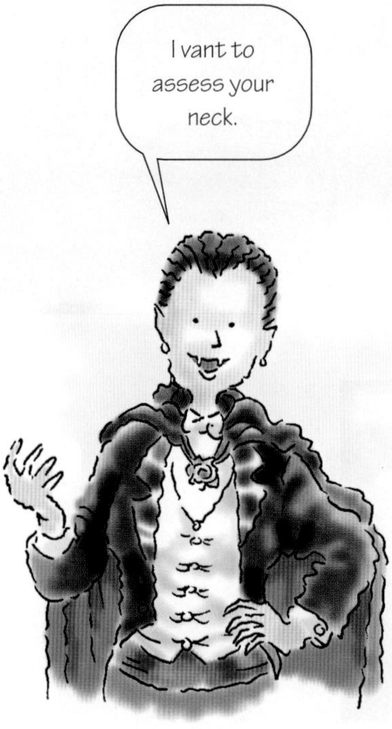
I vant to assess your neck.

Graves disease (toxic goiter)

Graves disease is the most common form of thyrotoxicosis, a metabolic imbalance that results from thyroid hormone overproduction. The classic features of Graves disease are an enlarged thyroid, nervousness, heat intolerance, weight loss despite increased appetite, sweating, frequent bowel movements, tremor, palpitations, and exophthalmos.

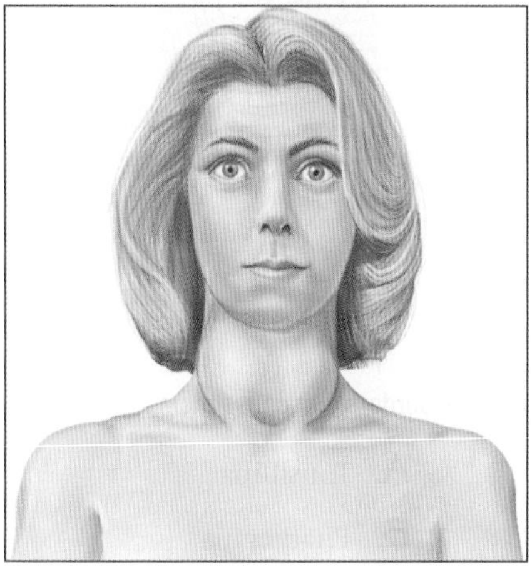

Toxic multinodular goiter

Common in the elderly, toxic multinodular goiter is a form of thyrotoxicosis that involves overproduction of thyroid hormone by one or more autonomously functioning nodules within a diffusely enlarged gland. Multiple thyroid nodules can be felt on palpation.

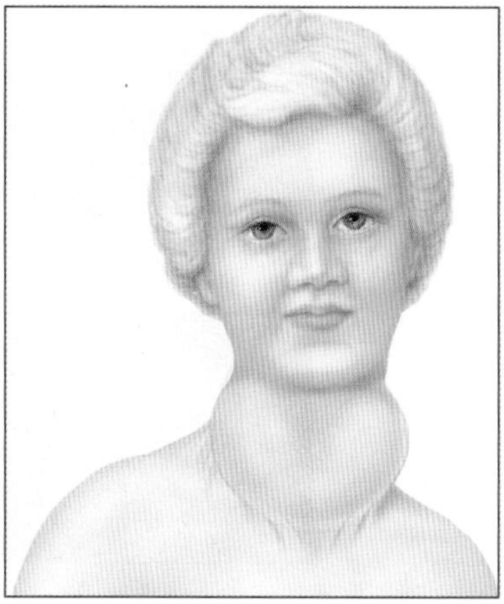

Q&A

Able to label?

Identify the neck structures indicated on this illustration.

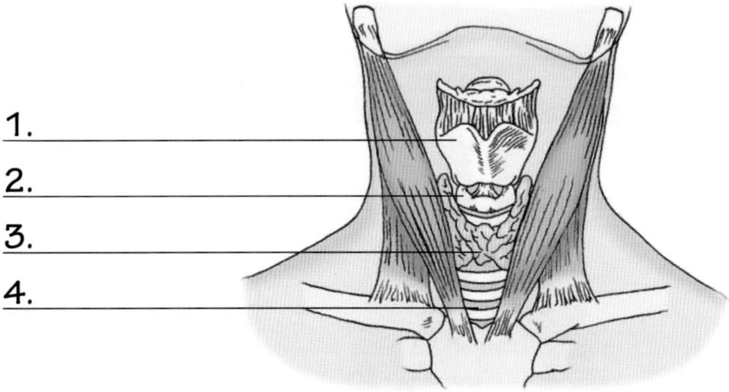
1. ______
2. ______
3. ______
4. ______

Matchmaker

Match the throat abnormalities shown here with the disorders that cause them.

1. ______

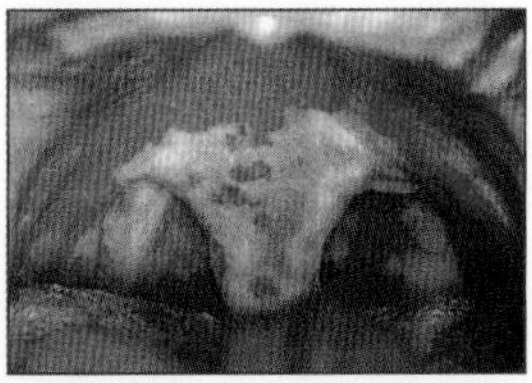

2. ______

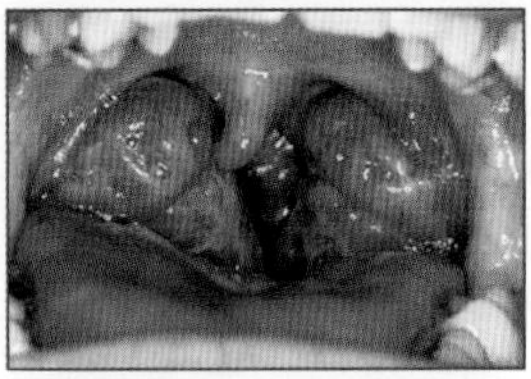

3. ______

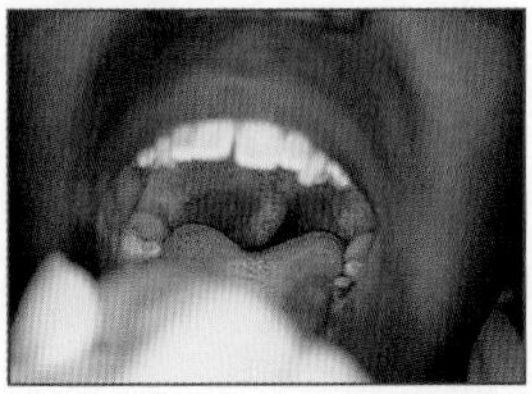

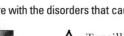

A. Tonsillitis

B. Pharyngitis

C. Diphtheria

Answers: Able to label? 1. Thyroid cartilage, 2. Cricoid cartilage, 3. Thyroid gland, 4. Trachea; Matchmaker 1. C, 2. A, 3. B.

Selected References

Barbara, D. W., Ronan, K. P., Maddox, D. E., & Warner, M. A. (2013). Perioperative angioedema: Background, diagnosis, and management. *Journal of Clinical Anesthesia, 25*, 335–343.

Chan, N. J., & Soliman, A. M. (2015). Angiotensin converting enzyme inhibitor-related angioedema: Onset, presentation, and management. *Annals of Otology, Rhinology & Laryngology, 124*, 89–96.

Hoyer, C., Hill, M. R., & Kaminski, E. R. (2012). Angio-oedema: An overview of differential diagnosis and clinical management. *Continuing education in Anaesthesia, Critical Care & Pain, 12*, 307–311.

Shepherd, A. B. (2013). Assessment and management of acute sore throat. *Nurse Prescribing, 11*, 549–553

Watkins, J. (2014). Diagnosing rashes, part 12: Lip lesions. *Practice Nursing, 25*, 557–566.

Watkins, J. (2014, September). Diagnosing rashes, part 11: Lip sores (cheilitis). *Practice Nursing, 25*, 440–445.

Chapter 5

Respiratory system

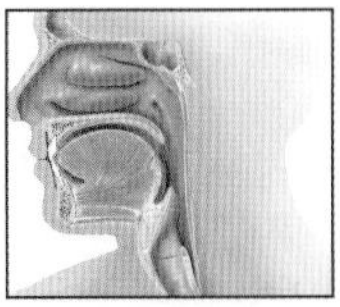
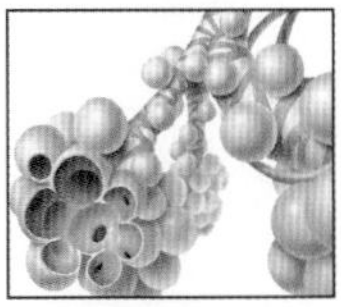
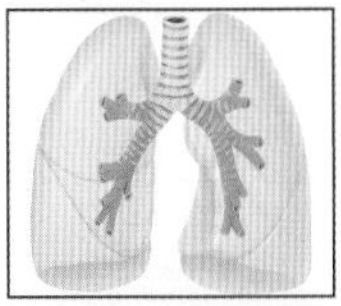
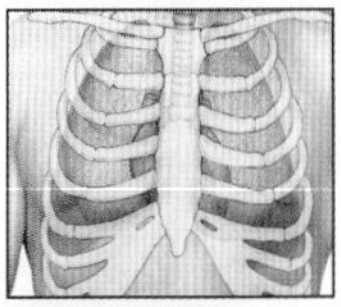
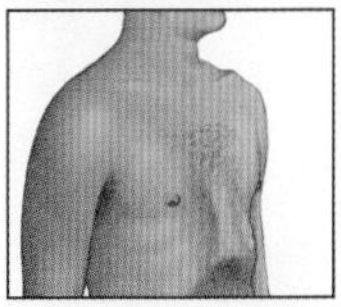
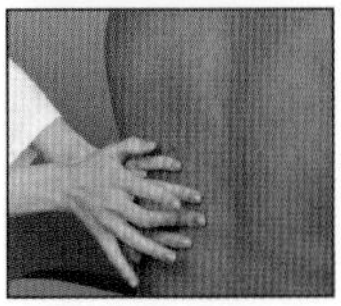
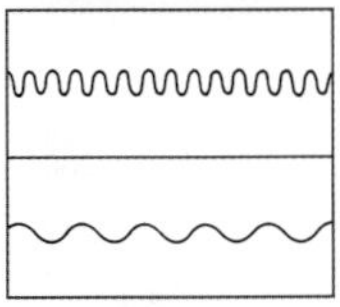
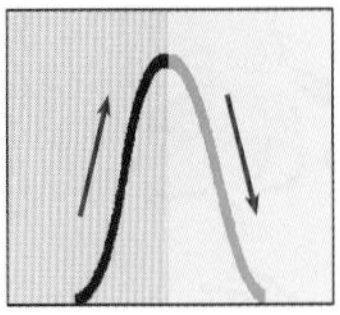
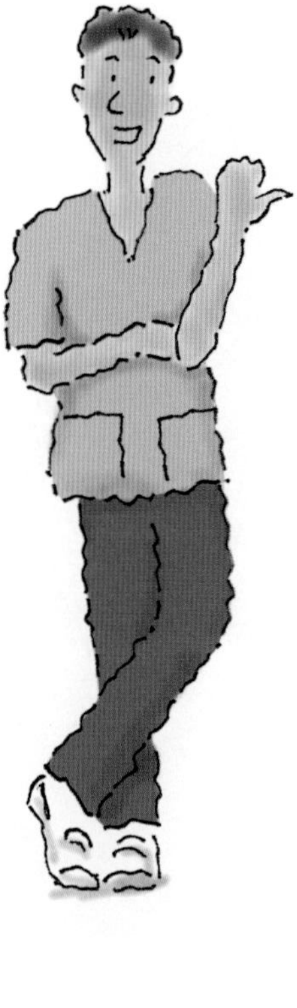

Anatomy

The structures of the respiratory system (the airways, lungs, bony thorax, respiratory muscles, and central nervous system) work together to deliver oxygen to the bloodstream and remove excess carbon dioxide from the body.

Upper airways

The upper airways include the nasopharynx (nose), oropharynx (mouth), laryngopharynx, and larynx. These structures warm, filter, and humidify inhaled air.

Lower airways

The lower airways begin with the trachea, or windpipe, which extends from the cricoid cartilage to the carina. The trachea then divides into the right and left mainstem bronchi, which continue to divide all the way down to the alveoli, the gas exchange units of the lungs.

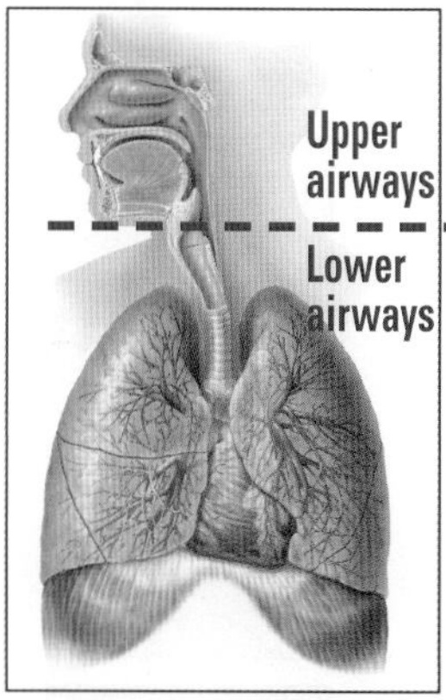
Upper
airways
Lower
airways

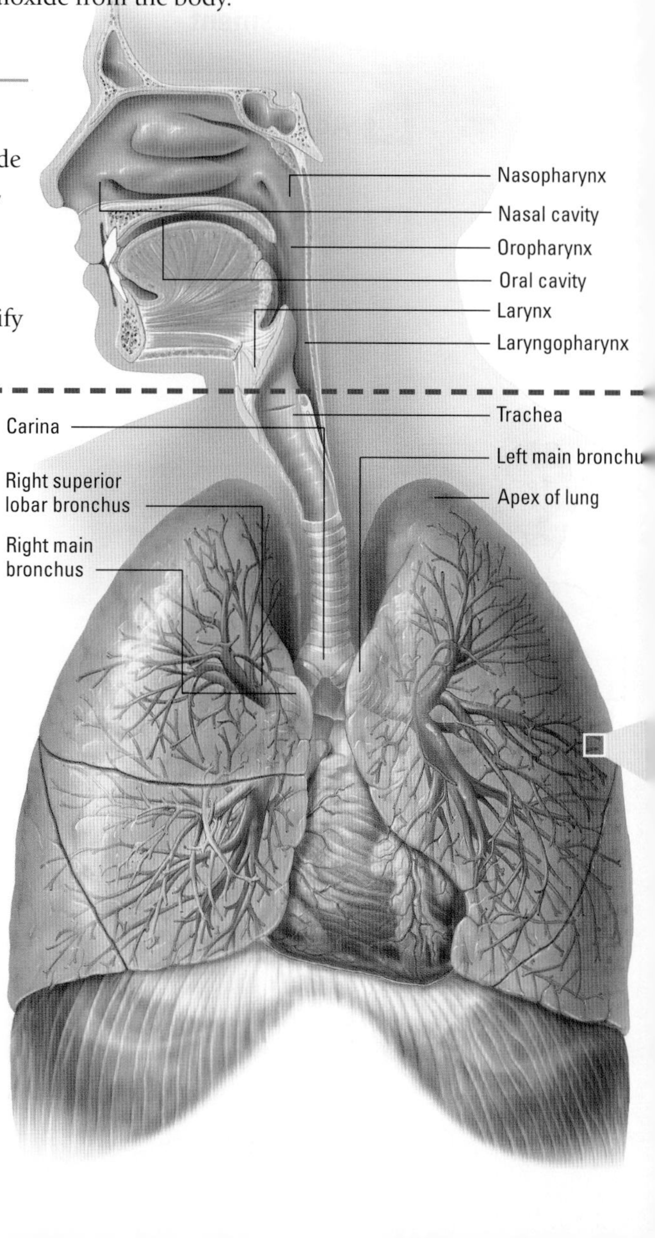
Nasopharynx
Nasal cavity
Oropharynx
Oral cavity
Larynx
Laryngopharynx
Carina
Trachea
Left main bronchu
Right superior
lobar bronchus
Apex of lung
Right main
bronchus

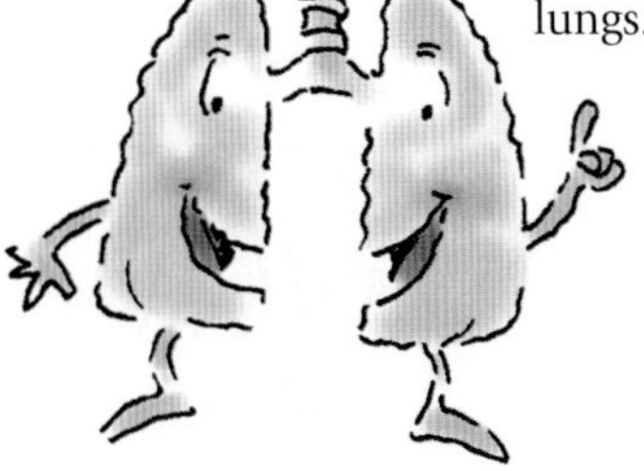

The larynx

The larynx houses the vocal cords. It's the transition point between the upper and lower airways. The epiglottis, a flap of tissue that closes over the top of the larynx when the patient swallows, protects the patient from aspirating food or fluid into the lower airways.

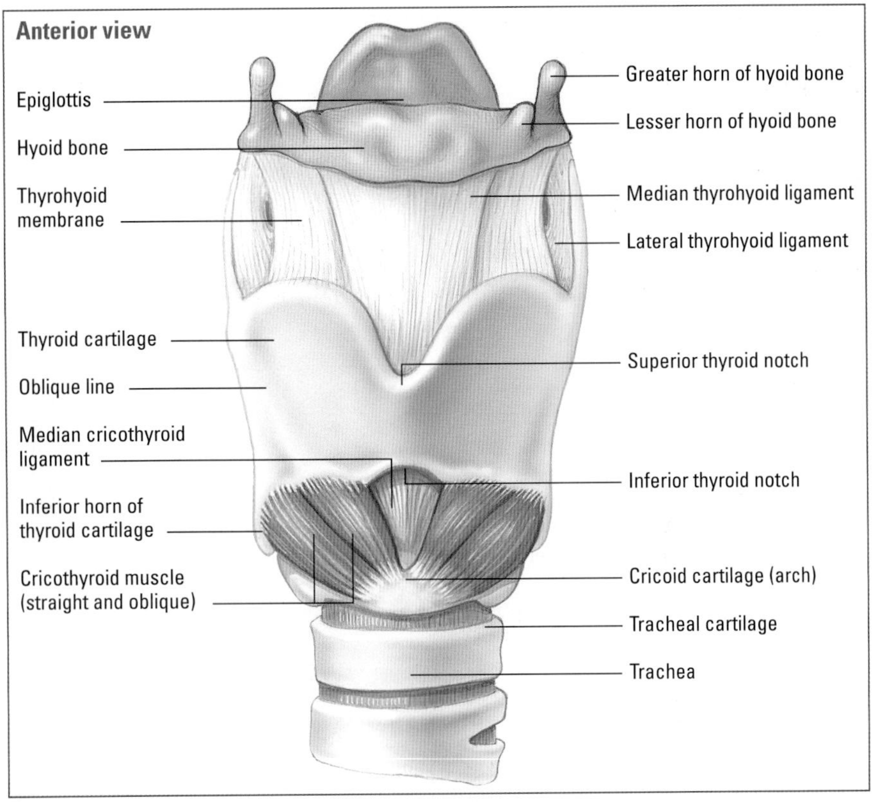
Anterior view
Epiglottis
Hyoid bone
Thyrohyoid membrane
Thyroid cartilage
Oblique line
Median cricothyroid ligament
Inferior horn of thyroid cartilage
Cricothyroid muscle (straight and oblique)
Greater horn of hyoid bone
Lesser horn of hyoid bone
Median thyrohyoid ligament
Lateral thyrohyoid ligament
Superior thyroid notch
Inferior thyroid notch
Cricoid cartilage (arch)
Tracheal cartilage
Trachea

Lower airways

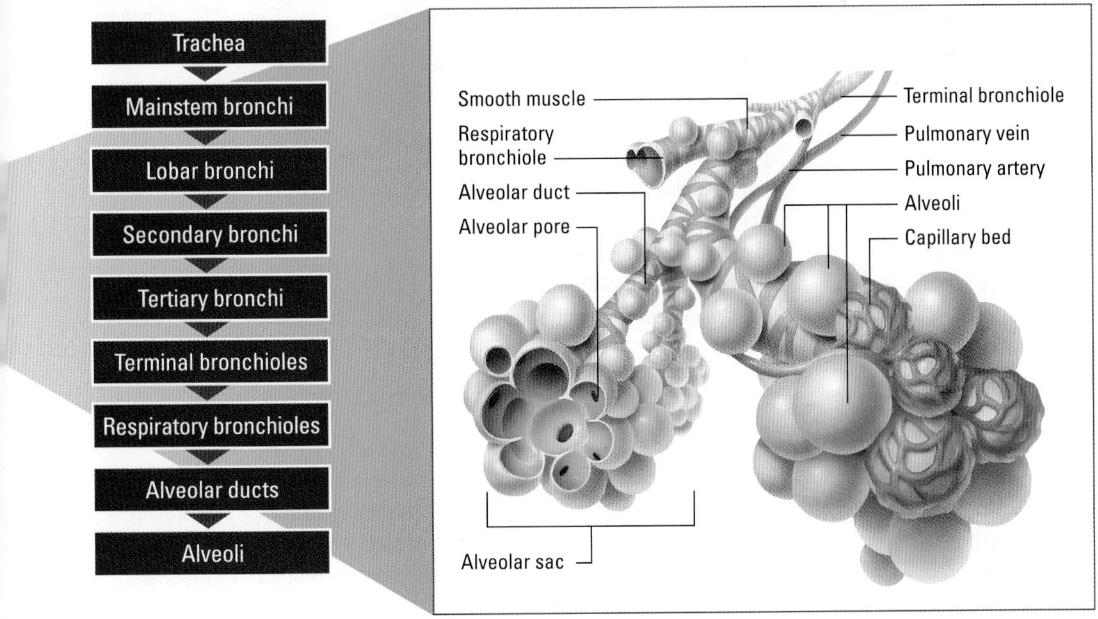
Trachea
Mainstem bronchi
Lobar bronchi
Secondary bronchi
Tertiary bronchi
Terminal bronchioles
Respiratory bronchioles
Alveolar ducts
Alveoli
Smooth muscle
Respiratory bronchiole
Alveolar duct
Alveolar pore
Alveolar sac
Terminal bronchiole
Pulmonary vein
Pulmonary artery
Alveoli
Capillary bed

Lungs

The right lung has three lobes: upper, middle, and lower. The left lung is smaller and has only an upper and a lower lobe. The lungs share space in the thoracic cavity with the heart and great vessels, the trachea, the esophagus, and the bronchi. The space between the lungs is called the *mediastinum*.

Thorax

The bony thorax includes the clavicles, sternum, scapula, 12 sets of ribs, and 12 thoracic vertebrae.

Respiratory muscles

The diaphragm and the external intercostal muscles are the primary muscles used in breathing. They contract when the patient inhales and relax when the patient exhales. Accessory inspiratory muscles include the trapezius, sternocleidomastoid, and scalenes, which combine to elevate the scapulae, clavicles, sternum, and upper ribs.

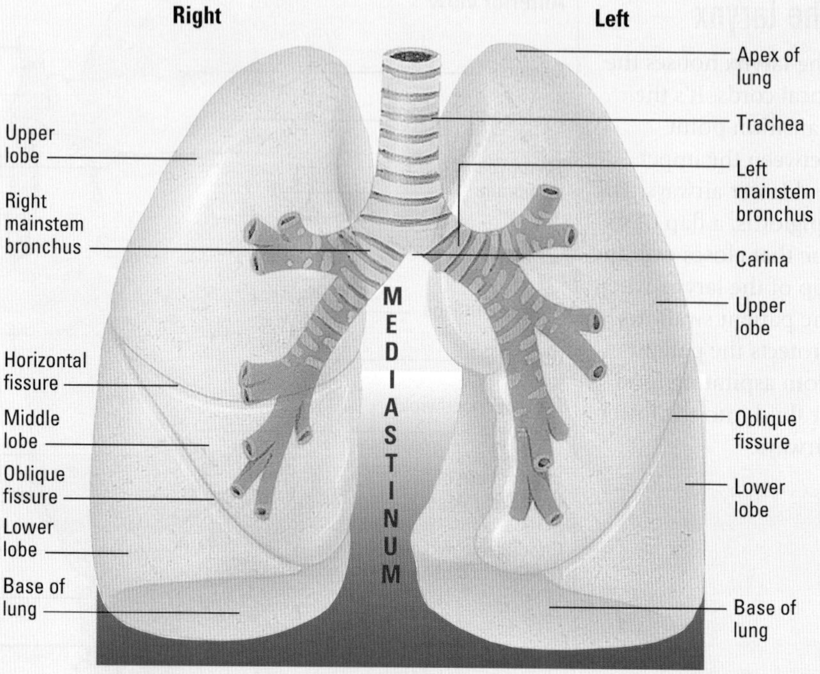
Right
Left
Apex of lung
Trachea
Left mainstem bronchus
Carina
Upper lobe
Oblique fissure
Lower lobe
Base of lung
Upper lobe
Right mainstem bronchus
Horizontal fissure
Middle lobe
Oblique fissure
Lower lobe
Base of lung
MEDIASTINUM

Pleurae

Each lung is wrapped in a lining called the *visceral pleura.* All areas of the thoracic cavity that come in contact with the lungs are lined with parietal pleura. A small amount of pleural fluid fills the area between the two layers of the pleura and allows the layers to slide smoothly over each other as the chest expands and contracts.

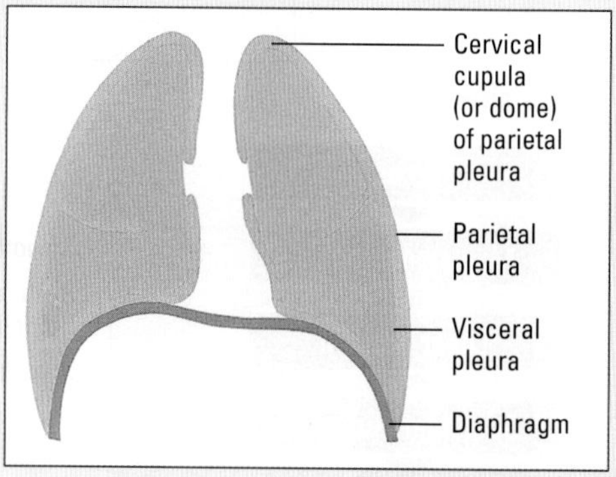
Cervical cupula (or dome) of parietal pleura
Parietal pleura
Visceral pleura
Diaphragm

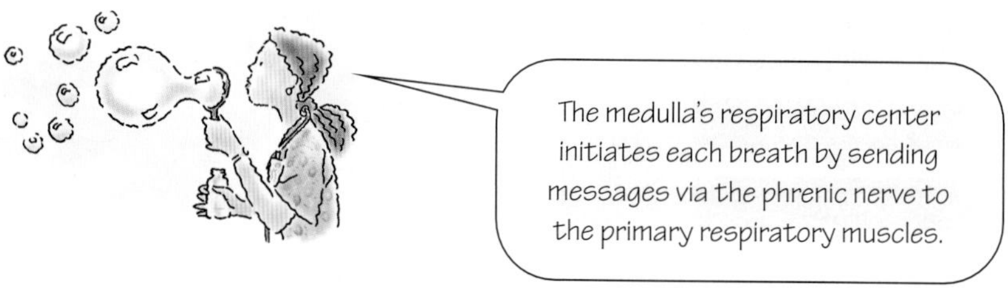
The medulla's respiratory center initiates each breath by sending messages via the phrenic nerve to the primary respiratory muscles.

Assessment

Begin your respiratory assessment by first observing the patient's general appearance. Then use inspection, palpation, percussion, and auscultation to perform a physical examination.

Examine the back of the chest first, comparing one side with the other. Then examine the front of the chest using the same sequence. Observe the chest from the side as well. The diameter of the thorax should be greater from side to side than from front to back.

Respiratory assessment landmarks

These illustrations show the anterior and posterior landmarks of the respiratory system. You can use these landmarks to help describe the locations of your assessment findings.

Anterior view

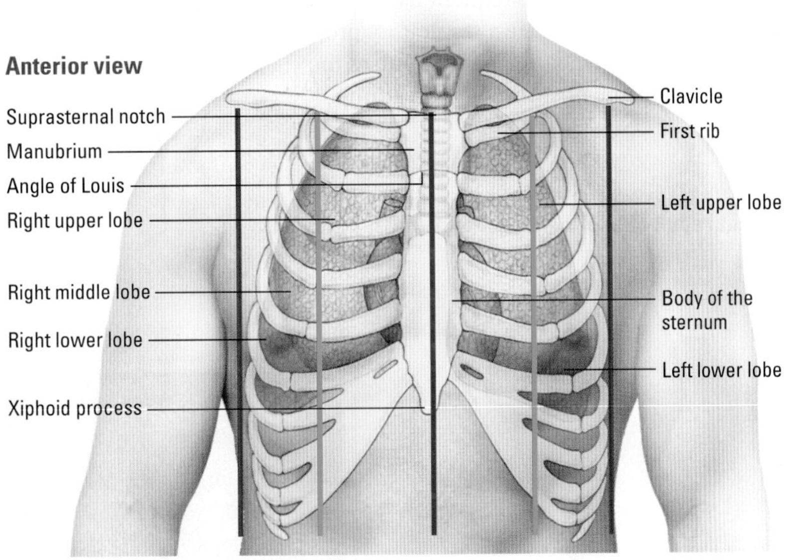
Suprasternal notch
Manubrium
Angle of Louis
Right upper lobe
Right middle lobe
Right lower lobe
Xiphoid process
Clavicle
First rib
Left upper lobe
Body of the sternum
Left lower lobe

Posterior view

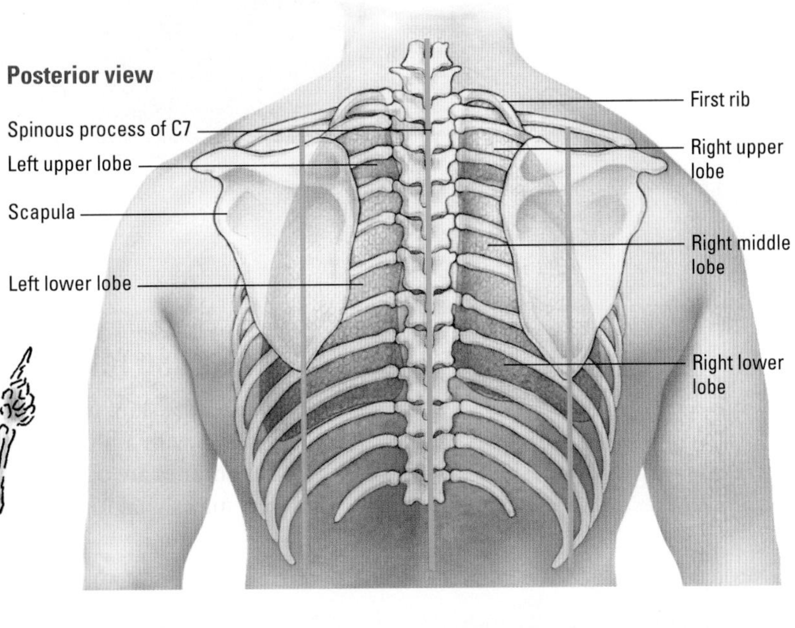
Spinous process of C7
Left upper lobe
Scapula
Left lower lobe
First rib
Right upper lobe
Right middle lobe
Right lower lobe

Inspecting the chest

Inspect for chest-wall symmetry. Note masses or scars that indicate trauma or surgery.

Landmark lines key

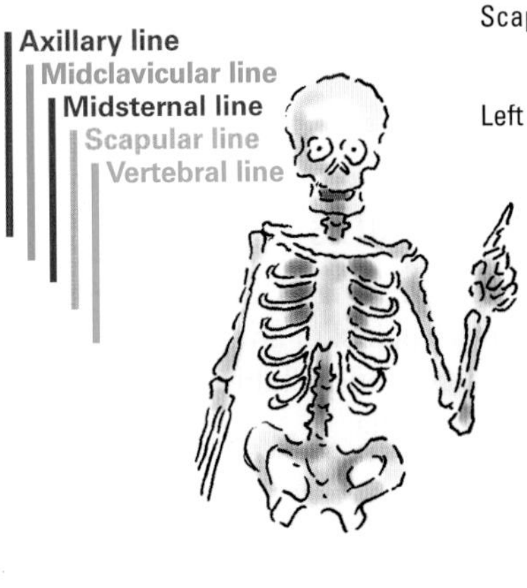
Axillary line
Midclavicular line
Midsternal line
Scapular line
Vertebral line

Respiratory rate and pattern

Count the number of breaths for a full minute. Adults normally breathe at a rate of 12 to 20 breaths/minute. An infant's breathing rate may reach 40 breaths/minute. The respiratory pattern should be even, coordinated, and regular, with occasional sighs (long, deep breaths).

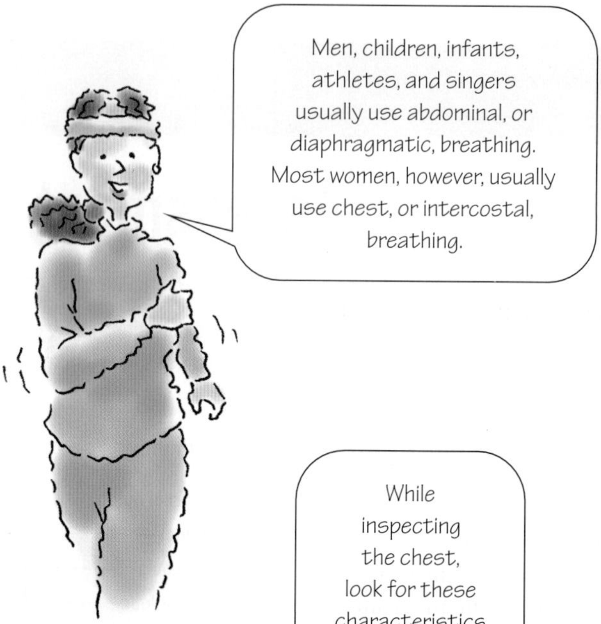
Men, children, infants, athletes, and singers usually use abdominal, or diaphragmatic, breathing. Most women, however, usually use chest, or intercostal, breathing.

Accessory muscle use

Observe the diaphragm and the intercostal muscles with breathing. Frequent use of accessory muscles may indicate a respiratory problem, particularly when the patient purses the lips and flares the nostrils when breathing.

Normal adult chest

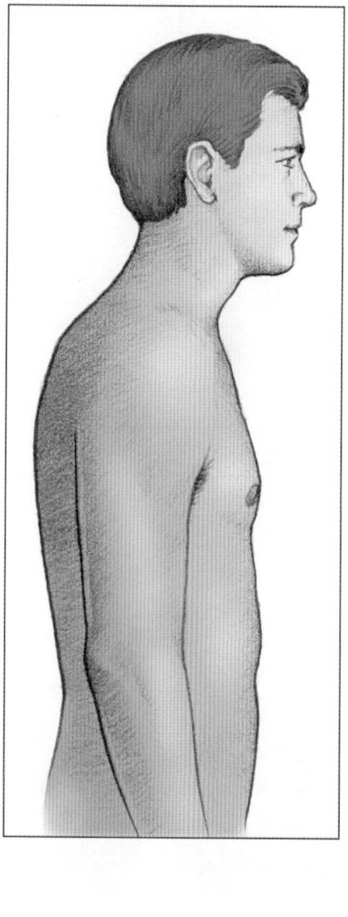

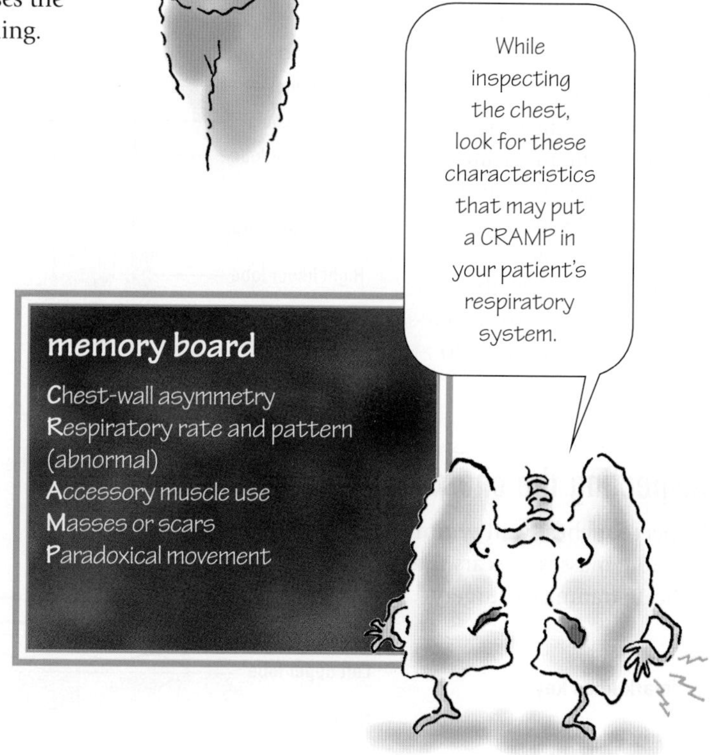
While inspecting the chest, look for these characteristics that may put a CRAMP in your patient's respiratory system.
memory board
Chest-wall asymmetry
Respiratory rate and pattern (abnormal)
Accessory muscle use
Masses or scars
Paradoxical movement

Inspecting related structures

Inspect the skin, tongue, mouth, fingers, and nail beds. Patients with a bluish tint to their skin and mucous membranes are considered cyanotic. Clubbing of the fingers may signal long-term hypoxia.

Palpating the chest

The chest wall should feel smooth, warm, and dry. Gentle palpation shouldn't cause the patient pain. Pain may be caused by costochondritis, rib or vertebral fractures, or sore muscles as a result of protracted coughing. Crepitus, which feels like puffed rice cereal crackling under the skin, indicates that air is leaking from the airways or lungs. Also, palpate for tactile fremitus, palpable vibrations caused by the transmission of air through the bronchopulmonary system. Then, evaluate chest-wall symmetry and expansion.

Skill check

1 Place your palm (or palms) lightly over the thorax. Palpate for tenderness, alignment, bulging, and retractions of the chest and intercostal spaces. Assess the patient for crepitus (a crackling sensation in the skin with palpation), especially around drainage sites. Repeat this procedure on the patient's back.

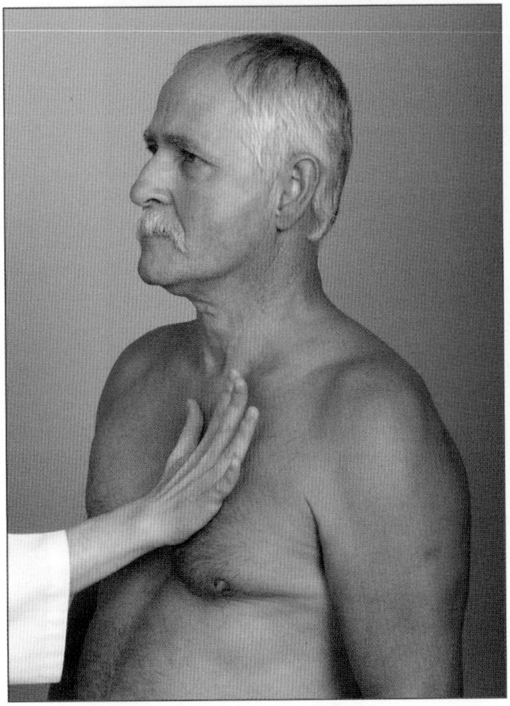

2 Use the pads of your fingers to palpate the front and back of the thorax. Pass your fingers over the ribs and any scars, lumps, lesions, or ulcerations. Note the skin temperature, turgor, and moisture. Also note tenderness or subcutaneous crepitus. The muscles should feel firm and smooth.

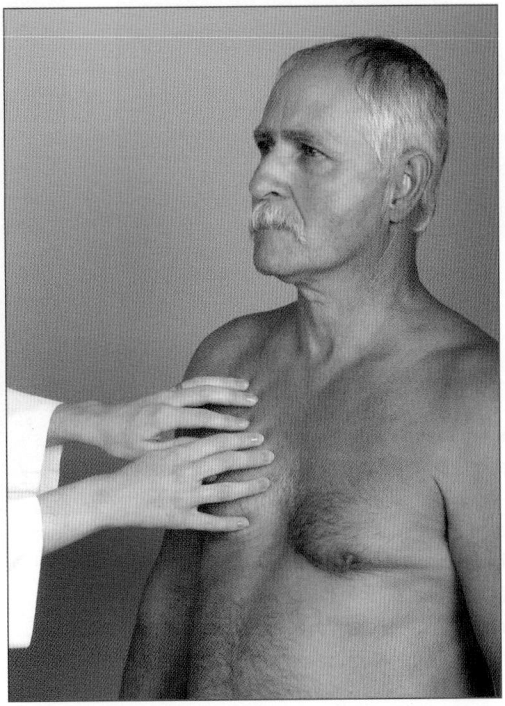

Skill check

Checking for tactile fremitus

Ask the patient to fold the arms across the chest. This movement shifts the scapulae out of the way. Lightly place your open palms on both sides of the patient's back, as shown, without touching the back with your fingers. Ask the patient to repeat the phrase "ninety-nine" loud enough to produce palpable vibrations. Then palpate the front of the chest using the same hand positions.

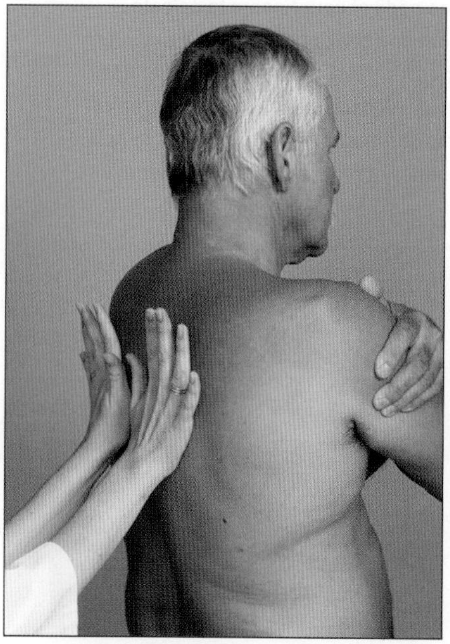

What the results mean

Vibrations that feel more intense on one side than the other indicate tissue consolidation on that side. Less intense vibrations may indicate emphysema, pneumothorax, or pleural effusion. Faint or no vibrations in the upper posterior thorax may indicate bronchial obstruction or a fluid-filled pleural space.

Evaluating chest-wall symmetry and expansion

Place your hands on the front of the chest wall with your thumbs touching each other at the second intercostal space. As the patient inhales deeply, watch your thumbs. They should separate simultaneously and equally to a distance several centimeters away from the sternum. Repeat the measurement at the fifth intercostal space.

The same measurement may be made on the back of the chest near the tenth rib. The patient's chest may expand asymmetrically if the patient has pleural effusion, atelectasis, pneumonia, or pneumothorax.

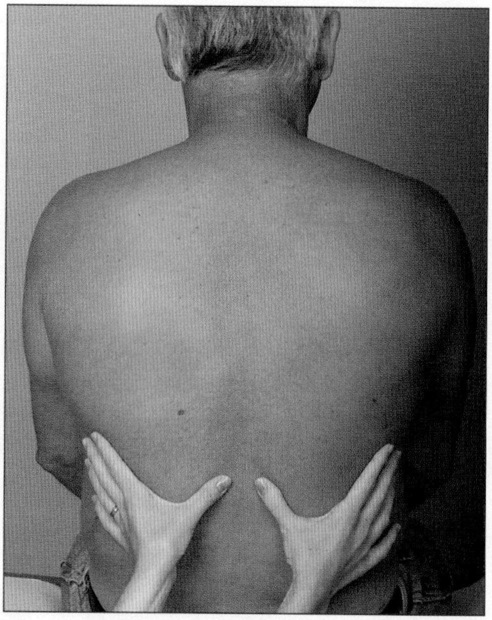

Percussing the chest

Chest percussion reveals the boundaries of the lungs and helps to determine whether the lungs are filled with air or fluid or solid material.

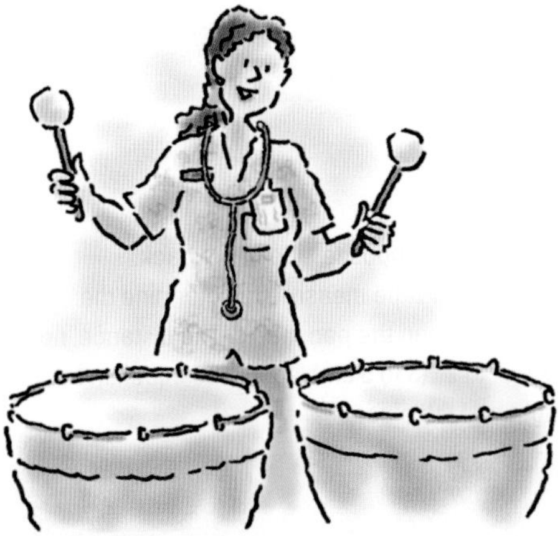

Percussion sounds

Sound	Description	Clinical significance
Flat	Short, soft, high-pitched, extremely dull, as found over the thigh	Consolidation, as in atelectasis and extensive pleural effusion
Dull	Medium in intensity and pitch, moderate length, thudlike, as found over the liver	Solid area, as in lobar pneumonia
Resonant	Long, loud, low-pitched, hollow	Normal lung tissue; bronchitis
Hyperresonant	Very loud, lower-pitched, as found over the stomach	Hyperinflated lung, as in emphysema or pneumothorax
Tympanic	Loud, high-pitched, moderate length, musical, drumlike, as found over a puffed-out cheek	Air collection, as in a large pneumothorax

Skill check

- Place your nondominant hand over the chest wall, pressing firmly with your middle finger.
- Position your dominant hand over your other hand.
- By flexing the wrist (not the elbow or upper arm) of your dominant hand, tap the middle finger of your nondominant hand with the middle finger of your dominant hand (as shown).
- Follow the standard percussion sequence over the front and back chest walls.

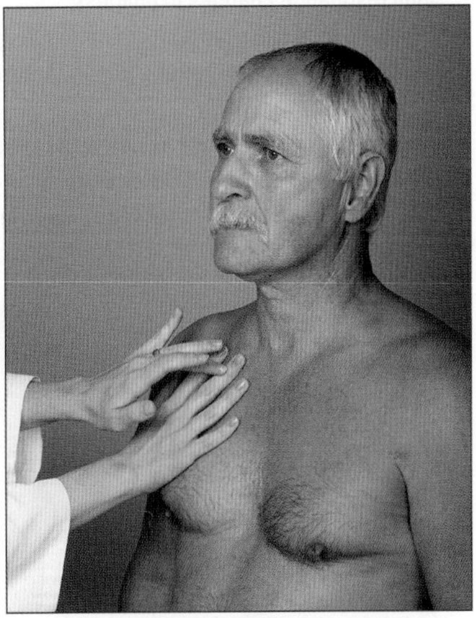

Diaphragmatic excursion

Percussion is also used to assess diaphragmatic excursion (the distance the diaphragm moves between inhalation and exhalation). Keep in mind that the diaphragm doesn't move as far in obese patients or patients with certain respiratory disorders.

Skill check

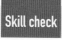

Measuring diaphragm movement

- Ask the patient to exhale.
- Percuss the back on one side to locate the upper edge of the diaphragm, the point at which normal lung resonance changes to dullness.
- Use a pen to mark the spot indicating the position of the diaphragm at full expiration on that side of the back.
- Ask the patient to inhale as deeply as possible.
- Percuss the back when the patient has breathed in fully until you locate the diaphragm. Use the pen to mark this spot as well.

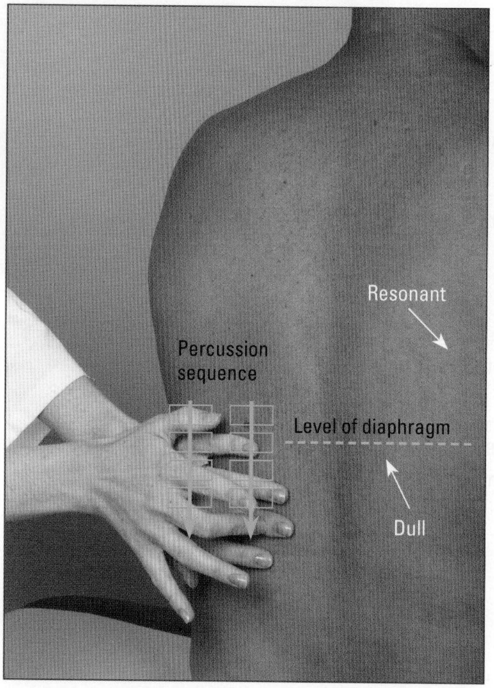
Resonant
Percussion sequence
Level of diaphragm
Dull

- Repeat on the opposite side of the back.
- Use a ruler or tape measure to determine the distance between the pen marks. The distance, normally 1¼″ to 2″ (3 to 5 cm), should be equal on both the right and left sides.

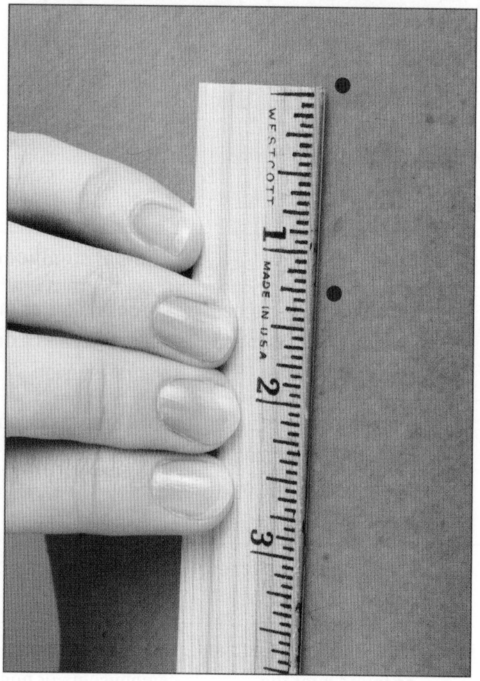
WESTCOTT
MADE IN U.S.A.

Auscultating the chest

As air moves through the bronchi, it creates sound waves that travel to the chest wall. The sounds produced by breathing change as air moves from larger airways to smaller airways. Sounds also change if they pass through fluid, mucus, or narrowed airways. Auscultation of these sounds helps you to determine the condition of the alveoli and surrounding pleura.

Classify each sound you hear according to its intensity, location, pitch, duration, and characteristic. Note whether the sound occurs when the patient inhales, exhales, or both.

Auscultation sequence

To distinguish between normal and adventitious breath sounds in the patient's lungs, press the diaphragm of the stethoscope firmly against the skin. Listen to a full inspiration and a full expiration at each site in the sequence shown. Remember to compare sound variations from one side to the other. Document adventitious sounds that you hear and include their locations.

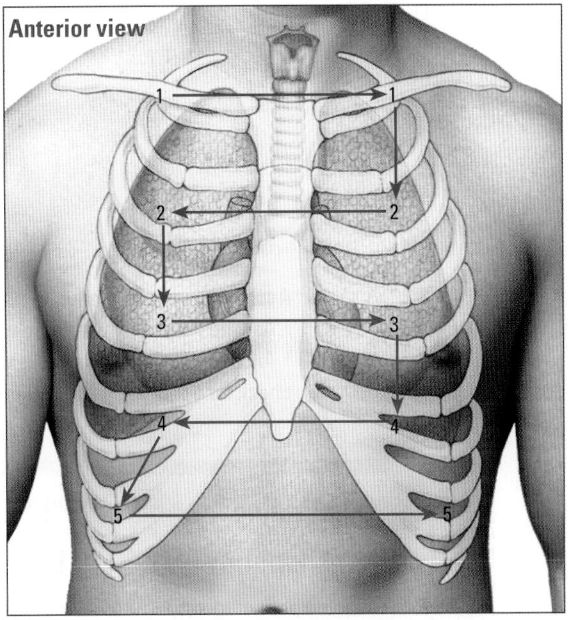
Anterior view
1
1
2
2
3
3
4
4
5
5

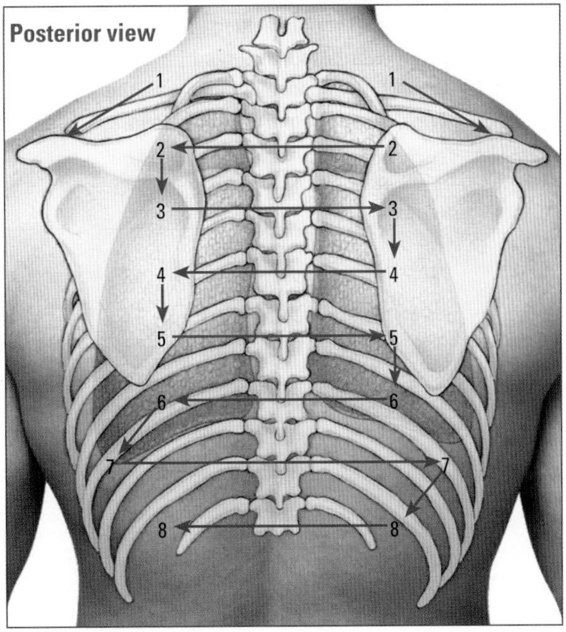
Posterior view
1
1
2
2
3
3
4
4
5
5
6
6
7
7
8
8

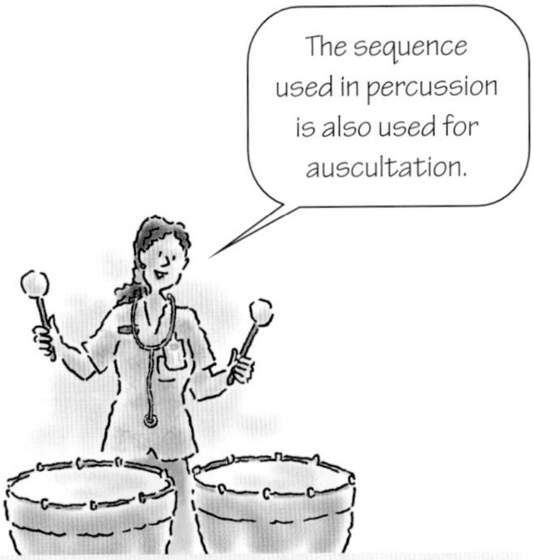
The sequence used in percussion is also used for auscultation.

Listen to these auscultation tips

- Have the patient breathe through the mouth; nose breathing alters the pitch of breath sounds.
- If the patient has abundant chest hair, mat it down with a damp washcloth so the hair doesn't make sounds like crackles.

Assessing voice sounds

Check the patient for vocal fremitus—voice sounds resulting from chest vibrations that occur as the patient speaks. Abnormal transmission of voice sounds may occur over consolidated areas. The most common abnormal voice sounds are bronchophony, egophony, and whispered pectoriloquy.

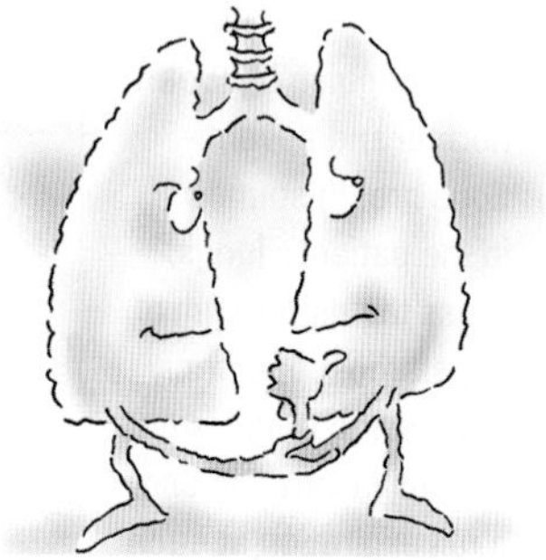

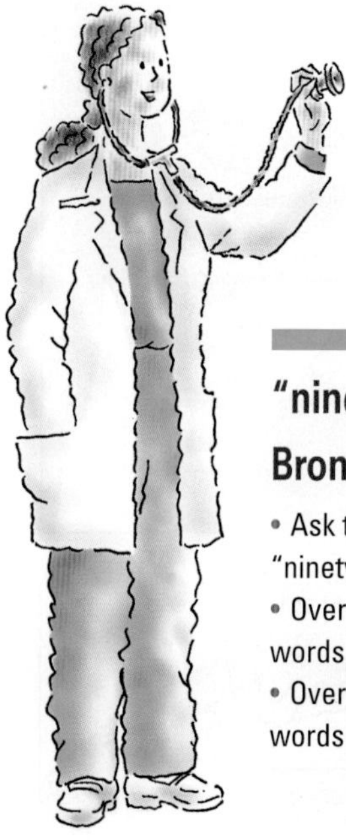

Assessing vocal fremitus

- Ask the patient to repeat the words below while you listen.
- Auscultate over an area where you heard abnormally located bronchial breath sounds to check for abnormal voice sounds.

"ninety-nine"

Bronchophony

- Ask the patient to say, "ninety-nine."
- Over normal lung tissue, the words sound muffled.
- Over consolidated areas, the words sound unusually loud.

"E"

Egophony

- Ask the patient to say "E."
- Over normal lung tissue, the sound is muffled.
- Over consolidated lung tissue, it will sound like the letter a.

"1, 2, 3"

Whispered pectoriloquy

- Ask the patient to whisper "1, 2, 3."
- Over normal lung tissue, the numbers will be almost indistinguishable.
- Over consolidated lung tissue, the numbers will be loud and clear.

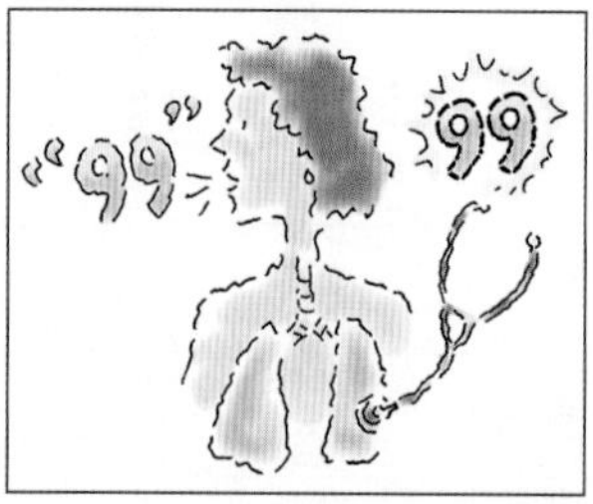
"99"
99

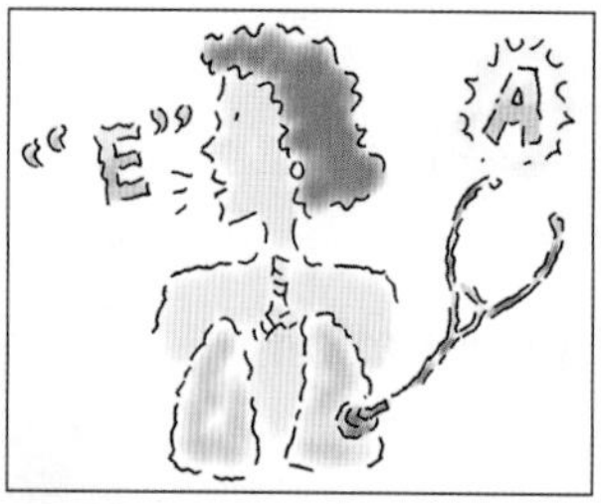
"E"
A

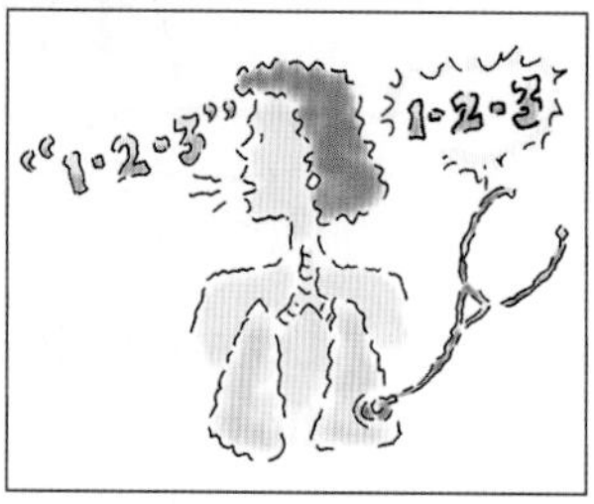
"1•2•3"
1•2•3

Locations of normal breath sounds

You'll hear four types of breath sounds over normal lungs. The type of sound you hear depends on where you listen. These illustrations show the normal locations of different types of breath sounds.

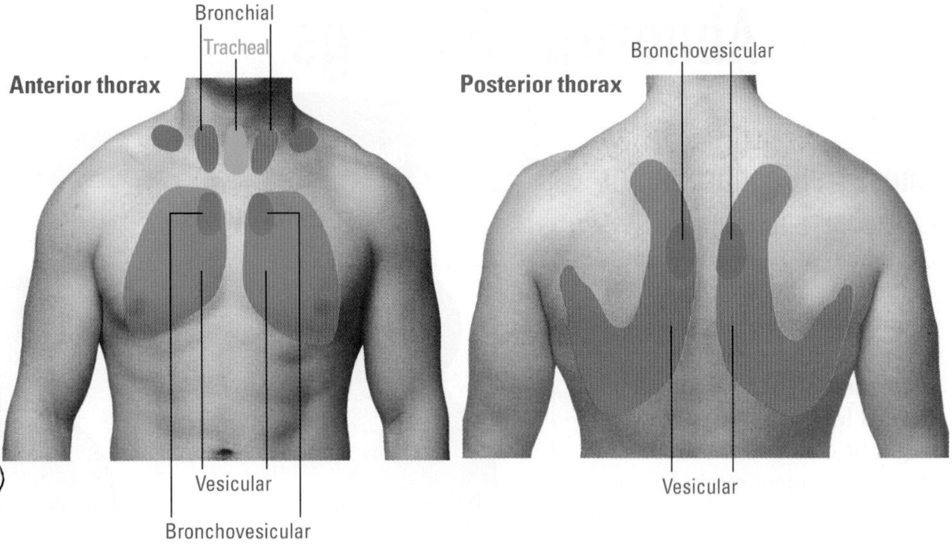
Anterior thorax
Bronchial
Tracheal
Vesicular
Bronchovesicular
Posterior thorax
Bronchovesicular
Vesicular

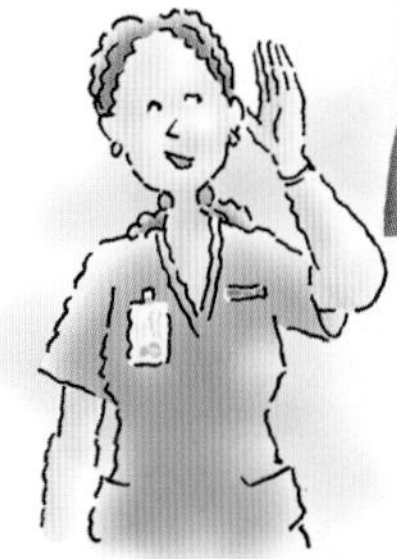

Qualities of normal breath sounds

Breath sound	Quality	Inspiration-expiration (I:E) ratio	Location		
Tracheal 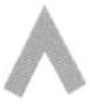	Harsh, high-pitched	I = E	Above supraclavicular notch, over the trachea	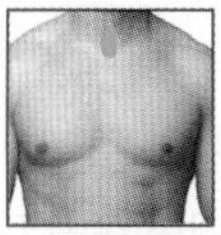	
Bronchial 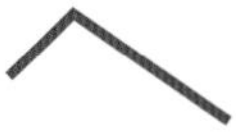	Loud, high-pitched	I < E	Just above clavicles on each side of the sternum, over the manubrium	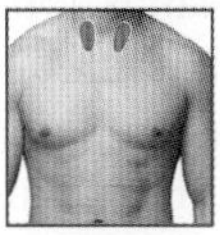	
Bronchovesicular 	Medium in loudness and pitch	I = E	Next to sternum, between scapulae	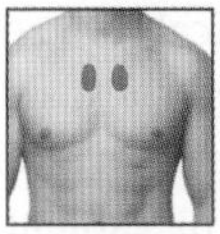	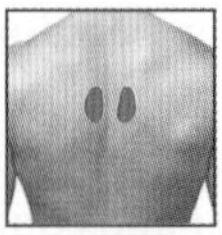
Vesicular 	Soft, low-pitched	I > E	Remainder of lungs	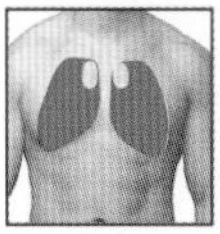	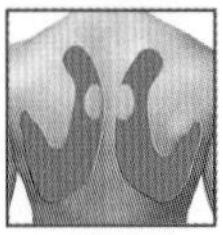

Abnormal findings

Chest-wall abnormalities

Chest-wall abnormalities may be congenital or acquired. As you examine a patient for chest-wall abnormalities, keep in mind that a patient with a deformity of the chest wall might have completely normal lungs and that the lungs might be cramped within the chest. The patient might have a smaller-than-normal lung capacity and limited exercise tolerance and may more easily develop respiratory failure from a respiratory tract infection.

Paradoxical movement

Paradoxical (uneven) movement of the chest wall is abnormal. It can occur as a result of chest-wall injury, such as multiple rib fractures or blunt force trauma to the chest. With spontaneous breathing, paradoxical movement occurs on the injured chest side, which collapses during inspiration and expands during exhalation.

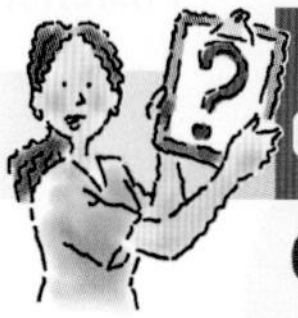
?

Outside the norm

Chest deformities

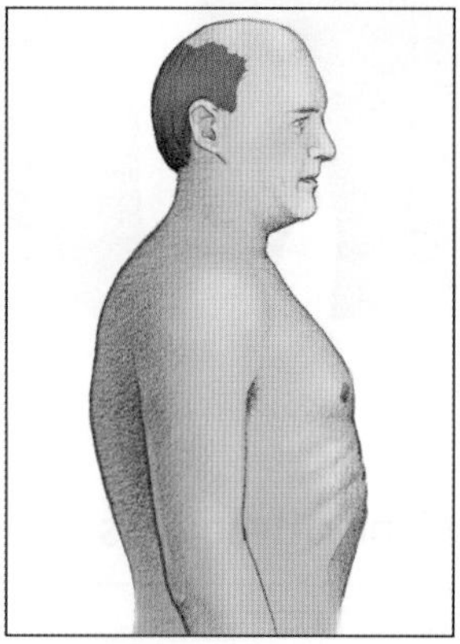

Barrel chest

Increased anteroposterior diameter

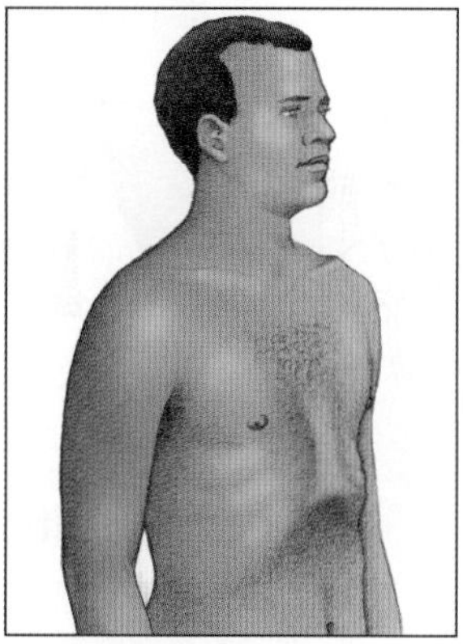

Funnel chest (pectus excavatum)

Depressed lower sternum

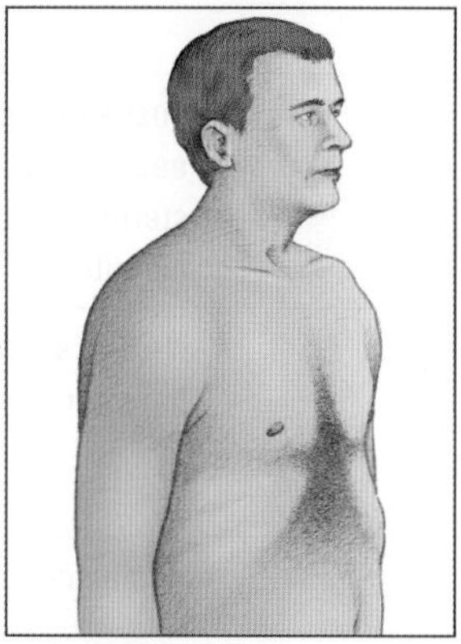

Pigeon chest (pectus carinatum)

Anteriorly displaced sternum

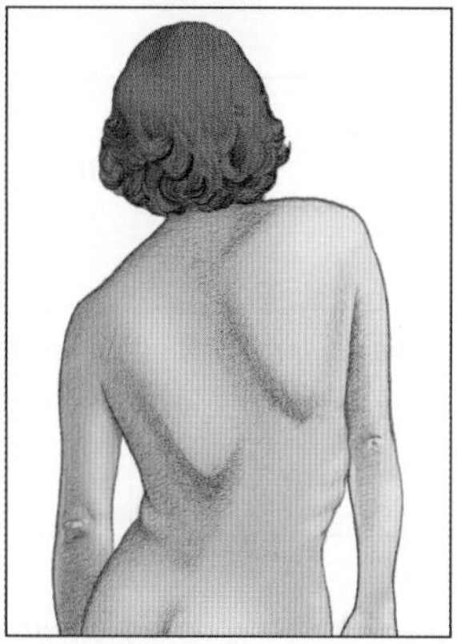

Thoracic kyphoscoliosis

Raised shoulder and scapula, thoracic convexity, and flared interspaces

Abnormal respiratory patterns

Common abnormal respiratory patterns include tachypnea, bradypnea, apnea, hyperpnea, Kussmaul respirations, Cheyne-Stokes respirations, and Biot respirations.

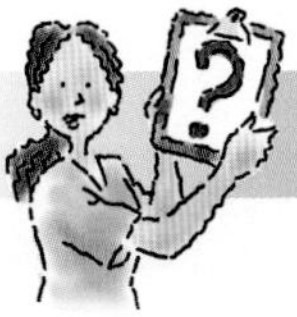
?

Outside the norm

Tachypnea
Shallow breathing with increased respiratory rate

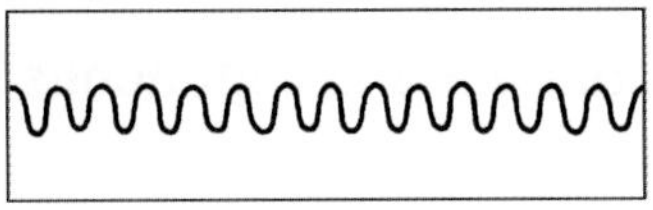

Bradypnea
Slower rate of breathing; may be periodic

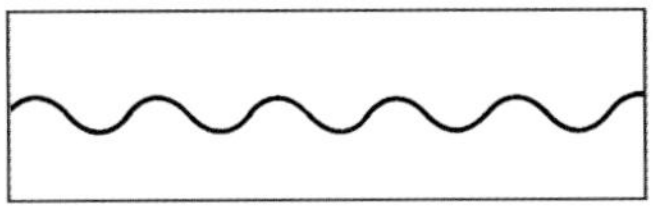

Apnea
Absence of breathing; may be periodic

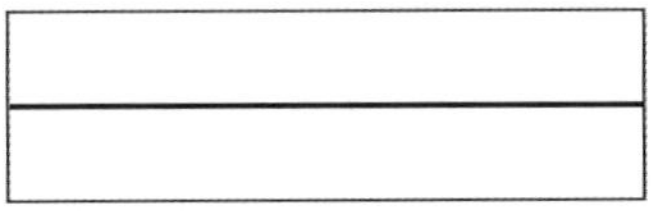

Hyperpnea
Increased depth of breathing

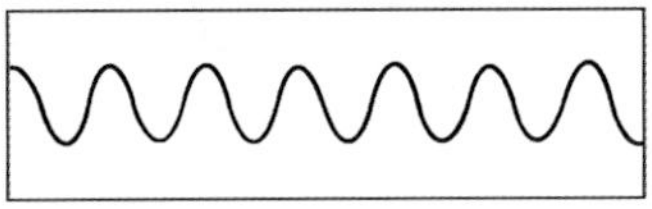

Kussmaul respirations
Rapid, deep breathing without pauses; in adults, more than 20 breaths/minute; breathing usually sounds labored with deep breaths that resemble sighs.

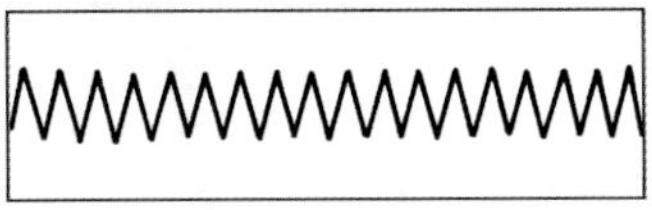

Cheyne-Stokes respirations
Breaths that gradually become faster and deeper than normal, then slower, and alternate with periods of apnea

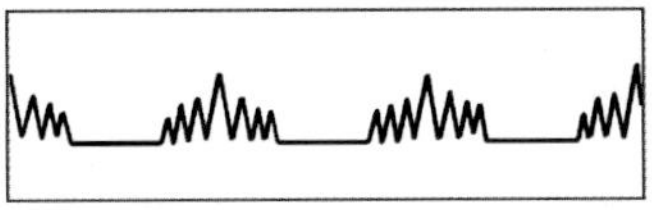

Biot respirations
Rapid, deep breathing with abrupt pauses between each breath; equal depth to each breath

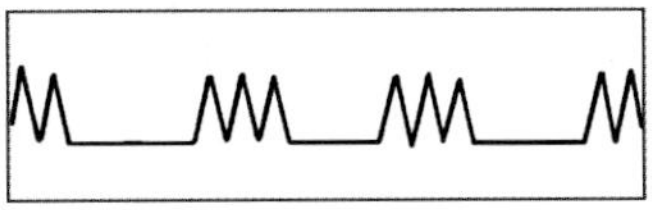

Grading dyspnea

To assess dyspnea (shortness of breath) as objectively as possible, ask your patient to briefly describe how various activities affect his breathing. Then, document his response using this grading system:

Grade 0	Not troubled by breathlessness except with strenuous exercise
Grade 1	Troubled by shortness of breath when hurrying on a level path or walking up a slight hill
Grade 2	Walks more slowly on a level path than people of the same age because of breathlessness or has to stop to breathe when walking on a level path at own pace
Grade 3	Stops to breathe after walking approximately 100 yards (91 m) on a level path
Grade 4	Too breathless to leave the house or breathless when dressing or undressing

Abnormal breath sounds

If you hear a sound in an area other than where you would expect to hear it, consider the sound abnormal. For example, if you hear bronchial or bronchovesicular breath sounds in an area where you would normally hear vesicular breath sounds, then the alveoli and small bronchioles in that area might be filled with fluid or exudate, as occurs in pneumonia and atelectasis.

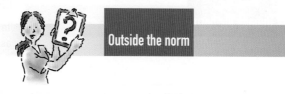

Outside the norm

Discontinuous and continuous adventitious breath sounds

The characteristics of some discontinuous and continuous adventitious breath sounds are compared in the chart below. Note the timing of each sound during inspiration and expiration on the corresponding graphs.

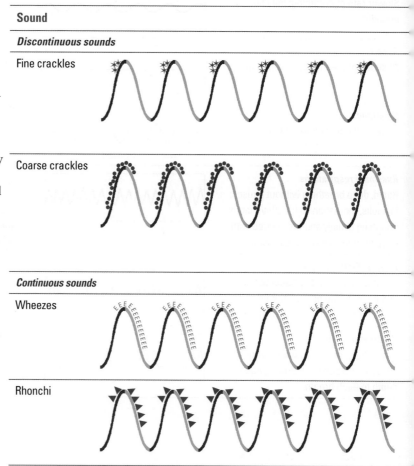

Sound	
Discontinuous sounds	
Fine crackles	
Coarse crackles	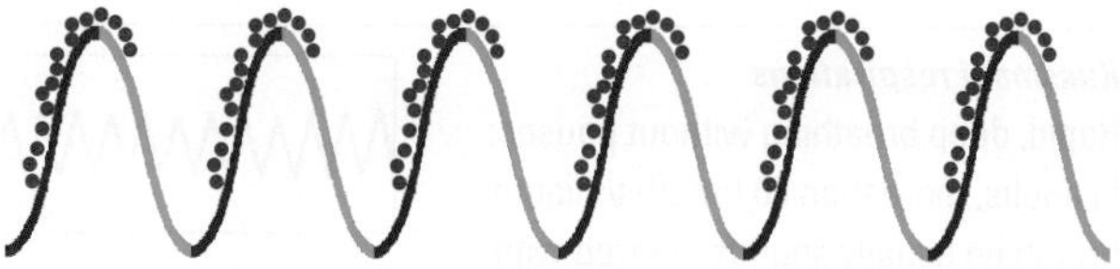
Continuous sounds	
Wheezes	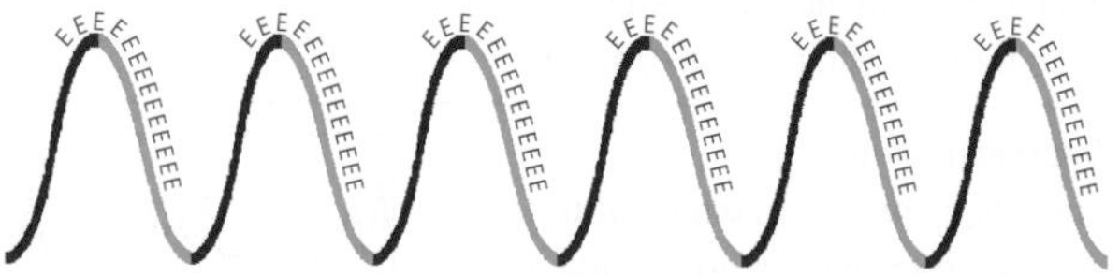
Rhonchi	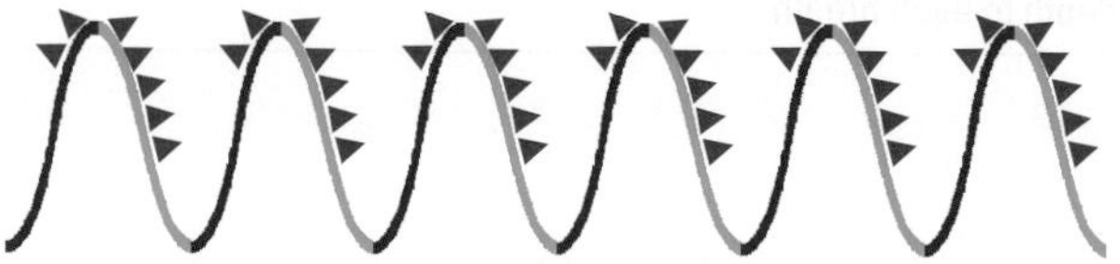

Adventitious sounds

Other breath sounds, called *adventitious sounds,* are abnormal no matter where you hear them in the lungs. These sounds, which are superimposed on normal breath sounds, include fine and coarse crackles, wheezes, rhonchi, stridor, and pleural friction rub.

Stridor is a loud, high-pitched crowing sound, usually heard without a stethoscope during auscultation. It's caused by upper airway obstruction.

Pleural friction rub is a low-pitched, grating, rubbing sound heard on inspiration and expiration. It's caused by pleural inflammation.

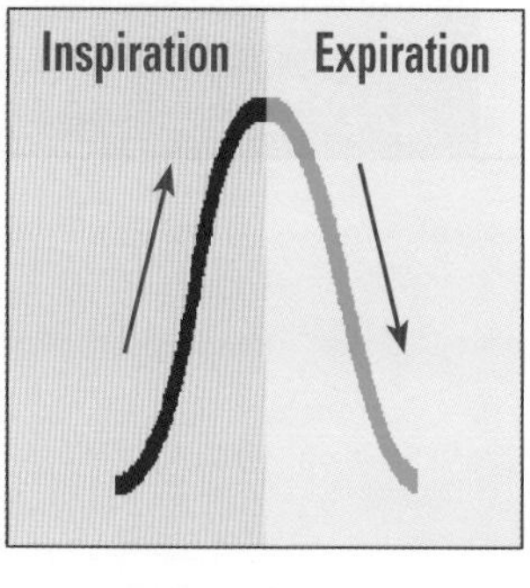
Inspiration
Expiration

Characteristics
• Intermittent • Nonmusical • Soft • High-pitched • Short, cracking, popping sounds • Heard during inspiration
• Intermittent • Nonmusical • Loud • Low-pitched • Bubbling, gurgling sounds • Heard during early inspiration and possibly during expiration
• Musical • High-pitched • Squeaky, whistling sounds • Predominantly heard during expiration but may also occur during inspiration
• Musical • Low-pitched • Snoring, moaning sounds • Heard during both inspiration and expiration but are more prominent during expiration

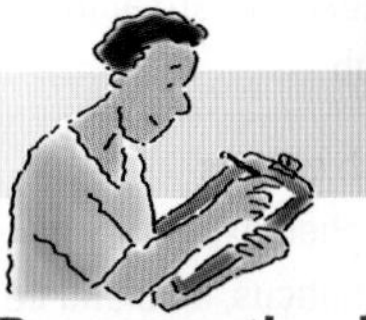

Take note

Documenting breath sounds

4/1/2010	1830	Pt. c/o shortness of breath and dizziness after walking from the bathroom to the bed. Skin cool and dry, color pale, lips and nail beds pink. Bilateral breath sounds with fine crackles in right lower and middle lobes. Respirations easy and regular without use of accessory muscles. BP 130/90, P 88/minute, RR 28/minute. Oxygen saturation 92% on room air. Dr. Ryan notified at 1820 and pt. placed on nasal O_2 at 4 L/minute and 12-lead ECG obtained. Wife at bedside.
		Linda Martin, RN

Auscultation findings for common disorders

Disorder	Auscultation findings
Asbestosis	• Bronchial breath sounds in both lung bases • High-pitched crackles heard at the end of inspiration • Pleural friction rub
Asthma	• Diminished breath sounds • Musical, high-pitched expiratory polyphonic wheezes • With status asthmaticus, loud and continuous random monophonic wheezes, along with prolonged expiration and possible silent chest if severe
Atelectasis	• High-pitched, hollow, tubular bronchial breath sounds, crackles, and wheezes • Fine, high-pitched, late inspiratory crackles • Bronchophony, egophony, and whispered pectoriloquy when right upper lobe is affected
Bronchiectasis	• Profuse, low-pitched crackles heard during mid inspiration
Chronic obstructive pulmonary disease (COPD)	• Diminished, low-pitched breath sounds • Sonorous or sibilant wheezes • Inaudible bronchophony, egophony, and whispered pectoriloquy • Prolonged expiration • Fine inspiratory crackles

(continued)

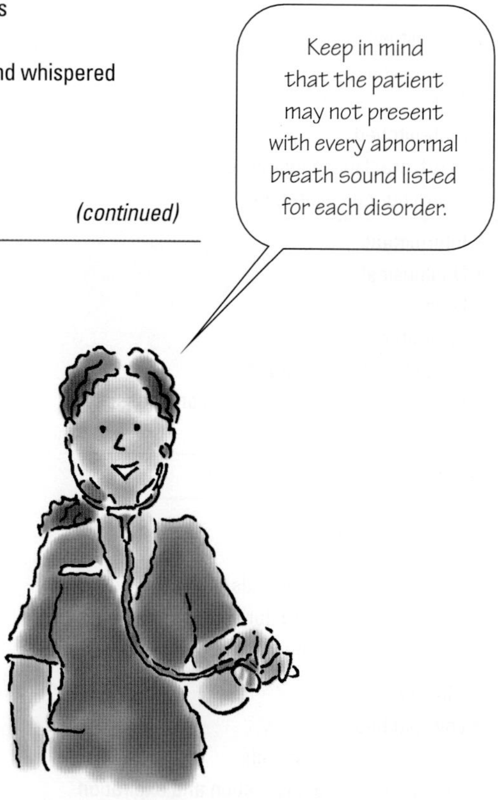
Keep in mind that the patient may not present with every abnormal breath sound listed for each disorder.

Auscultation findings for common disorders *(continued)*

Disorder	Auscultation findings
Pleural effusion	• Absent or diminished low-pitched breath sounds • Occasionally loud bronchial breath sounds • Normal breath sounds on contralateral side • Bronchophony, egophony, and whispered pectoriloquy at upper border of pleural effusion
Pneumonia	• High-pitched, tubular bronchial breath sounds over affected area during inspiration and expiration • Bronchophony, egophony, and whispered pectoriloquy • Late inspiratory crackles not affected by coughing or position changes
Pneumothorax	• Absent or diminished low-pitched breath sounds • Inaudible bronchophony, egophony, and whispered pectoriloquy • Normal breath sounds on contralateral side
Upper airway obstruction	• Stridor • Decreased or absent breath sounds • Wheezing

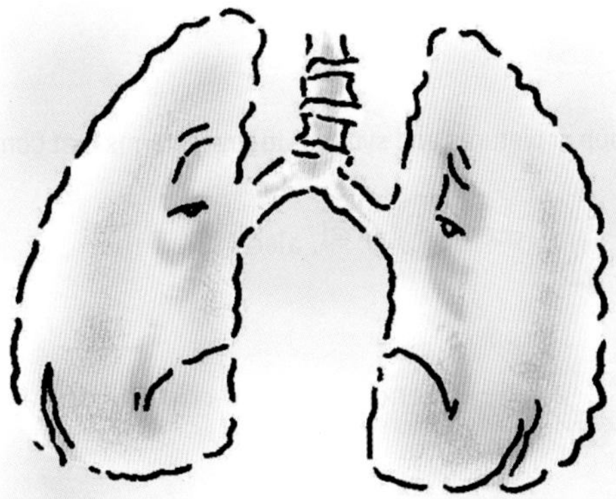

Q&A

Able to label?

Identify the respiratory structures indicated on this illustration.

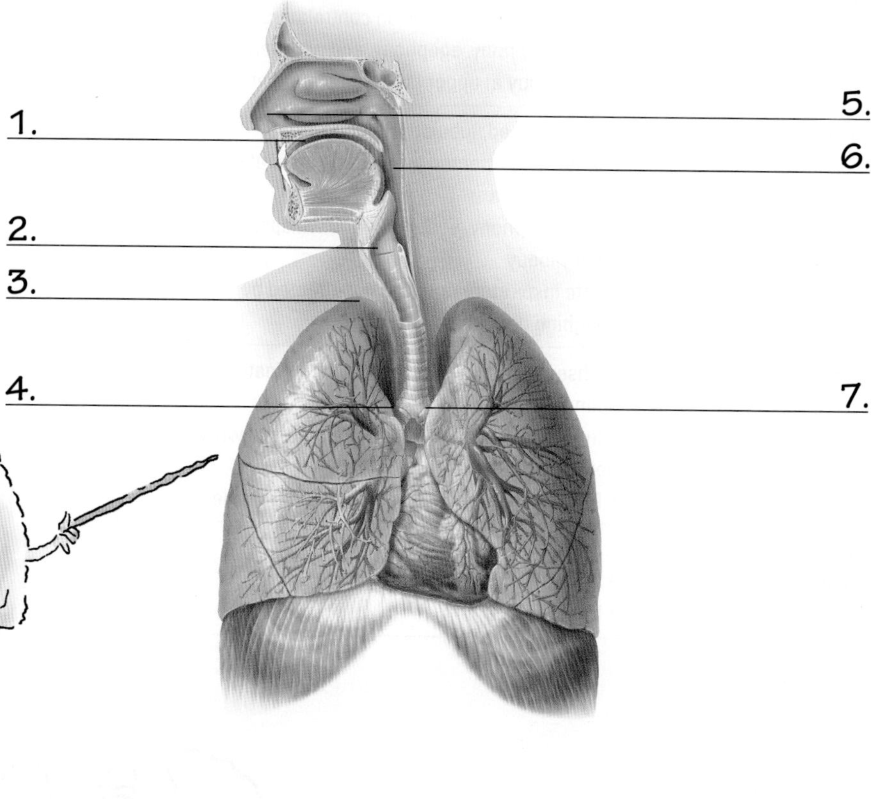
1.
2.
3.
4.
5.
6.
7.

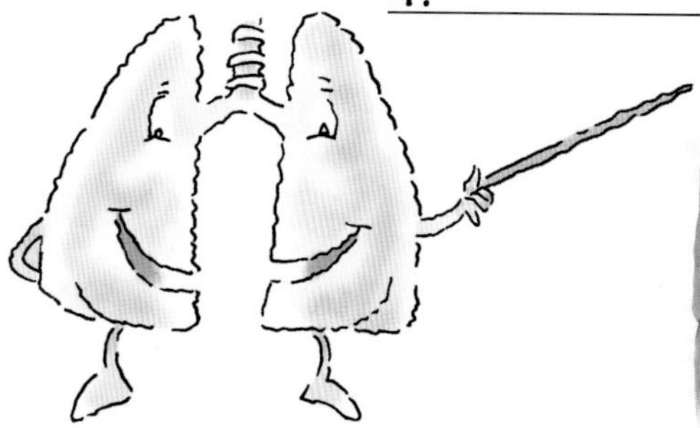

Rebus riddle

Sound out each group of pictures and symbols to reveal terms that complete these two sentences about respiratory anatomy.

1. The  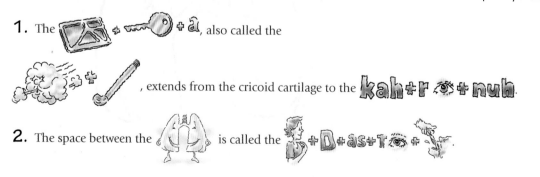, also called the , extends from the cricoid cartilage to the 
kah+r + nuh.

2. The space between the  is called the 
+D+as+T +.

Answers: Able to label? 1. Oral cavity, 2. Trachea, 3. Apex of lung, 4. Right mainstem bronchus, 5. Nasal cavity, 6. Oropharynx, 7. Left mainstem bronchus; Rebus riddle 1. The trachea, also called the windpipe, extends from the cricoid cartilage to the carina. 2. The space between the lungs is called the mediastinum.

Selected References

Buttaro, T. M., Trybulski, J., Bailey, P., & Sandburg-Cook, J. (2013). *Primary care: A collaborative practice* (4th ed.). St. Louis, MO: Elsevier Mosby.

Goroll, A. H., & Mulley, A. G. (2014). *Primary care medicine: Office evaluation and management of the adult patient* (7th ed.). China: Wolters Kluwer.

Chapter 6

Cardiovascular system

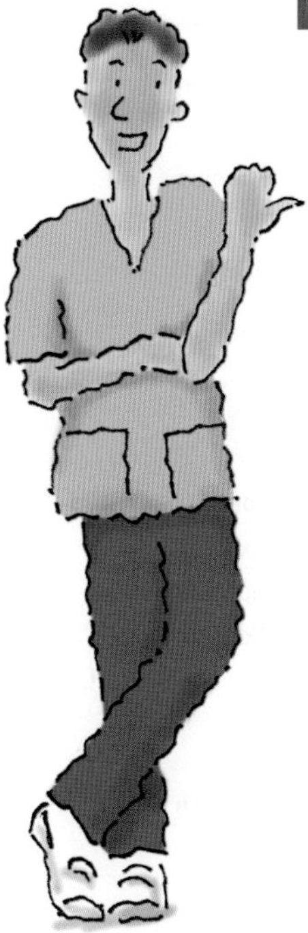
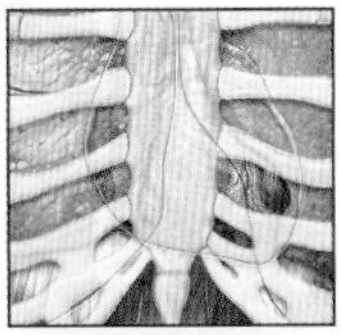
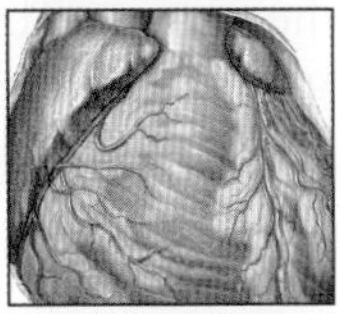
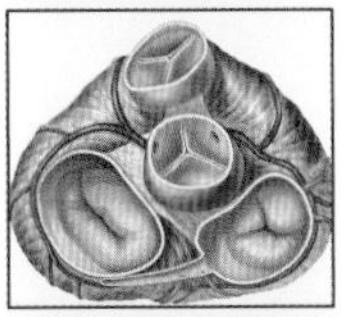
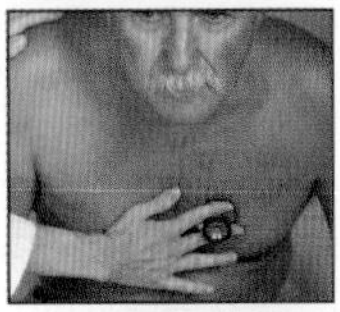
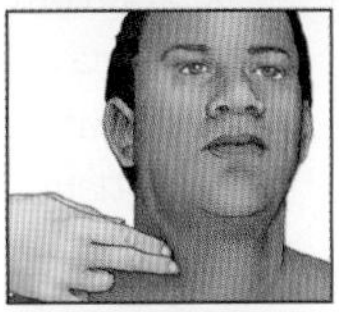
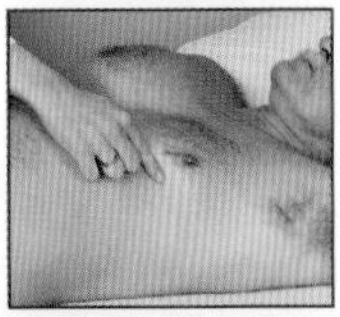
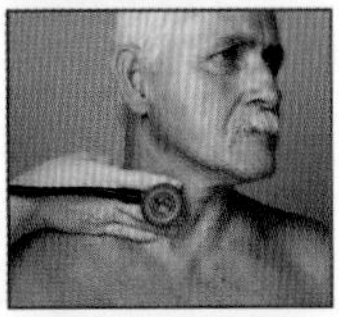
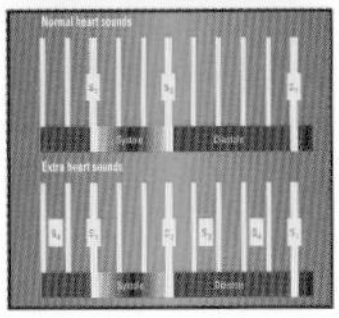

Anatomy of the heart

The heart is a hollow, muscular organ encased and cushioned in its own serous membrane, the pericardium. The heart is about the size of a closed fist. It's located between the lungs in the mediastinum, behind and to the left of the sternum. The heart spans the area from the second to the fifth intercostal space. Its right border aligns with the right border of the sternum. The left border aligns with the left midclavicular line.

The heart's location

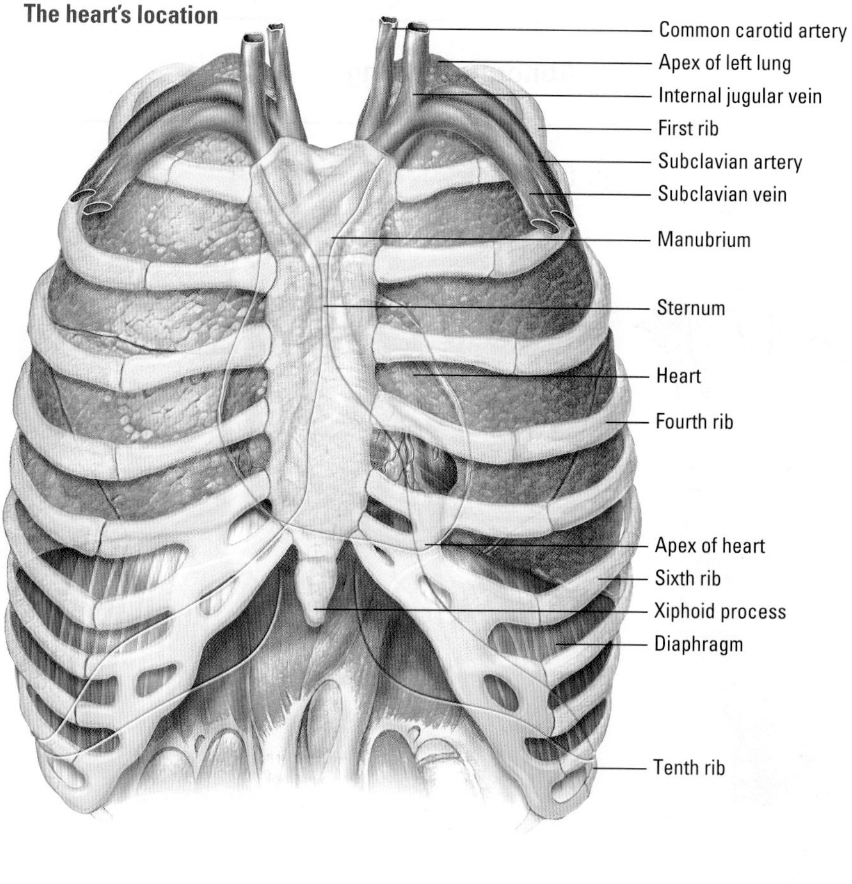
Common carotid artery
Apex of left lung
Internal jugular vein
First rib
Subclavian artery
Subclavian vein
Manubrium
Sternum
Heart
Fourth rib
Apex of heart
Sixth rib
Xiphoid process
Diaphragm
Tenth rib

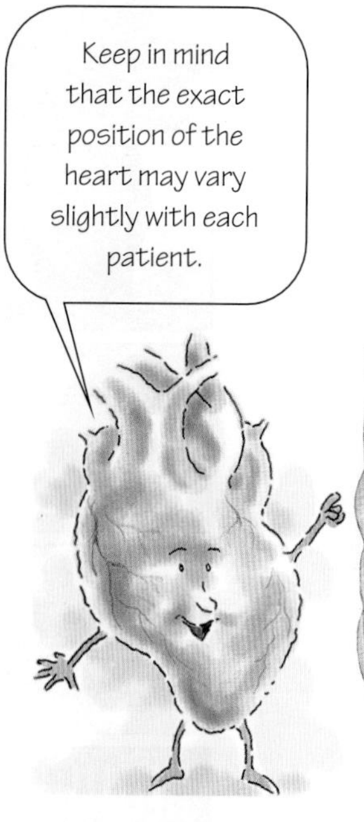
Keep in mind that the exact position of the heart may vary slightly with each patient.

Pericardium

The pericardium is a thin sac with an inner, or visceral, layer that forms the epicardium and an outer, or parietal, layer that protects the heart. The space between the two layers (the pericardial space) contains 10 to 30 ml of serous fluid, which lubricates and cushions the surface of the heart and prevents friction between the layers as the heart pumps.

Layers of the heart wall

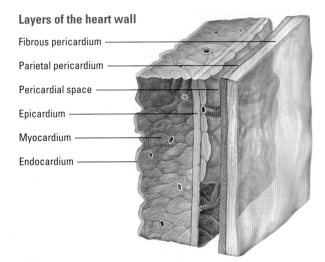

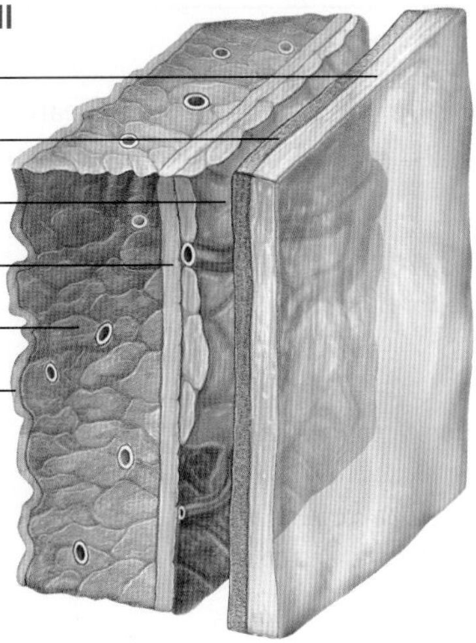
Fibrous pericardium
Parietal pericardium
Pericardial space
Epicardium
Myocardium
Endocardium

Atria and ventricles

The heart has four chambers—two atria and two ventricles—separated by a cardiac septum. The upper atria have thin walls and serve as reservoirs for blood. They also boost the amount of blood moving into the lower ventricles, which fill primarily by gravity. The left ventricle pumps blood against a much higher pressure than does the right ventricle, so its wall is two and one-half times thicker.

Structures of the heart

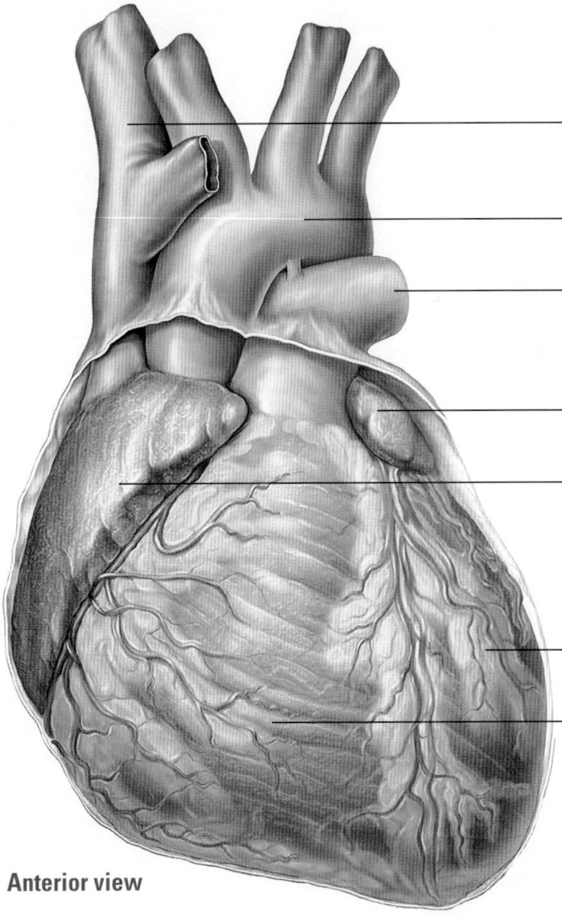
Superior vena cava
Aortic arch
Pulmonary artery
Left atrium
Right atrium
Left ventricle
Right ventricle

Anterior view

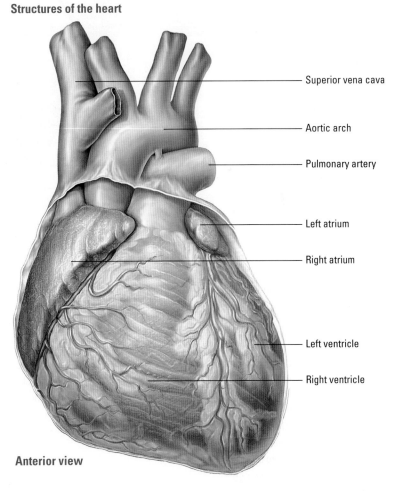

Vessels

Leading into and out of the heart are the great vessels: the inferior vena cava, the superior vena cava, the aorta, the pulmonary artery, and four pulmonary veins.

Cardiac circulation

1

Deoxygenated venous blood returns to the right atrium through the superior vena cava, inferior vena cava, and coronary sinus.

2

Blood in the right atrium empties into the right ventricle passively; once the pressure in the right ventricle exceeds the pressure in the right atrium, the tricuspid valve closes. The ventricle then contracts.

3

Blood is ejected through the pulmonic valve into the pulmonary artery and then travels to the lungs to be oxygenated.

4

From the lungs, oxygenated blood travels to the left atrium through the pulmonary veins.

5

The left atrium empties the blood into the left ventricle passively; once the pressure in the left ventricle exceeds the pressure in the left atrium, the mitral valve will close. The left ventricle contracts and pumps the blood through the aortic valve into the aorta and throughout the body.

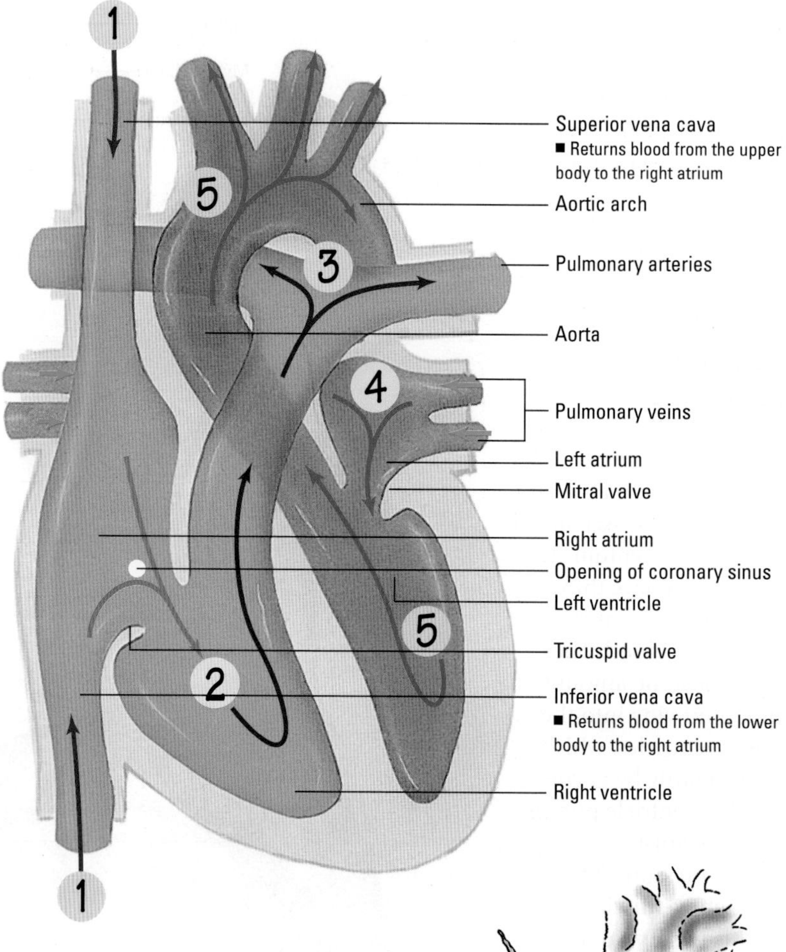
1
5
3
4
2
5
1
Superior vena cava
■ Returns blood from the upper body to the right atrium
Aortic arch
Pulmonary arteries
Aorta
Pulmonary veins
Left atrium
Mitral valve
Right atrium
Opening of coronary sinus
Left ventricle
Tricuspid valve
Inferior vena cava
■ Returns blood from the lower body to the right atrium
Right ventricle

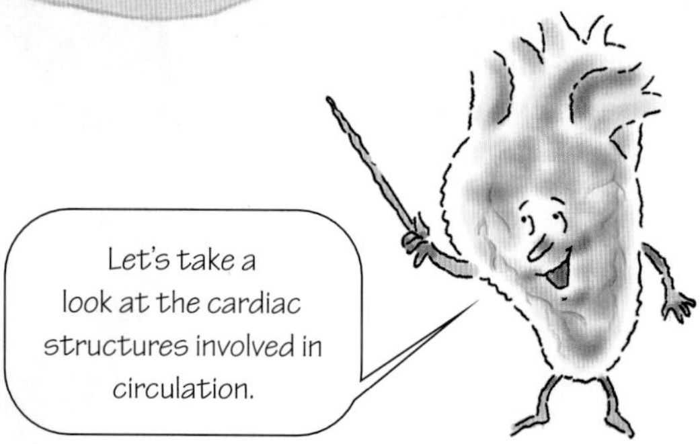
Let's take a look at the cardiac structures involved in circulation.

Valves

Valves in the heart keep blood flowing in only one direction through the heart. Healthy valves open and close passively as pressure changes within the four heart chambers.

On the cusp

Each valve's leaflets, or cusps, are anchored to the heart wall by cords of fibrous tissue. Those cords, called *chordae tendineae*, are controlled by papillary muscles. The valves' cusps maintain tight closure. The tricuspid valve has three cusps. The mitral valve has two. The semilunar valves each have three cusps.

Locating the heart valves

Valves between the atria and ventricles are called *atrioventricular valves often referred* to as *AV valves* and include the tricuspid valve on the right side of the heart and the mitral valve on the left. The pulmonic valve (between the right ventricle and pulmonary artery) and the aortic valve (between the left ventricle and the aorta) are called *semilunar valves*.

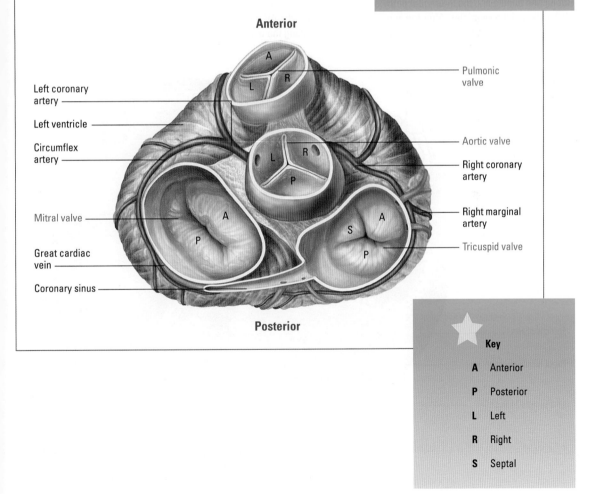

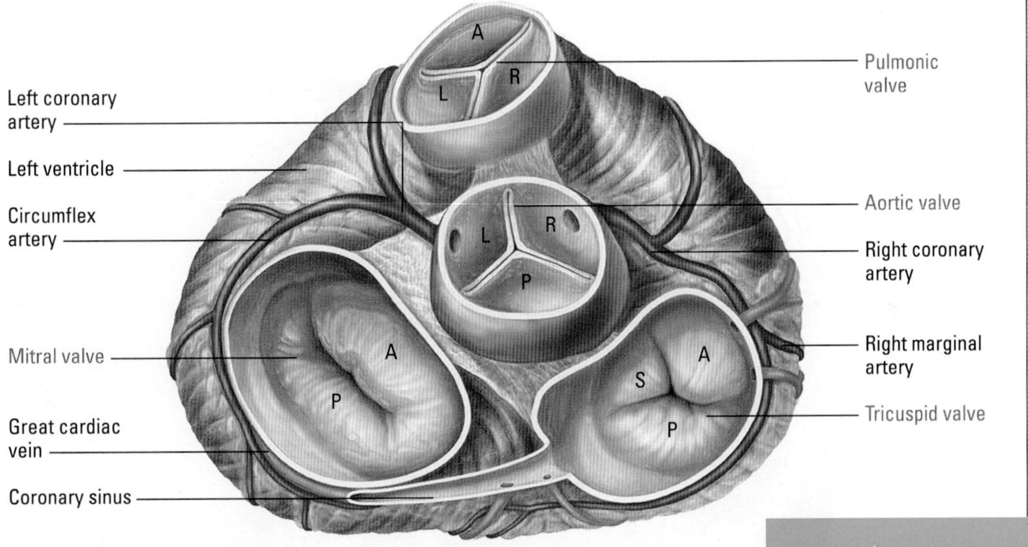

Anterior
A
R
L
Pulmonic valve
Left coronary artery
Left ventricle
Circumflex artery
L
R
P
Aortic valve
Right coronary artery
Mitral valve
A
P
S
A
P
Right marginal artery
Tricuspid valve
Great cardiac vein
Coronary sinus
Posterior

Key

A Anterior

P Posterior

L Left

R Right

S Septal

Physiology of the heart

Contractions of the heart occur in a rhythm—called the *cardiac cycle*—and are regulated by impulses that normally begin at the sinoatrial (SA) node.

Cardiac conduction

The heart's conduction system begins with the heart's primary pacemaker, the SA node. When an impulse leaves the SA node, it travels through the atria along Bachmann bundle and the internodal pathways on its way to the atrioventricular (AV) node and the ventricles. After the impulse passes through the AV node, it travels to the ventricles, first down the bundle of His, then along the bundle branches, and, finally, down the Purkinje fibers.

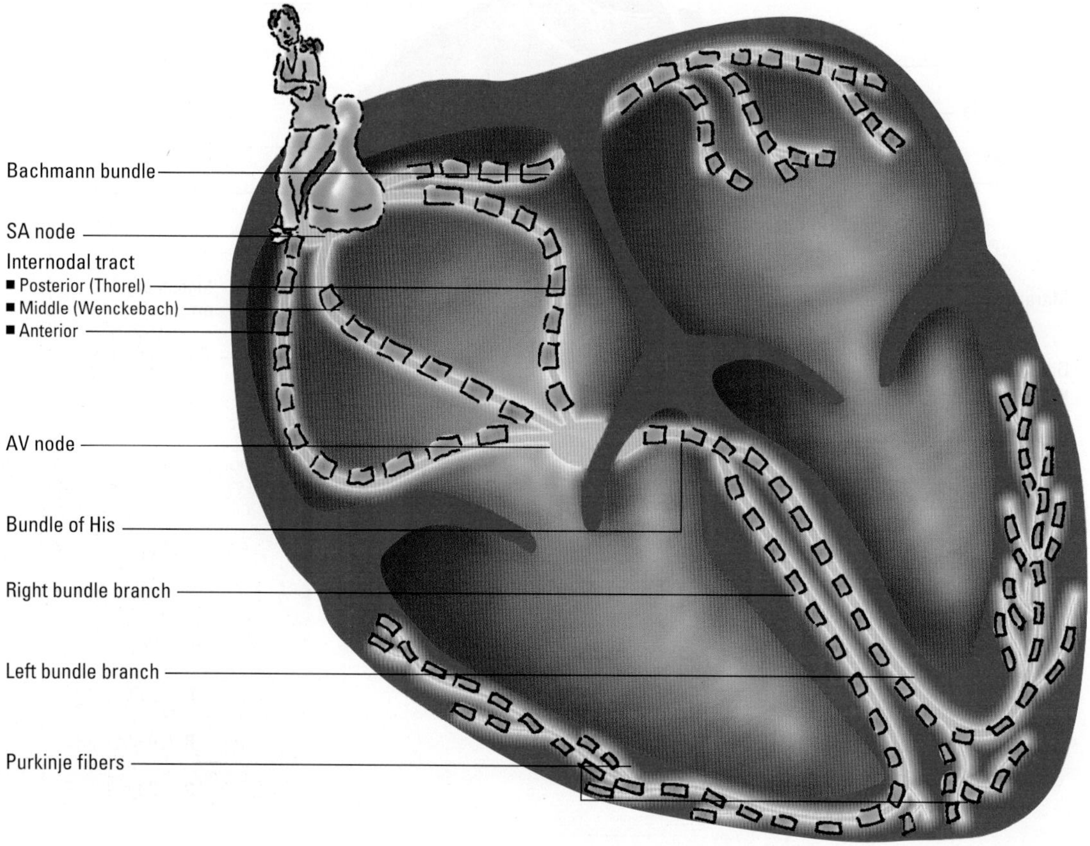
Bachmann bundle
SA node
Internodal tract
■ Posterior (Thorel)
■ Middle (Wenckebach)
■ Anterior
AV node
Bundle of His
Right bundle branch
Left bundle branch
Purkinje fibers

Anatomy of the vascular system

The vascular system delivers oxygen, nutrients, and other substances to the body's cells and removes the waste products of cellular metabolism. The peripheral vascular system consists of a network of about 60,000 miles of arteries, arterioles, capillaries, venules, and veins that's constantly filled with about 5 L of blood, which circulates to and from every functioning cell in the body.

A look at the cardiac cycle

The cardiac cycle consists of *systole*, the period when the heart contracts and sends blood on its outward journey, and *diastole*, the period when the heart relaxes and fills with blood.

1. Atrial systole
The atria contract, emptying blood into the ventricles. As pressure within the ventricles rises, the mitral and tricuspid valves snap shut, producing the first heart sound, S_1.

2. Ventricular systole
Shortly after atrial systole, the ventricles contract, ejecting blood from the heart to the lungs and the rest of the body. At the end of ventricular contraction, the aortic and pulmonic valves snap shut, producing the second heart sound, S_2.

3. Diastole
Atria and ventricles relax and blood refills each chamber.

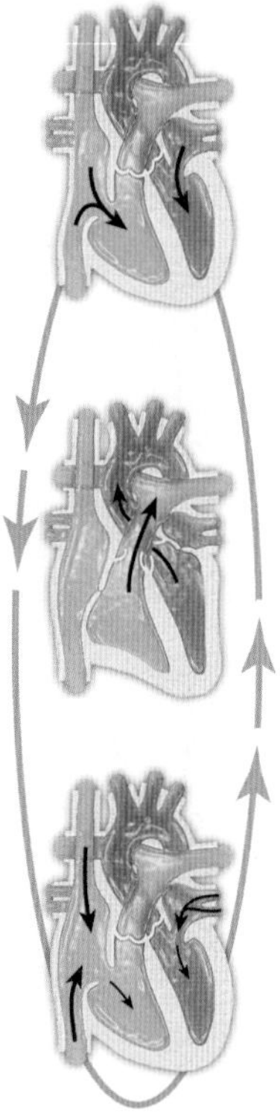

Arteries
Arteries carry blood away from the heart. Nearly all arteries carry oxygen-rich blood from the heart throughout the rest of the body. The only exception is the pulmonary artery, which carries oxygen-depleted blood from the right ventricle to the lungs. Arteries are thick-walled because they transport blood under high pressure.

Capillaries
The exchange of fluid, nutrients, and metabolic wastes between blood and cells occurs in the capillaries. This exchange can occur because capillaries are thin-walled and highly permeable. Arterioles constrict and dilate to control blood flow to the capillaries. Venules gather blood from the capillaries.

Veins
Veins carry blood toward the heart. Most carry oxygen-depleted blood, with the exception of the pulmonary veins, which carry oxygenated blood from the lungs to the left atrium. Veins serve as a large reservoir for circulating blood. The wall of a vein is thinner and more pliable than the wall of an artery. Veins contain valves at periodic intervals to prevent blood from flowing backward.

Major veins and arteries of the vascular system

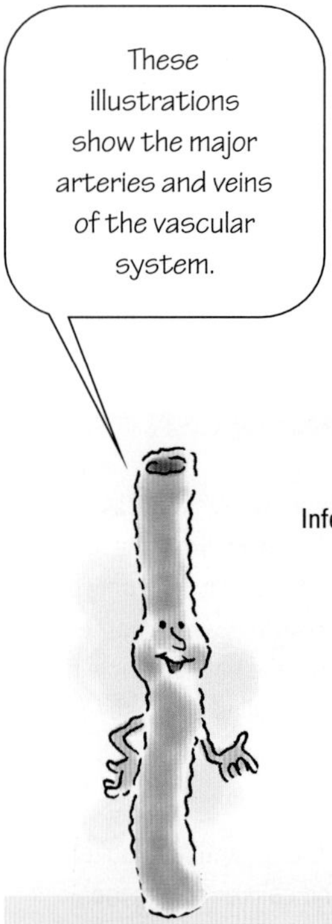
These illustrations show the major arteries and veins of the vascular system.

Major arteries

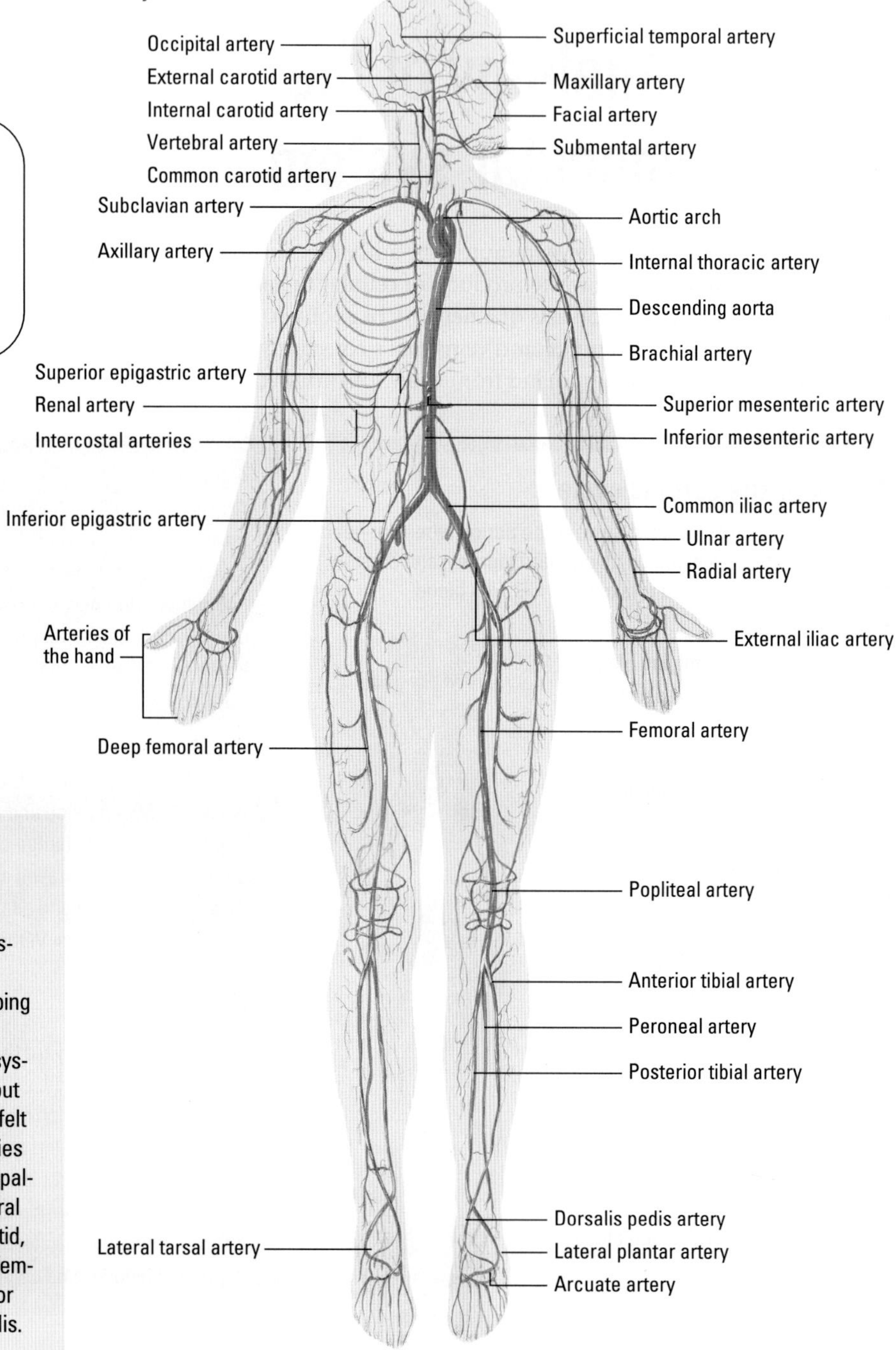
Occipital artery
External carotid artery
Internal carotid artery
Vertebral artery
Common carotid artery
Subclavian artery
Axillary artery
Superior epigastric artery
Renal artery
Intercostal arteries
Inferior epigastric artery
Arteries of the hand
Deep femoral artery
Lateral tarsal artery
Superficial temporal artery
Maxillary artery
Facial artery
Submental artery
Aortic arch
Internal thoracic artery
Descending aorta
Brachial artery
Superior mesenteric artery
Inferior mesenteric artery
Common iliac artery
Ulnar artery
Radial artery
External iliac artery
Femoral artery
Popliteal artery
Anterior tibial artery
Peroneal artery
Posterior tibial artery
Dorsalis pedis artery
Lateral plantar artery
Arcuate artery

Finger on the pulse

Arterial pulses are pressure waves of blood generated by the pumping action of the heart. All vessels in the arterial system have pulsations, but the pulsations can be felt only where an artery lies near the skin. You can palpate for these peripheral pulses: temporal, carotid, brachial, radial, ulnar, femoral, popliteal, posterior tibial, and dorsalis pedis.

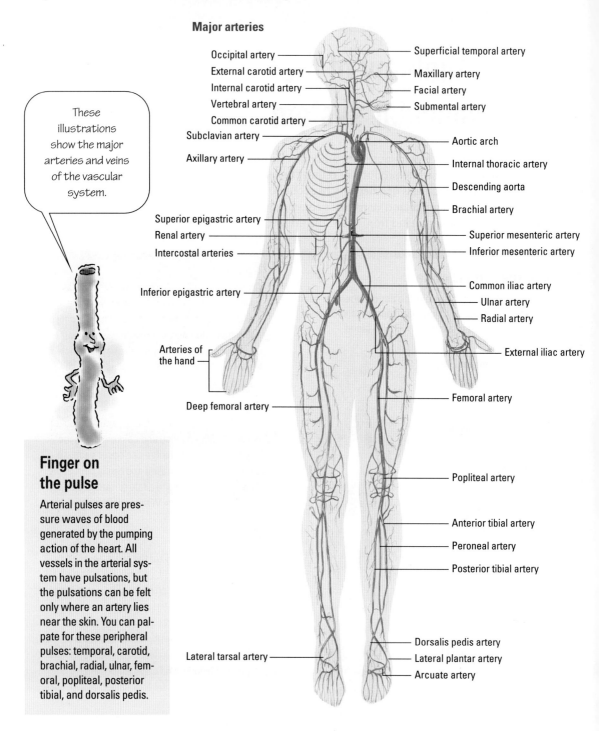

Major veins

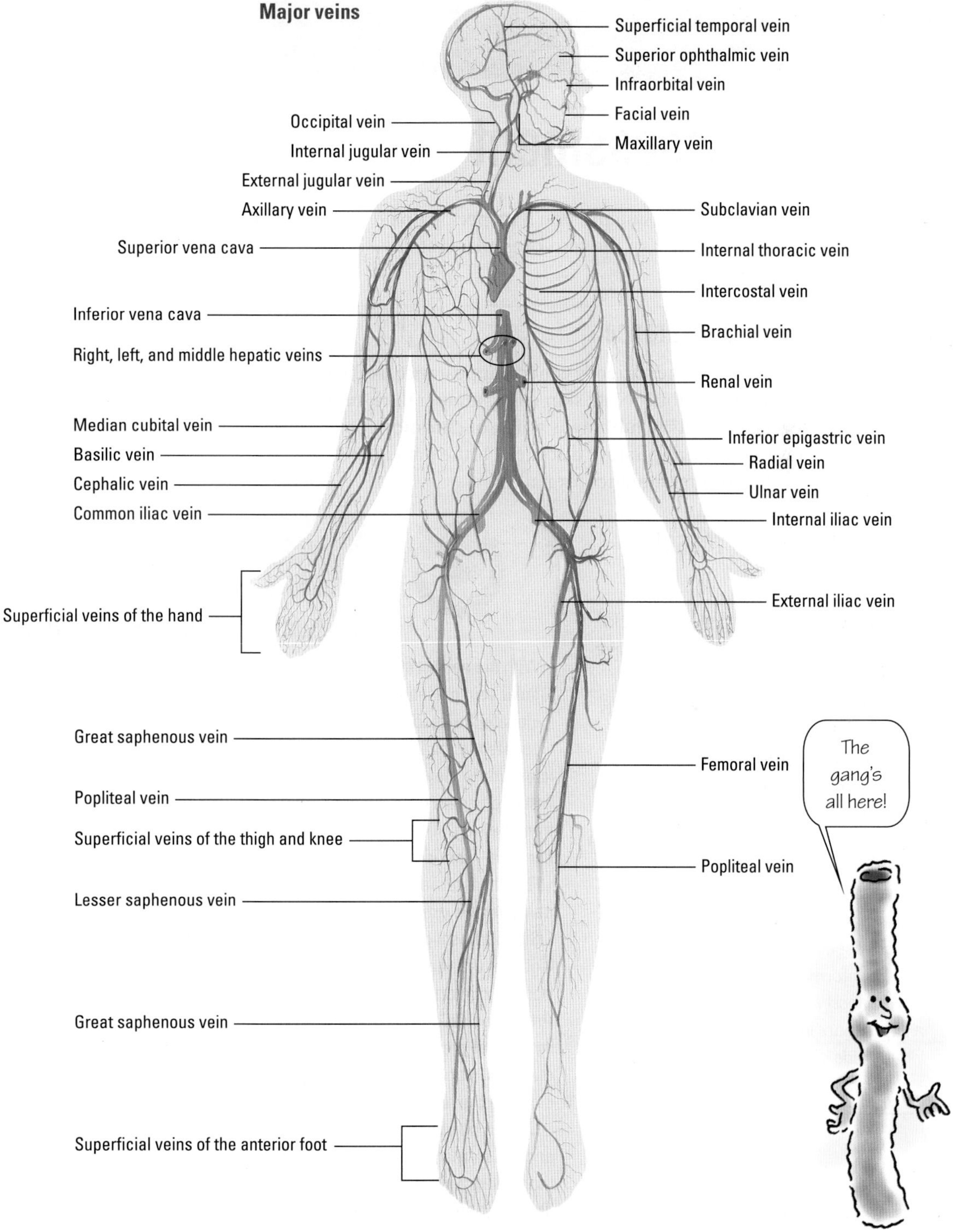
Superficial temporal vein
Superior ophthalmic vein
Infraorbital vein
Facial vein
Maxillary vein
Occipital vein
Internal jugular vein
External jugular vein
Axillary vein
Subclavian vein
Superior vena cava
Internal thoracic vein
Intercostal vein
Inferior vena cava
Brachial vein
Right, left, and middle hepatic veins
Renal vein
Median cubital vein
Inferior epigastric vein
Basilic vein
Radial vein
Cephalic vein
Ulnar vein
Common iliac vein
Internal iliac vein
Superficial veins of the hand
External iliac vein
Great saphenous vein
Femoral vein
Popliteal vein
Superficial veins of the thigh and knee
Popliteal vein
Lesser saphenous vein
Great saphenous vein
Superficial veins of the anterior foot
The gang's all here!

Assessment

As with assessment of other body systems, you'll inspect, palpate, percuss, and auscultate during your assessment of the cardiovascular system.

Assessing general appearance

First, take a moment to assess the patient's general appearance. Is the patient overly thin? Obese? Alert? Anxious? Note skin color, temperature, turgor, and texture. Are the fingers clubbed? (Clubbing is a sign of chronic hypoxia caused by a lengthy cardiovascular or respiratory disorder.) If the patient is dark skinned, inspect the mucous membranes for pallor.

Assessing the neck vessels

Inspection

Inspect the vessels in the patient's neck. The carotid artery should appear to have a brisk, localized pulsation. The internal jugular vein has a softer, undulating pulsation. Unlike the pulsation of the carotid artery, pulsation of the internal jugular vein changes in response to position and breathing. The vein normally protrudes when the patient is lying down and lies flat when standing.

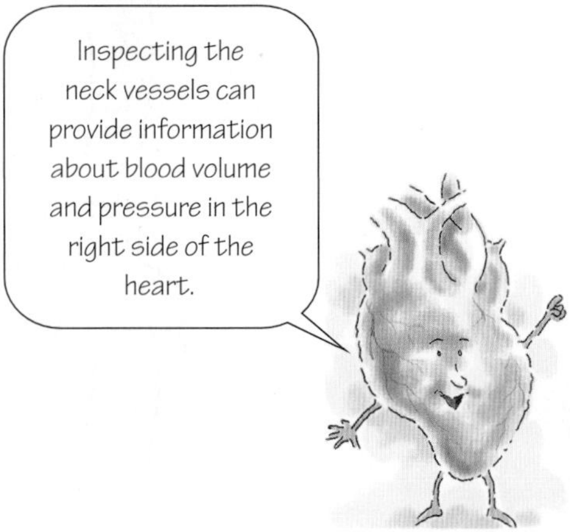
Inspecting the neck vessels can provide information about blood volume and pressure in the right side of the heart.

Skill check

Evaluating jugular vein distention

- With the patient in a supine position, position so that you can visualize jugular vein pulsations reflected from the right atrium.
- Elevate the head of the bed 30 to 45 degrees.
- Locate the angle of Louis (sternal notch). To do so, palpate the clavicles where they join the sternum (the suprasternal notch). Place your first two fingers on the suprasternal notch. Then, without lifting them from the skin, slide them down the sternum until you feel a bony protuberance—this is the angle of Louis.
- Find the internal jugular vein. (It indicates venous pressure more reliably than the external jugular vein.)
- Shine a flashlight across the patient's neck to create shadows that highlight the venous pulse. Be sure to distinguish jugular vein pulsations from carotid artery pulsations. You can do this by palpating the vessel: Arterial pulsations continue, whereas venous pulsations disappear with light finger pressure. Also, venous pulsations increase or decrease with changes in body position; arterial pulsations remain constant.
- Locate the highest point along the vein where you can see pulsations.
- Using a centimeter ruler, measure the distance between the high point and the sternal notch. Record this finding as well as the angle at which the patient was lying. A finding greater than 1¼″; to 1½″; (3 to 4 cm) above the sternal notch, with the head of the bed at a 45-degree angle, indicates jugular vein distention.

Palpation

To palpate the carotid artery, lightly place your index and middle fingers just medial to the trachea and below the angle of the jaw. The pulse should be regular in rhythm and have equal strength in the right and left carotid arteries. You shouldn't be able to detect any palpable vibrations, known as *thrills*. Don't palpate both carotid arteries at the same time or press too firmly. If you do, the patient may faint or become bradycardic.

Auscultation

Normally, you should hear no vascular sounds over the carotid arteries upon auscultation using the bell of the stethoscope. If you detect a blowing, swishing sound, this is a bruit that results from turbulent blood flow. A bruit can occur in patients with arteriosclerotic plaque formation.

Skill check

Auscultating the carotid artery

Lightly place the bell of the stethoscope over the carotid artery, first on one side of the trachea and then on the other. Ask the patient to hold the breath while you auscultate each artery. Doing so will help eliminate respiratory sounds that may interfere with your findings.

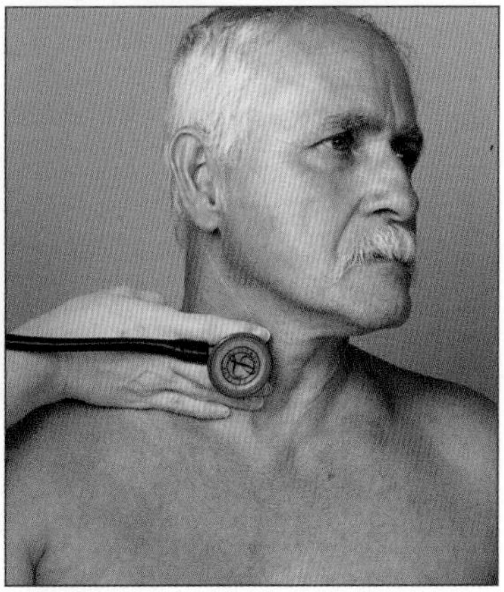

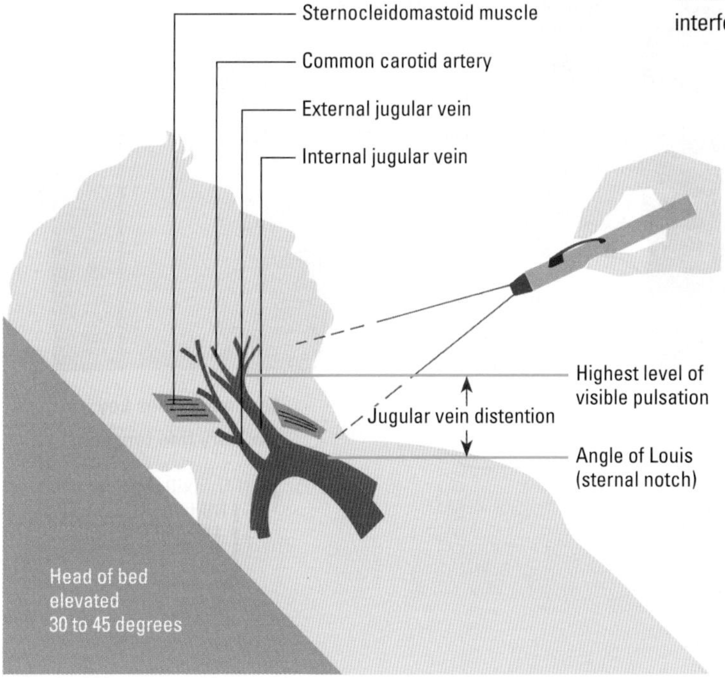
Sternocleidomastoid muscle
Common carotid artery
External jugular vein
Internal jugular vein
Highest level of visible pulsation
Jugular vein distention
Angle of Louis (sternal notch)
Head of bed elevated 30 to 45 degrees

Assessing the heart

Inspection

Inspect the chest. Note landmarks you can use to describe your findings as well as structures underlying the chest wall. Look for pulsations, symmetry of movement, retractions, or heaves (strong outward thrusts of the chest wall that occur during systole).

Note the location of the apical impulse. This is also usually the point of maximal impulse and should be located in the fifth intercostal space at or just medial to the left midclavicular line. You'll notice it more easily in children and in patients with thin chest walls. To find the apical impulse in a woman with large breasts, displace the breasts during the examination.

Cardiovascular landmarks

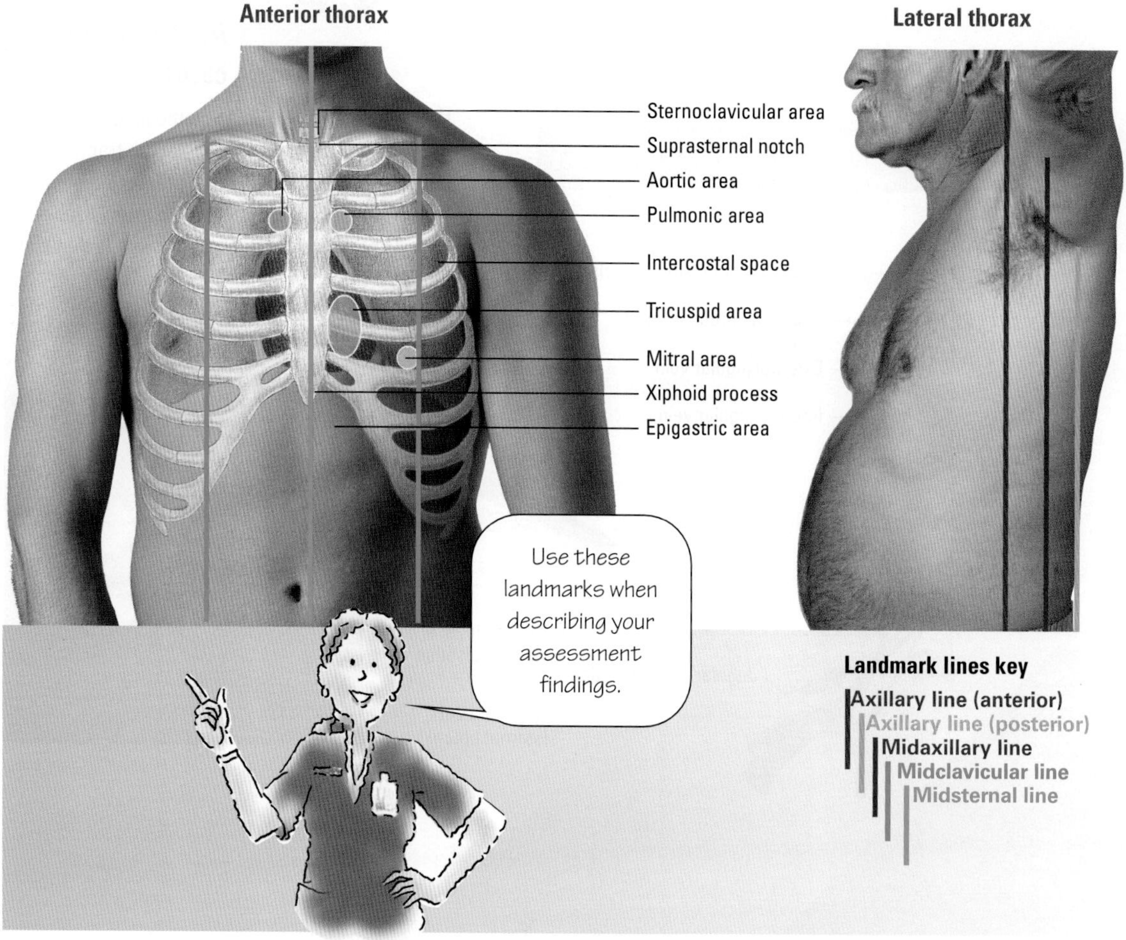
Anterior thorax
Sternoclavicular area
Suprasternal notch
Aortic area
Pulmonic area
Intercostal space
Tricuspid area
Mitral area
Xiphoid process
Epigastric area
Lateral thorax
Use these landmarks when describing your assessment findings.
Landmark lines key
Axillary line (anterior)
Axillary line (posterior)
Midaxillary line
Midclavicular line
Midsternal line

Palpation

Maintain a gentle touch when you palpate so that you won't obscure pulsations or similar findings. Follow a systematic palpation sequence covering the sternoclavicular, aortic, pulmonic, tricuspid, and epigastric areas.

Skill check

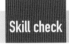

Palpating the apical impulse

To find the apical impulse, use the ball of your hand, then your fingertips, to palpate over the precordium. Note heaves or thrills, fine vibrations that feel like the purring of a cat.

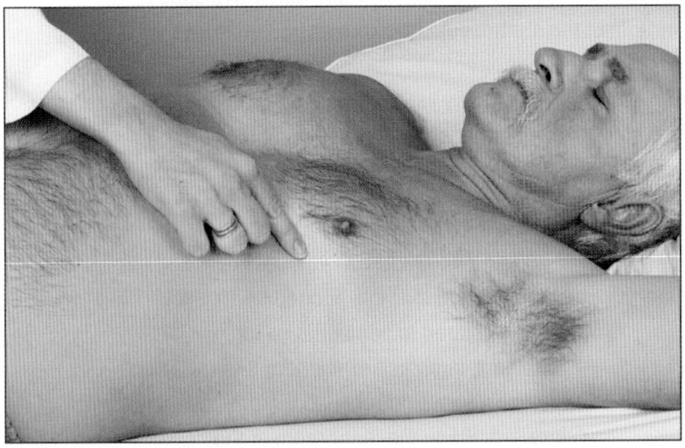

Percussion

Percuss at the anterior axillary line and continue toward the sternum along the fifth intercostal space. The sound changes from resonance to dullness over the left border of the heart, normally at the midclavicular line. The right border of the heart is usually aligned with the sternum and can't be percussed.

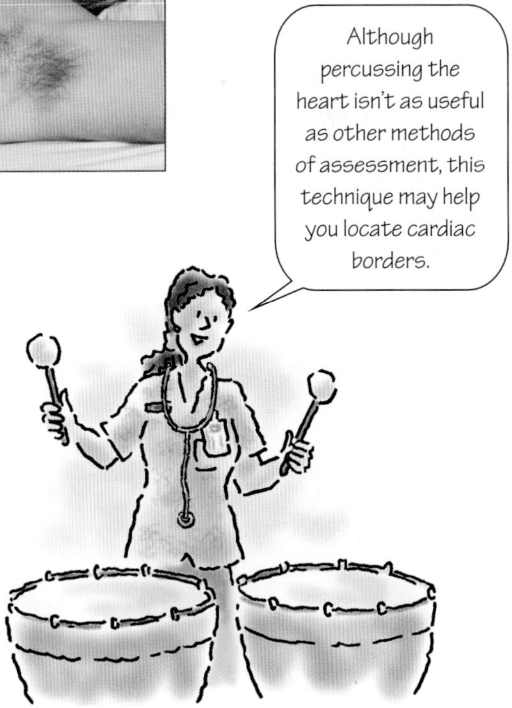
Although percussing the heart isn't as useful as other methods of assessment, this technique may help you locate cardiac borders.

Auscultation

Use a zigzag pattern over the precordium. Be sure to listen over the entire precordium, not just over the valves. Note the heart rate and rhythm. Identify the first and second heart sounds (S_1 and S_2) and then listen for adventitious sounds, such as third and fourth heart sounds (S_3 and S_4), murmurs, and pericardial friction rubs (scratchy, rubbing sounds).

Skill check

Positioning the patient for auscultation

Auscultate for heart sounds with the patient in three positions: lying in a supine position with the head of the bed raised 30 to 45 degrees, lying on the left side, and sitting up.

For the supine position, have the patient lie on the back with the head of the bed elevated 30 to 45 degrees. Begin auscultation at the aortic area. Listen over all heart valve sites and the entire precordium. Use the diaphragm of the stethoscope to listen as you go in one direction, and use the bell as you come back in the other direction.

If heart sounds are faint or if you hear abnormal sounds, try listening to them with the patient lying on the left side (left lateral recumbent position) or seated and leaning forward.

Left lateral recumbent

The left lateral recumbent position is best suited for hearing low-pitched sounds, such as mitral valve murmurs and extra heart sounds. To hear these sounds, place the bell of the stethoscope over the apical area, as shown.

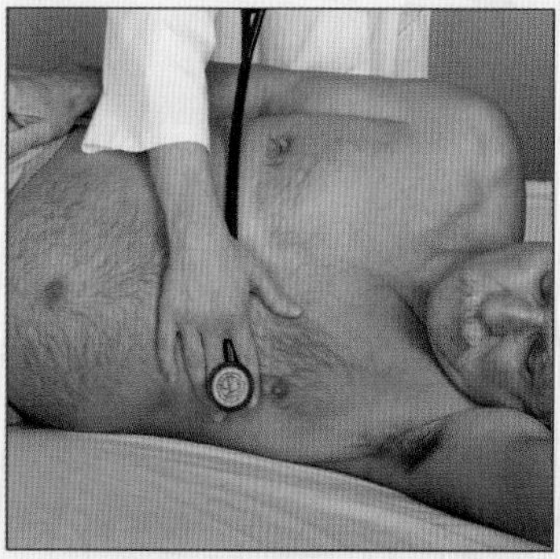

Leaning forward

To auscultate for high-pitched heart sounds related to semilunar valve problems, such as aortic and pulmonic valve murmurs, lean the patient forward. Place the diaphragm of the stethoscope over the aortic and pulmonic areas in the right and left second intercostal spaces, as shown.

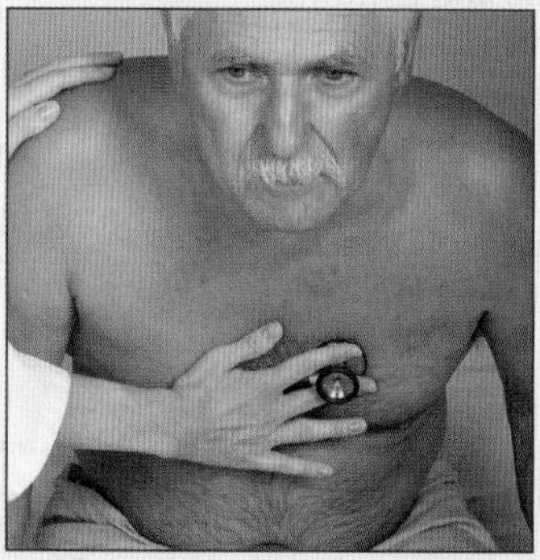

Auscultating for heart sounds

1

Begin auscultating over the **aortic area,** placing the stethoscope over the second intercostal space, along the right sternal border.

2

Then, move to the **pulmonic area,** located at the second intercostal space, at the left sternal border.

3

Next, assess the **tricuspid area,** which lies over the fourth and fifth intercostal spaces, along the left sternal border.

4

Finally, listen over the **mitral area,** located at the fifth intercostal space, near the midclavicular line.

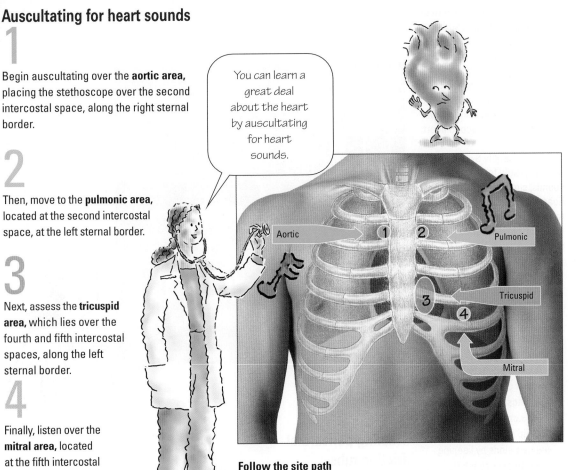

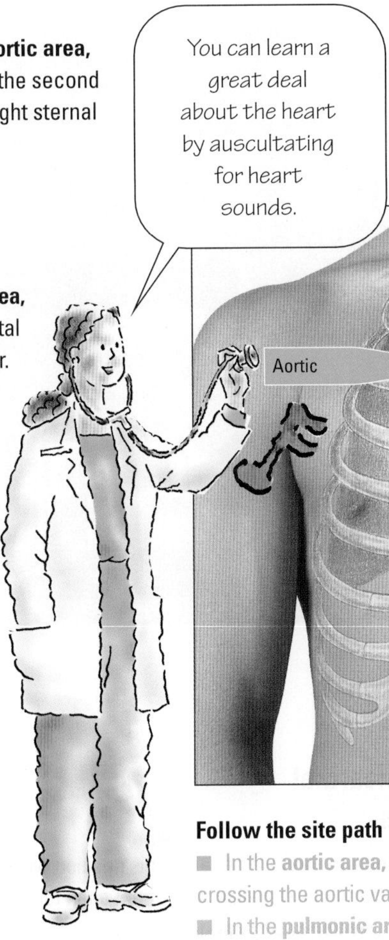
You can learn a great deal about the heart by auscultating for heart sounds.

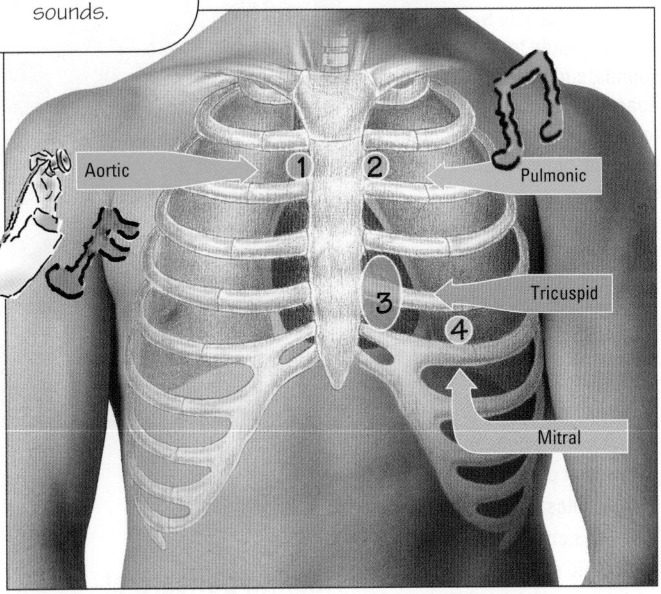
Aortic
1
2
Pulmonic
3
Tricuspid
4
Mitral

Follow the site path

- In the **aortic area,** blood moves from the left ventricle during systole, crossing the aortic valve and flowing through the aortic arch.
- In the **pulmonic area,** blood ejected from the right ventricle during systole crosses the pulmonic valve and flows through the main pulmonary artery.
- In the **tricuspid area,** sounds reflect movement from the right atrium across the tricuspid valve, filling the right ventricle during diastole.
- In the **mitral area,** also called the *apical area,* sounds represent blood flow across the mitral valve and left ventricular filling during diastole.

Heart sounds

Systole is the period of ventricular contraction. As pressure in the ventricles increases, the mitral and tricuspid valves snap closed. This closure produces the first heart sound, S_1. At the end of ventricular contraction, the aortic and pulmonic valves snap shut. This produces the second heart sound, S_2.

Always identify S_1 and S_2, and then listen for adventitious sounds, such as third and fourth heart sounds (S_3 and S_4). Also listen for murmurs, which sound like vibrating, blowing, or rumbling sounds.

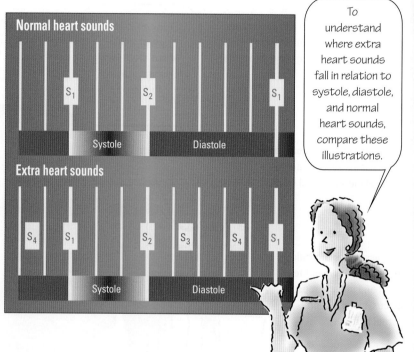

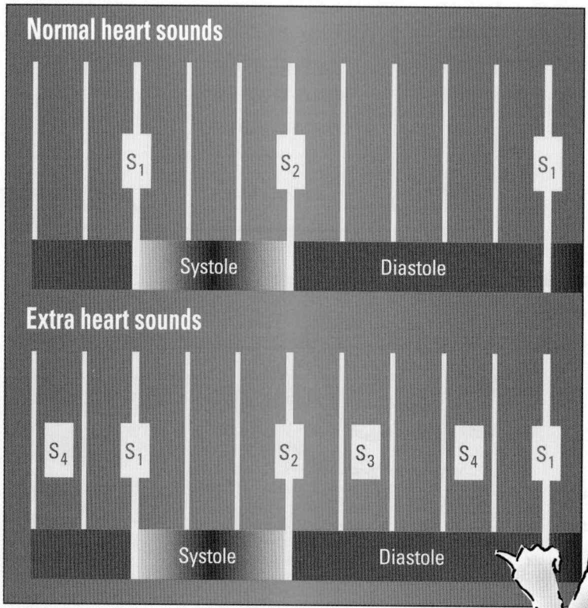
Normal heart sounds
S_1
S_2
S_1
Systole
Diastole
Extra heart sounds
S_4
S_1
S_2
S_3
S_4
S_1
Systole
Diastole

To understand where extra heart sounds fall in relation to systole, diastole, and normal heart sounds, compare these illustrations.

Auscultation tips

- Concentrate as you listen for each sound.
- Avoid auscultating through clothing or wound dressings because these items can block sound.
- Avoid picking up extraneous sounds by keeping the stethoscope tubing off the patient's body and other surfaces.
- Until you become proficient at auscultation, explain to the patient that listening to his or her chest for a long period doesn't mean that anything is wrong.
- Ask the patient to breathe normally and to hold the breath periodically to enhance sounds that may be difficult to hear.

Hearing pericardial friction rubs

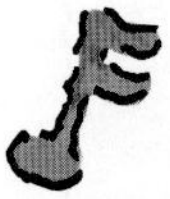

- Have the patient lean forward because this position will bring the heart closer to the chest wall. If the patient can't tolerate leaning forward, position sitting upright.
- Ask the patient to exhale, and then listen with the diaphragm of the stethoscope over the third intercostal space on the left side of the chest.
- If you suspect a rub but have trouble hearing one, ask the patient to hold the breath.
- A friction rub may be heard during atrial systole, ventricular systole, or ventricular diastole. As a result, the sounds produced by the rub may coincide with the first or second heart sound.
- To differentiate a pericardial friction rub from a pleural friction rub, ask the patient to hold the breath. The sound from a pericardial friction rub persists, but the sound from a pleural friction rub ceases.

Assessing the vascular system

Inspection

Start by making general observations. Are the arms equal in size? Are the legs symmetrical? Then note skin color, body hair distribution, and lesions, scars, clubbing, and edema of the extremities. If the patient is confined to bed, check the sacrum for swelling. Examine the fingernails and toenails for abnormalities.

Palpation

First, assess skin temperature, texture, and turgor. Then, assess capillary refill in the nail beds on the fingers and toes. Refill time should be no more than 3 seconds or long enough to say "capillary refill." Palpate the patient's arms and legs for temperature and edema. Then palpate arterial pulses.

Skill check

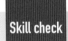

Palpating arterial pulses

Palpate for arterial pulses by gently pressing with the pads of your index and middle fingers. Start at the top of the patient's body at the temporal artery and work your way down. Palpate for the pulse on each side, comparing pulse volume and symmetry. All pulses should be regular in rhythm and equal in strength.

Carotid pulse

Lightly place your fingers just lateral to the trachea and below the jaw angle. Never palpate both carotid arteries at the same time.

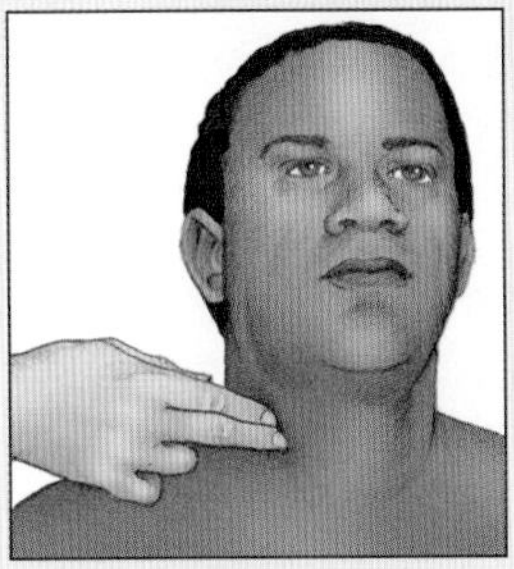

Brachial pulse

Position your fingers medial to the biceps tendon.

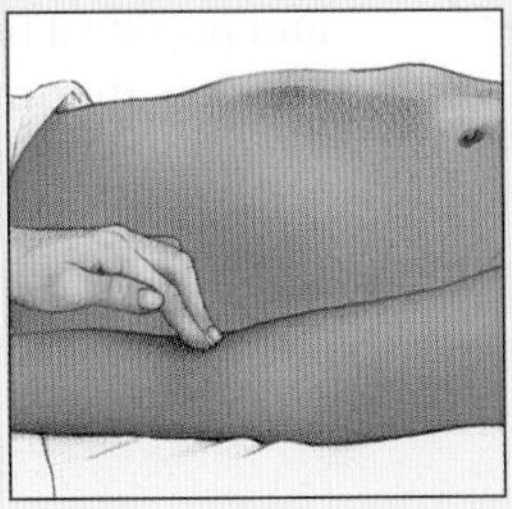

Radial pulse

Apply gentle pressure to the medial and ventral side of the wrist, just below the base of the thumb.

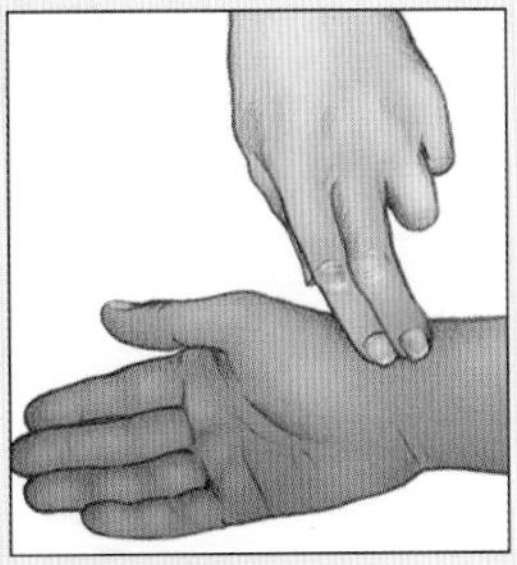

Femoral pulse

Press relatively hard at a point inferior to the inguinal ligament. For an obese patient, palpate in the crease of the groin, halfway between the pubic bone and the hip bone.

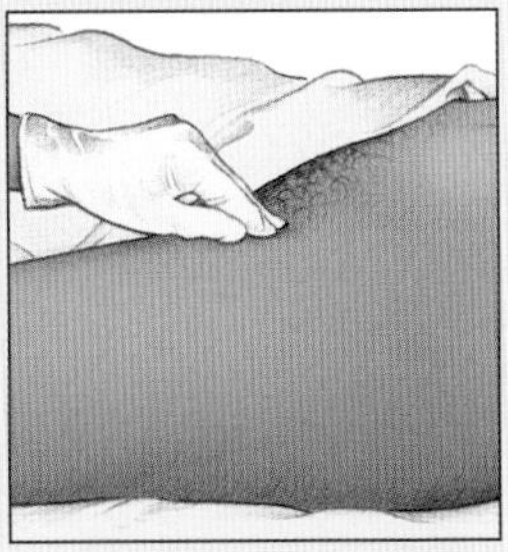

(*continued*)

Popliteal pulse

Press firmly in the popliteal fossa at the back of the knee.

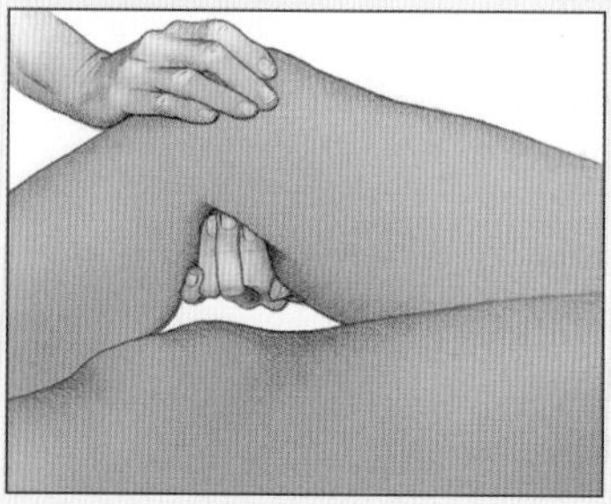

Posterior tibial pulse

Apply pressure behind and slightly below the malleolus of the ankle.

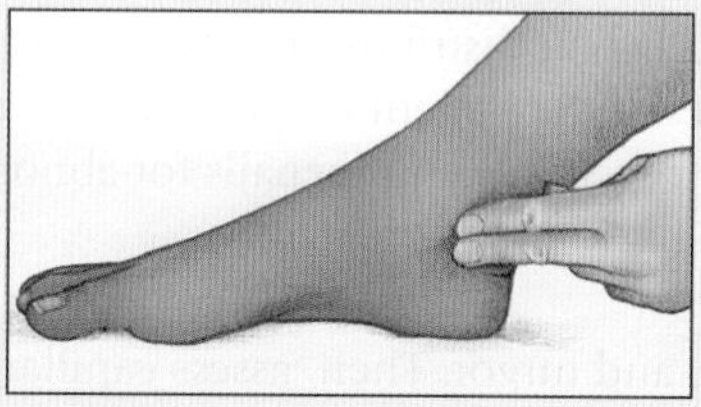

Dorsalis pedis pulse

Place your fingers on the medial dorsum of the foot while the patient points the toes down. The pulse is difficult to palpate here and may seem to be absent in healthy patients.

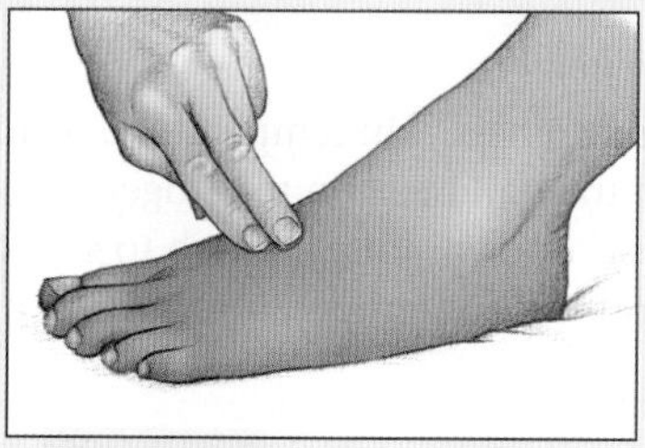

Grading pulses

Pulses are graded on a four-point scale.

4+ = bounding

3+ = increased

2+ = normal

1+ = weak

0 = absent

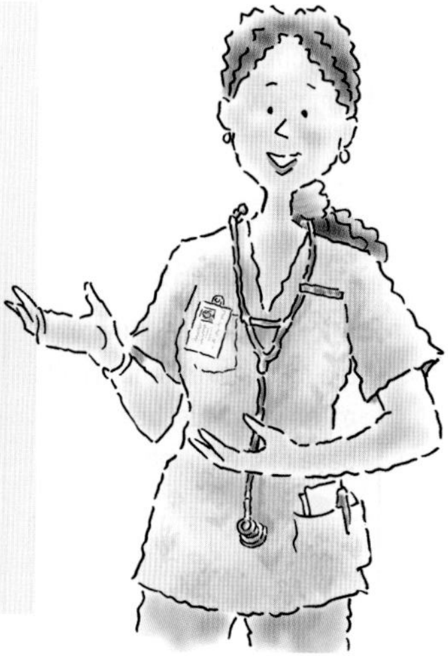

Auscultation

Using the bell of the stethoscope, follow the palpation sequence and auscultate over each artery. Assess the upper abdomen for abnormal pulsations, which could indicate the presence of an abdominal aortic aneurysm. Finally, auscultate for the femoral and popliteal pulses, checking for a bruit or other abnormal sounds.

Abnormal findings

Skin and hair abnormalities

Warm skin may indicate conditions causing fever or increased cardiac output. Absence of body hair on the arms or legs may indicate diminished arterial blood flow to these areas. Cyanosis, pallor, or cool skin may indicate poor cardiac output and tissue perfusion.

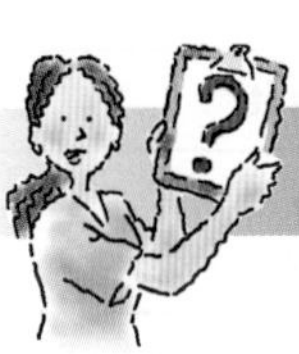

Outside the norm

Cyanosis and pallor

Cyanosis and pallor may indicate poor cardiac output and tissue perfusion.

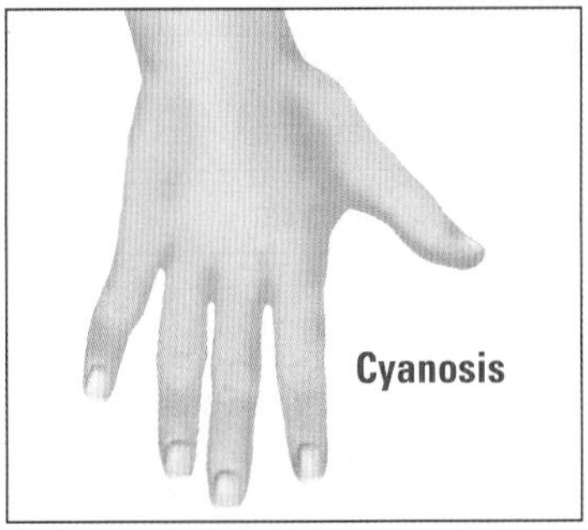
Cyanosis

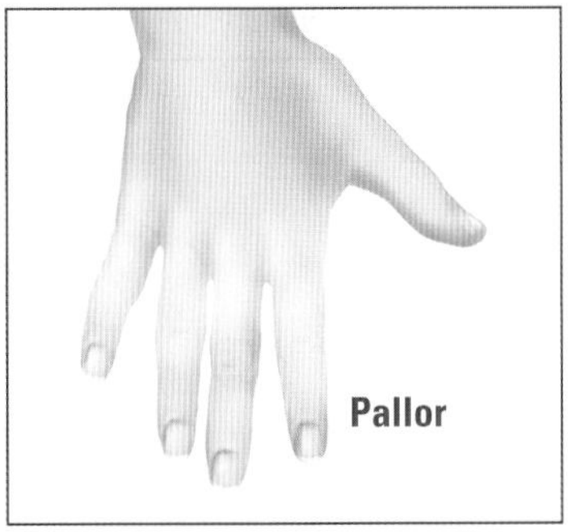
Pallor

Arterial and venous insufficiency

Arterial insufficiency

In a patient with arterial insufficiency, pulses may be decreased or absent. The skin is cool, pale, and shiny; hair loss occurs in the area; and the patient may have pain in the legs and feet. Ulcerations typically occur in the area around the toes, and the foot usually turns deep red when dependent. Nails may be thick and ridged.

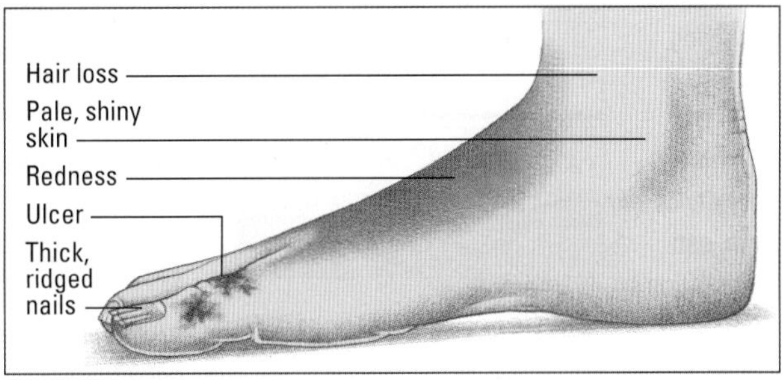
Hair loss
Pale, shiny skin
Redness
Ulcer
Thick, ridged nails

Chronic venous insufficiency

In a patient with chronic venous insufficiency, ulcerations develop around the ankle. Pulses are present but may be difficult to find because of edema. The foot may become cyanotic when dependent.

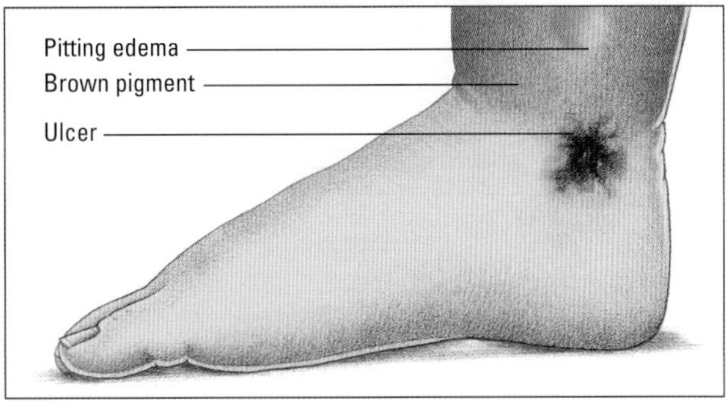
Pitting edema
Brown pigment
Ulcer

Edema

Swelling, or edema, may indicate heart failure or venous insufficiency. Right-sided heart failure may cause swelling in the lower legs. Edema may also result from varicosities or thrombophlebitis.

Abnormal pulsations

A weak arterial pulse may indicate decreased cardiac output or increased peripheral vascular resistance; both point to arterial atherosclerotic disease. Strong or bounding pulsations usually occur in a patient with a condition that causes increased cardiac output, such as hypertension, hypoxia, anemia, exercise, or anxiety. A thrill usually suggests a valvular dysfunction.

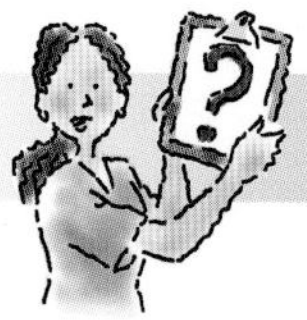

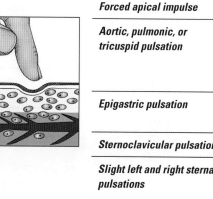

Outside the norm

Edema

Edema may be pitting or nonpitting. To differentiate between the two, press your finger against a swollen area for 5 seconds and then quickly remove it.

Pitting edema
With pitting edema, pressure forces fluid into the underlying tissues, causing an indentation that slowly fills. To determine the severity of pitting edema, estimate the indentation's depth in centimeters: 1+, 2+, 3+, or 4+.

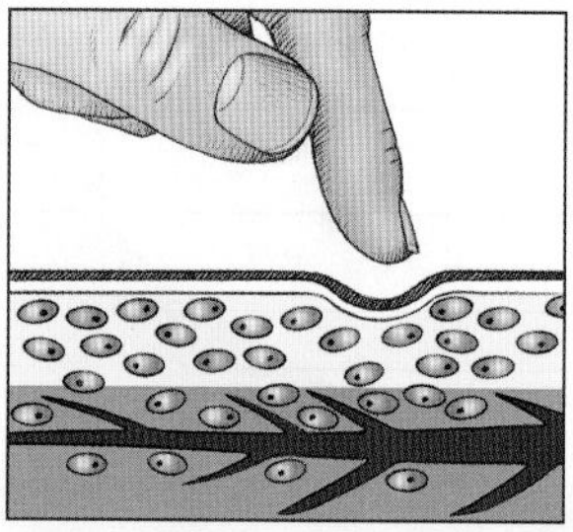

Nonpitting edema
With nonpitting edema, pressure leaves no indentation because fluid has coagulated in the tissues. Typically, the skin feels unusually tight and firm.

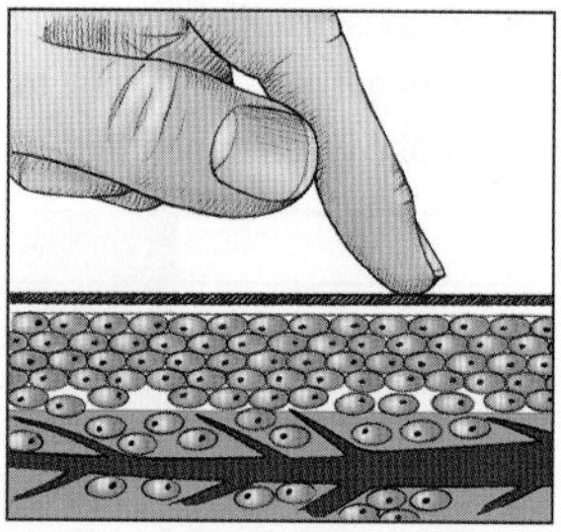

Abnormal pulsation	What causes it
Displaced apical impulse	• Heart failure • Hypertension
Forced apical impulse	• Increased cardiac output
Aortic, pulmonic, or tricuspid pulsation	• Valvular disease • Heart chamber enlargement • Aortic aneurysm (aortic pulsation only)
Epigastric pulsation	• Heart failure • Aortic aneurysm
Sternoclavicular pulsation	• Aortic aneurysm
Slight left and right sternal pulsations	• Anemia • Anxiety • Increased cardiac output • Thin chest wall
Sternal border heave	• Right ventricular hypertrophy • Ventricular aneurysm

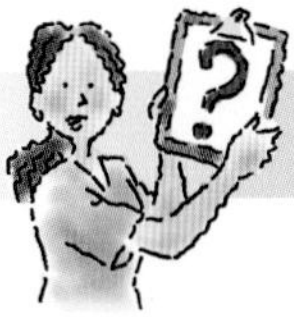

Outside the norm

Abnormal pulses

These waveforms illustrate abnormal arterial pulses.

Weak pulse
A weak pulse has a decreased amplitude with a slower upstroke and downstroke. Possible causes of a weak pulse include increased peripheral vascular resistance, as occurs in cold weather or with severe heart failure, and decreased stroke volume, as occurs with hypovolemia or aortic stenosis.

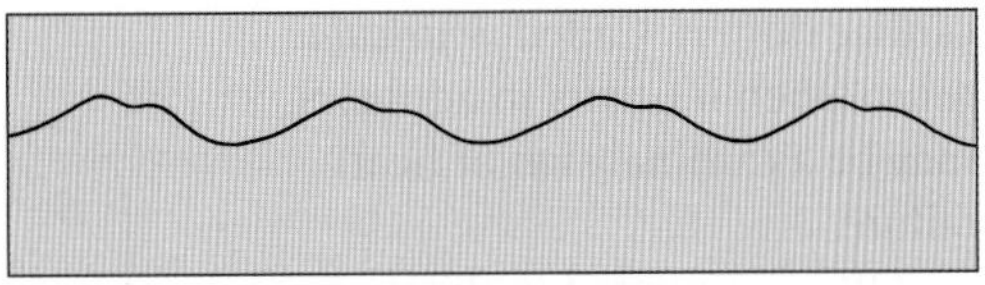

Bounding pulse
A bounding pulse has a sharp upstroke and downstroke with a pointed peak. The amplitude is elevated. Possible causes of a bounding pulse include increased stroke volume, as with aortic insufficiency, or stiffness of arterial walls, as with aging.

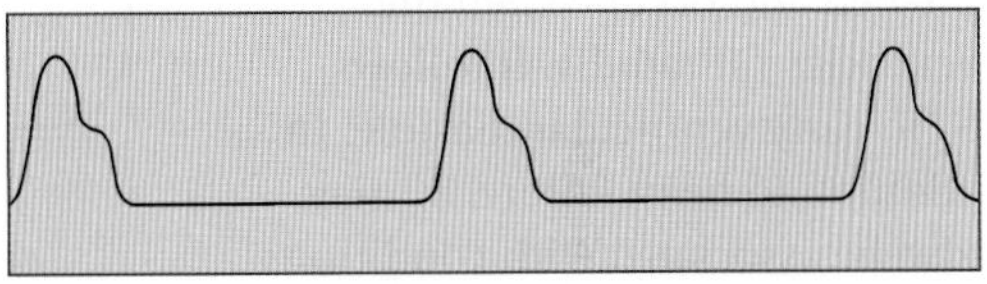

Pulsus alternans
Pulsus alternans has a regular, alternating pattern of a weak and a strong pulse. This pulse is associated with left-sided heart failure.

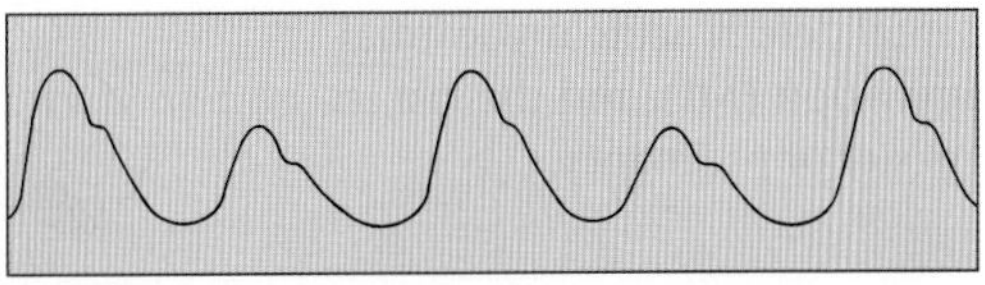

Pulsus bigeminus
Pulsus bigeminus is similar to pulsus alternans but occurs at irregular intervals. This pulse is caused by premature atrial or ventricular beats.

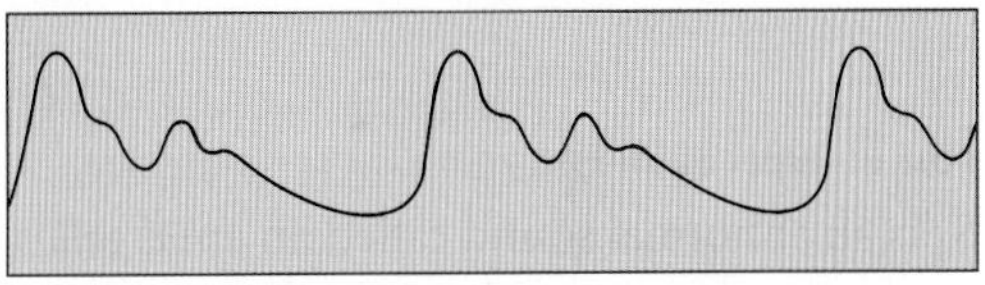

Pulsus paradoxus
Pulsus paradoxus has increases and decreases in amplitude associated with the respiratory cycle. Marked decreases occur when the patient inhales. Pulsus paradoxus is associated with pericardial tamponade, advanced heart failure, and constrictive pericarditis.

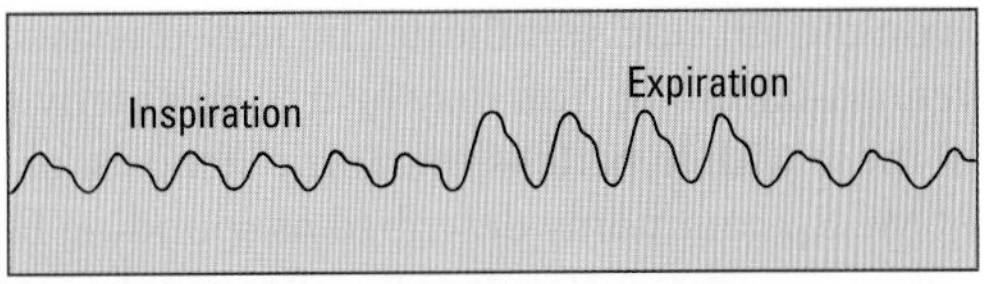
Inspiration
Expiration

Pulsus bisferiens
Pulsus bisferiens shows an initial upstroke, a subsequent downstroke, and then another upstroke during systole. Pulsus bisferiens is caused by aortic stenosis and aortic insufficiency.

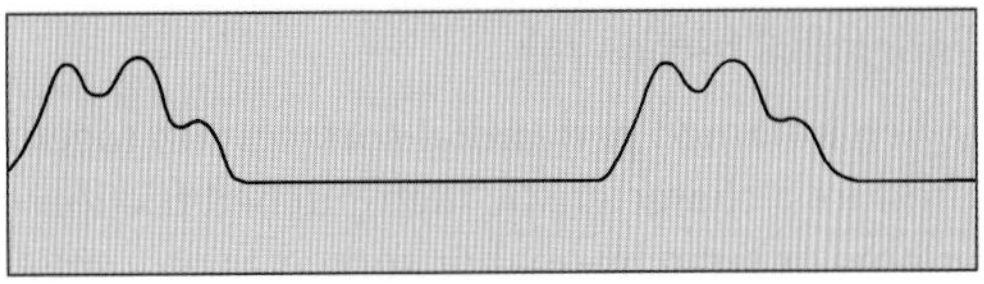

Abnormal heart sounds

Third heart sound

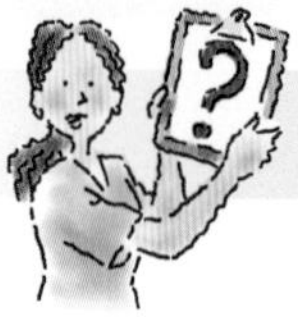

S_3 is a normal finding in children and young adults; however, an abnormal S_3 is commonly heard in patients with high cardiac output. Called *ventricular gallop* when it occurs in adults, S_3 may be a cardinal sign of heart failure.

Often compared to the y sound in "Ken-tuck-y," S_3 is low-pitched and occurs when the ventricles fill rapidly. It follows S_2 in early ventricular diastole. In addition to heart failure, S_3 may also be associated with conditions such as pulmonary edema, atrial septal defect, acute myocardial infarction (MI), and the last trimester of pregnancy.

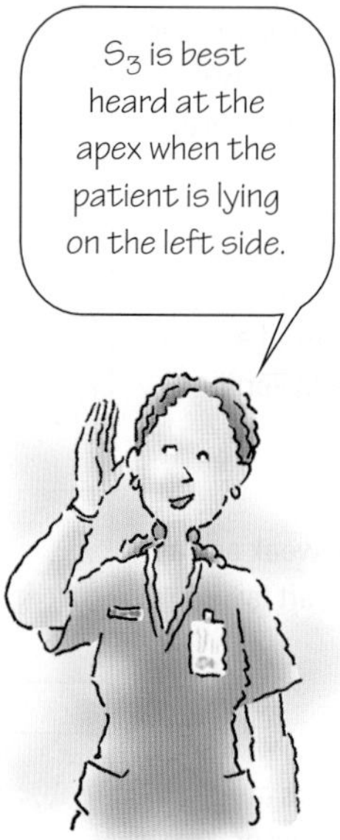
S_3 is best heard at the apex when the patient is lying on the left side.

Fourth heart sound

S_4 is an abnormal sound called an *atrial gallop* that's heard over the tricuspid or mitral areas when the patient is on the left side. It indicates increased resistance to ventricular filling. You may hear S_4 in elderly patients or in those with hypertension, aortic stenosis, or a history of MI. S_4, commonly described as sounding like "Ten-nes-see," occurs just before S_1, after atrial contraction.

Pericardial friction rub

When inflamed pericardial surfaces rub together, they produce a characteristic high-pitched friction noise of grating or scratchy quality known as *pericardial friction rub*. A classic sign of inflammation of the pericardium (pericarditis), a pericardial friction rub may result from a viral or bacterial infection, radiation therapy to the chest, or cardiac trauma.

Outside the norm

Abnormal heart sounds

Whenever auscultation reveals an abnormal heart sound, try to identify the sound and its timing in the cardiac cycle. Knowing those characteristics can help you identify the possible cause for the sound. Use this chart to put all that information together.

Abnormal heart sound
Accentuated S_1
Diminished S_1
Split S_1 (mitral and tricuspid components to the S_1 sound)
Accentuated S_2
Diminished or inaudible S_2
Persistent S_2 split (aortic and pulmonic components to the S_2 sound)
Reversed or paradoxical S_2 split that appears during exhalation and disappears during inspiration
S_3 (ventricular gallop)
S_4 (atrial or presystolic gallop)
Pericardial friction rub (grating or leathery sound at the left sternal border; usually muffled, high-pitched, and transient)

Timing	Possible causes
Beginning of systole	Mitral stenosis or fever
Beginning of systole	Mitral insufficiency, heart block, or severe mitral insufficiency with a calcified, immobile valve
Beginning of systole	Right bundle-branch block (BBB) or premature ventricular contractions
End of systole	Pulmonary or systemic hypertension
End of systole	Aortic or pulmonic stenosis
End of systole	Delayed closure of the pulmonic valve, usually from overfilling of the right ventricle, causing prolonged systolic ejection time
End of systole	Delayed ventricular stimulation, left BBB, or prolonged left ventricular ejection time
Early diastole	Overdistention of the ventricles during the rapid-filling segment of diastole or mitral insufficiency or ventricular failure (normal in children and young adults)
Late diastole	Pulmonic stenosis, hypertension, coronary artery disease, aortic stenosis, or forceful atrial contraction due to resistance to ventricular filling late in diastole (resulting from left ventricular hypertrophy)
Throughout systole and diastole	Pericardial inflammation

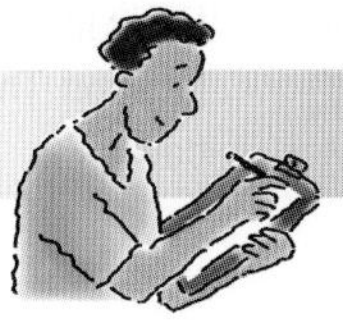

Take note

Documenting heart sounds

4/03/10	1530	Pt. alert and oriented to time, place, and person. Skin warm and dry; lips and nail beds pink. Reports SOB with ambulation to the bathroom. Denies SOB at rest. Denies chest pain. Has occasional dry cough. Bilateral breath sounds with scattered bibasilar crackles. S_3 sound heard on auscultation, no JVD, 2+ pitting edema both ankles. Nasal O_2 at 2 L/minute. Call placed to Dr. Anderson's office at 1520.
		Russ Wallace, RN

Murmurs

If you identify a heart murmur, listen closely to determine its timing in the cardiac cycle. Then determine its other characteristics: quality (blowing, musical, harsh, or rumbling), pitch (medium, high, or low), and location (where the murmur sounds the loudest). Use a standard, six-level grading scale to describe the intensity (loudness) of the murmur.

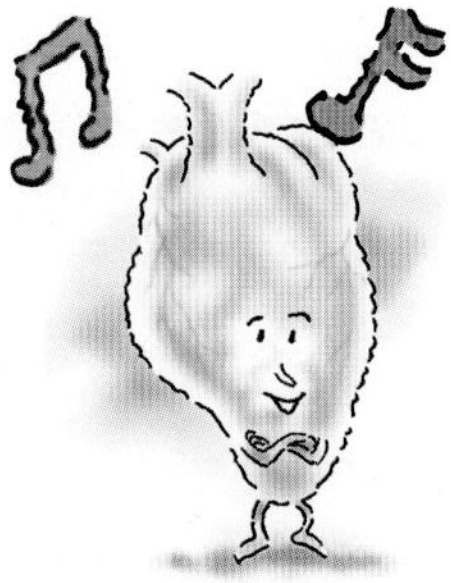

Murmur grading

Grade 1—barely audible, even to the trained ear

Grade 2—clearly audible

Grade 3—moderately loud

Grade 4—loud with palpable thrill

Grade 5—very loud with a palpable thrill; can be heard when the stethoscope has only partial contact with the chest

Grade 6—extremely loud with a palpable thrill; can be heard with the stethoscope lifted just off the chest wall

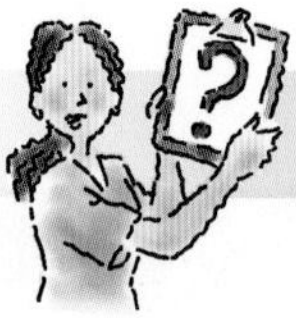

Outside the norm

Heart murmurs

Heart murmurs are described according to their timing, quality and pitch, and location. This chart outlines the various types of murmurs and their possible causes.

Timing	Quality and pitch	Location	Possible causes
Midsystolic (systolic ejection)	Harsh, rough with medium to high pitch	Pulmonic	Pulmonic stenosis
	Harsh, rough with medium to high pitch	Aortic and suprasternal notch	Aortic stenosis
Holosystolic (pansystolic)	Harsh with high pitch	Tricuspid	Ventricular septal defect
	Blowing with high pitch	Mitral, lower left sternal border	Mitral insufficiency
	Blowing with high pitch	Tricuspid	Tricuspid insufficiency
Early diastolic	Blowing with high pitch	Midleft sternal edge (not aortic area)	Aortic insufficiency
	Blowing with high pitch	Pulmonic	Pulmonic insufficiency
Middiastolic to late diastolic	Rumbling with low pitch	Apex	Mitral stenosis
	Rumbling with low pitch	Tricuspid, lower right sternal border	Tricuspid stenosis

Murmur configurations

Configurations, or patterns, refer to changes in murmur intensity.

Crescendo

A crescendo murmur becomes progressively louder.

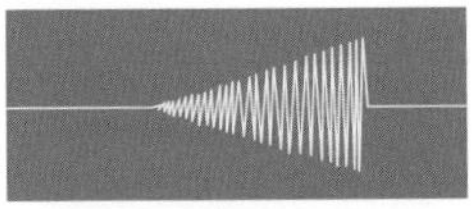

Decrescendo

A decrescendo murmur becomes progressively softer.

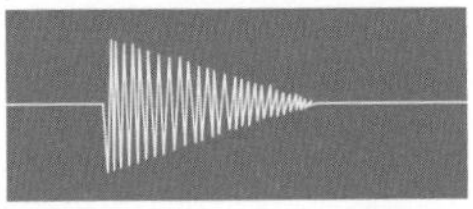

Crescendo-decrescendo

A crescendo-decrescendo murmur (also called diamond-shaped hair) peaks in intensity and then decreases again.

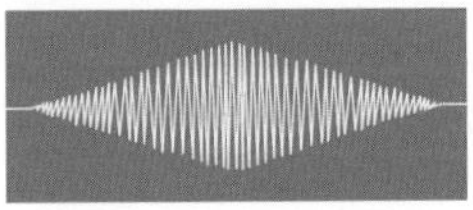

Plateau-shaped

A plateau-shaped murmur remains equal in intensity.

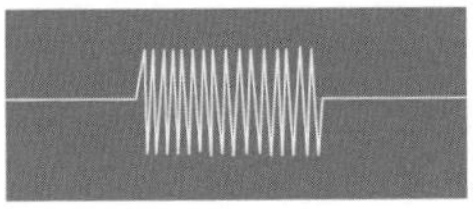

Bruits

A murmur-like sound of vascular (rather than cardiac) origin is called a *bruit*. If you hear a bruit during arterial auscultation, the patient may have occlusive arterial disease or an arteriovenous fistula. A carotid bruit may suggest carotid artery stenosis. Various high cardiac output conditions—such as anemia, hyperthyroidism, and pheochromocytoma—may also cause bruits.

Vascular abnormalities

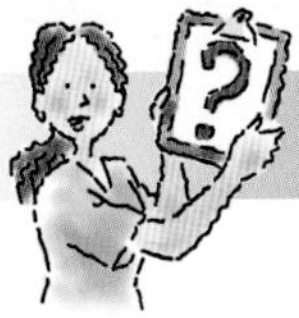

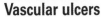

Outside the norm

Vascular ulcers

Venous ulcers

Venous ulcers result from venous hypertension. These ulcers, the most commonly occurring lower leg ulcers, are typically found around the ankle, as shown.

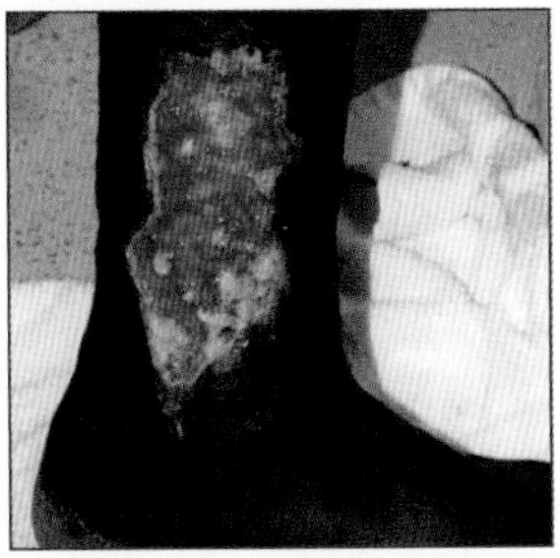

Lymphatic ulcers

Lymphatic ulcers result from lymphedema, in which the capillaries are compressed by thickened tissue, which occludes blood flow to the skin. Lymphatic ulcers are extremely difficult to treat because of the reduced blood flow. This photo shows a patient with lymphedema of the leg and a large lymphatic ulcer.

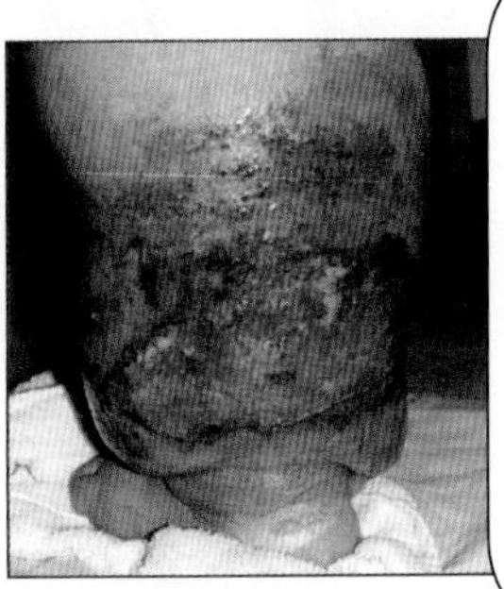

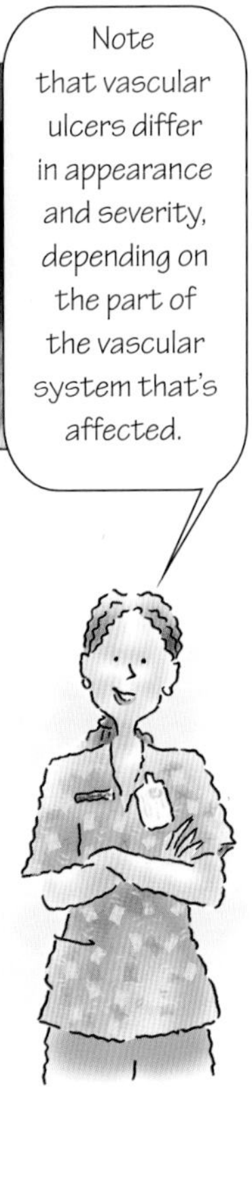
Note that vascular ulcers differ in appearance and severity, depending on the part of the vascular system that's affected.

Arterial ulcers

Arterial ulcers result from arterial occlusive disease caused by insufficient blood flow to tissue due to arterial insufficiency. They're commonly found at the distal ends of arterial branches, especially at the tips of the toes, the corners of nail beds, or over bony prominences, as shown.

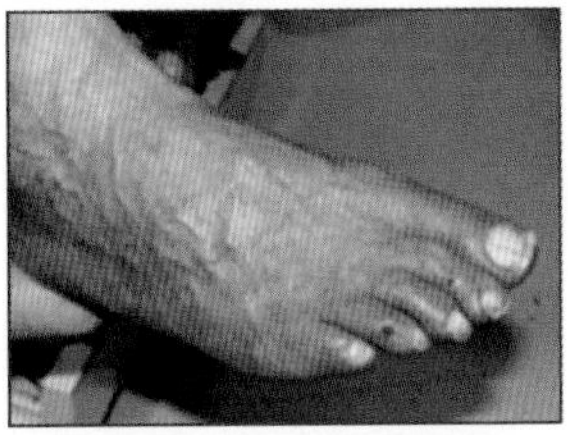

Q&A

Able to label?

Identify the arteries that can be palpated for peripheral pulses.

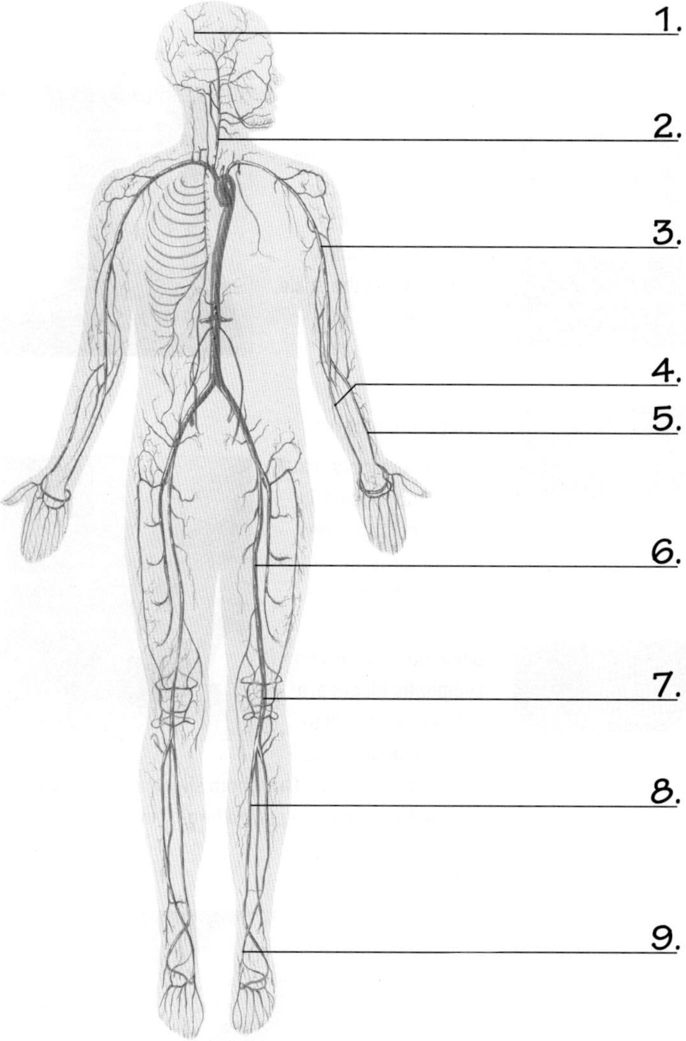
1.
2.
3.
4.
5.
6.
7.
8.
9.

Rebus riddle

Sound out each group of pictures and symbols to reveal information about normal physiology of the heart.

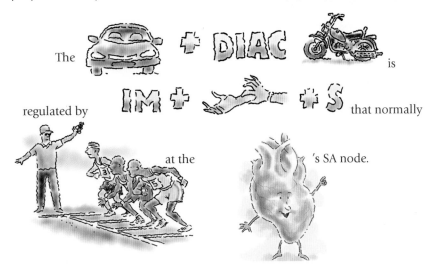
The
+ DIAC
is
regulated by
IM +
+ S
that normally
at the
's SA node.

Answers: Able to label? 1. Superficial temporal, 2. Carotid, 3. Brachial, 4. Ulnar, 5. Radial, 6. Femoral, 7. Popliteal, 8. Posterior tibial, 9. Dorsalis pedis; Rebus riddle The cardiac cycle is regulated by impulses that normally start at the heart's SA node.

Selected References

Aaronson, P. L. (2013). *The cardiovascular system at a glance* (4th ed.). Malden, MA:Wiley-Blackwell.

Lippincott. (2011). *Professional guide to pathophysiology* (3rd ed.). Philadelphia, PA: Wolters Kluwer.

Vorvick, L. J. (2013). "Cardiovascular System." [Online]. Accessed April 2015 via the web at https://www.nlm.nih.gov/medlineplus/ency/anatomyvideos/000023.htm

Woods, S. L., et al. (2010). *Cardiac nursing* (6th ed.). Philadelphia, PA: Wolters Kluwer.

Chapter 7

Breasts and axillae

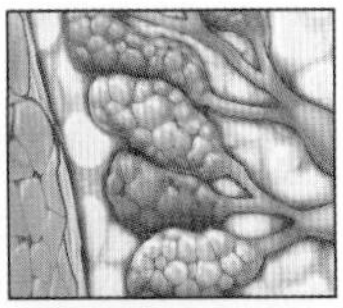

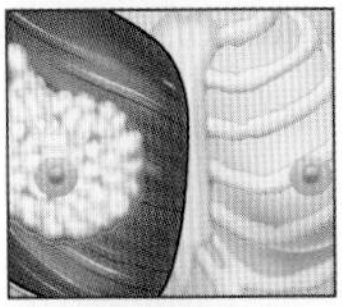

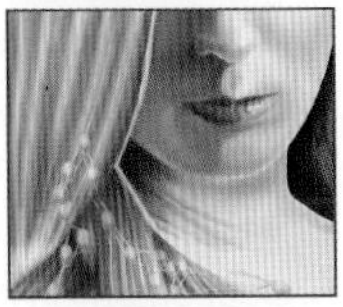

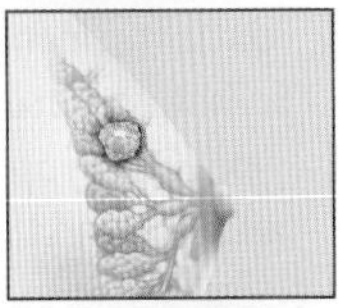

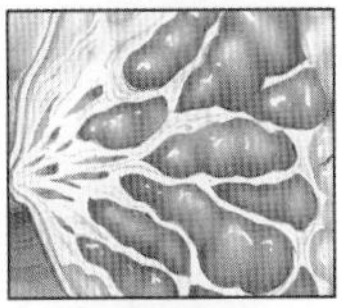

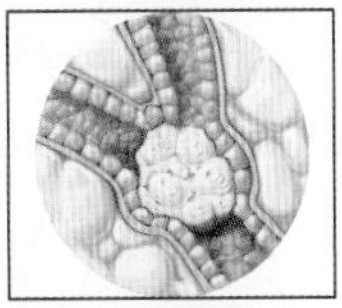

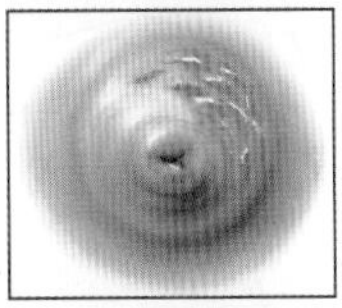

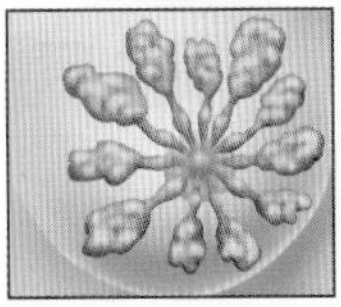

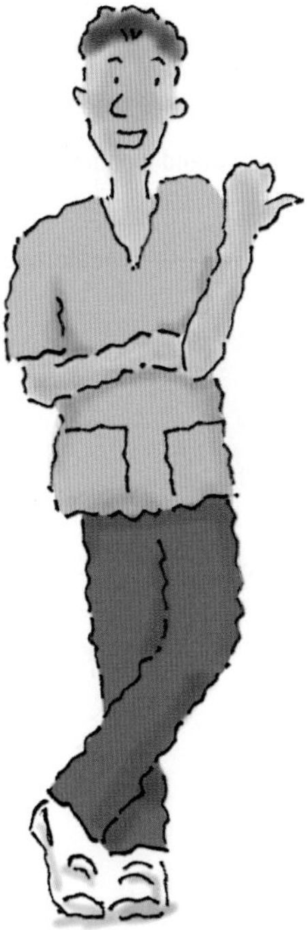

Anatomy

The breasts, also called *mammary glands* in women, lie on the anterior chest wall. They're located vertically between the second or third and the sixth or seventh ribs over the pectoralis major muscle and the serratus anterior muscle and horizontally between the sternal border and the midaxillary line.

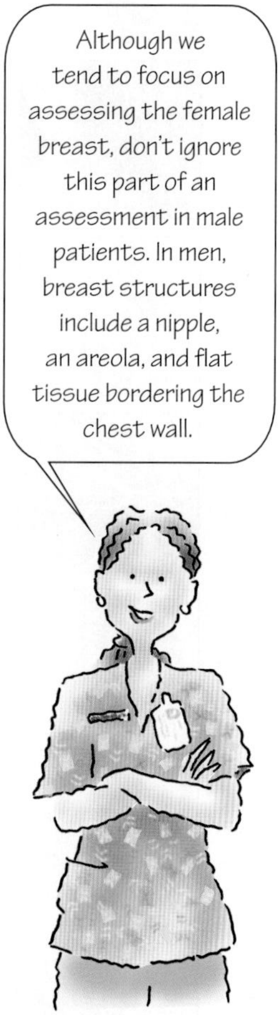
Although we tend to focus on assessing the female breast, don't ignore this part of an assessment in male patients. In men, breast structures include a nipple, an areola, and flat tissue bordering the chest wall.

Breast structures

Each breast has a centrally located nipple of pigmented erectile tissue ringed by an areola that's darker than the adjacent tissue. Sebaceous glands, also called *Montgomery tubercles*, are scattered on the areola surface, along with hair follicles.

Differences in areola pigmentation

The pigment of the nipple and areola varies among different races, getting darker as skin tone darkens. Caucasian patients have light-colored nipples and areolae, usually pink or light beige. People with darker complexions, such as African Americans and Asians, have medium brown to almost black nipples and areolae.

Normal breast anatomy

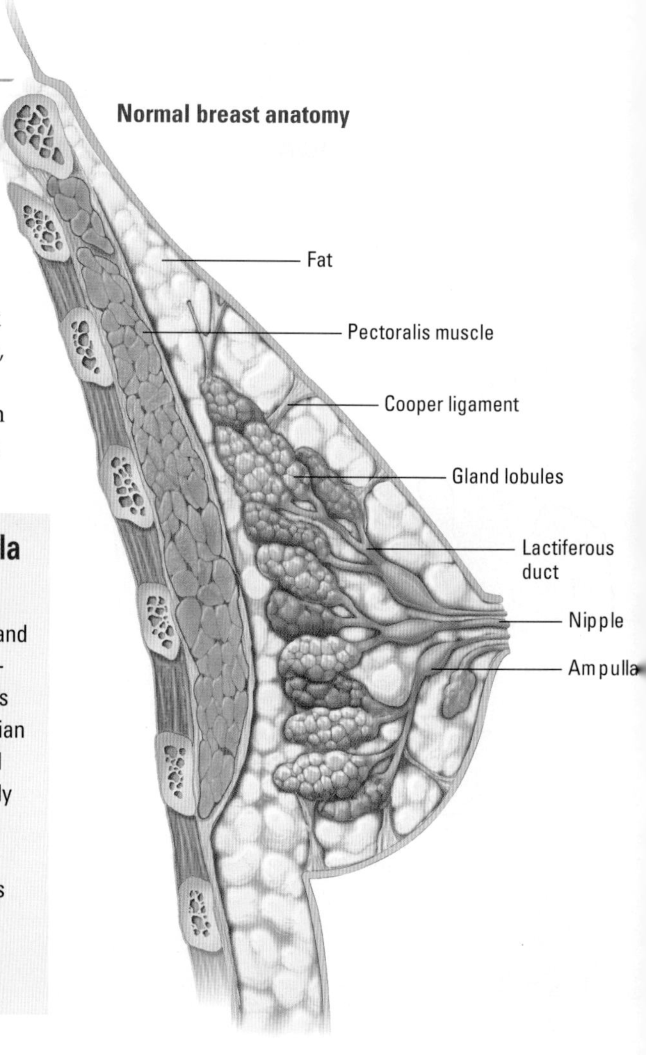
Fat
Pectoralis muscle
Cooper ligament
Gland lobules
Lactiferous duct
Nipple
Ampulla

What lies beneath

Beneath the skin are glandular, fibrous, and fatty tissues that vary in proportion with age, weight, gender, and other factors, such as pregnancy. A small triangle of tissue, called the *tail of Spence*, projects into the axilla. Attached to the chest wall musculature are fibrous bands, called *Cooper ligaments*, that support each breast.

Support structures of the breast

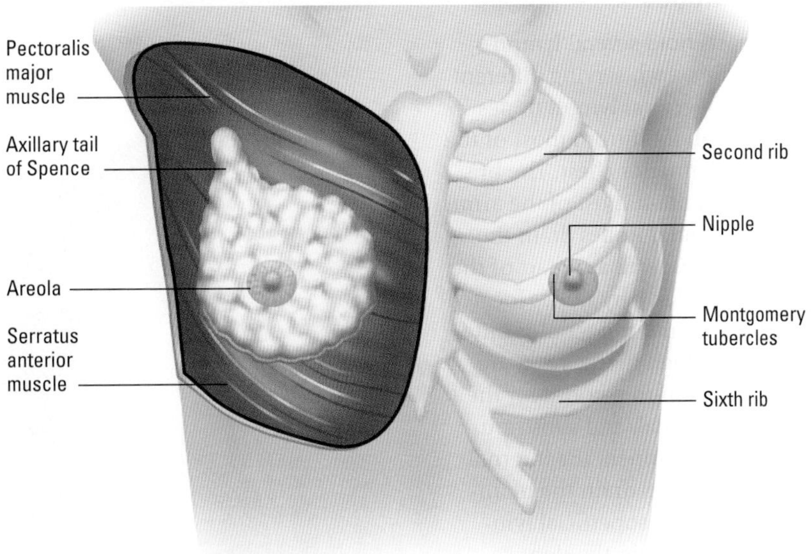
Pectoralis major muscle
Axillary tail of Spence
Areola
Serratus anterior muscle
Second rib
Nipple
Montgomery tubercles
Sixth rib

Lobes and ducts

In women, 12 to 25 glandular lobes containing alveoli that produce milk surround each breast. The lactiferous ducts from each lobe transport milk to the nipple.

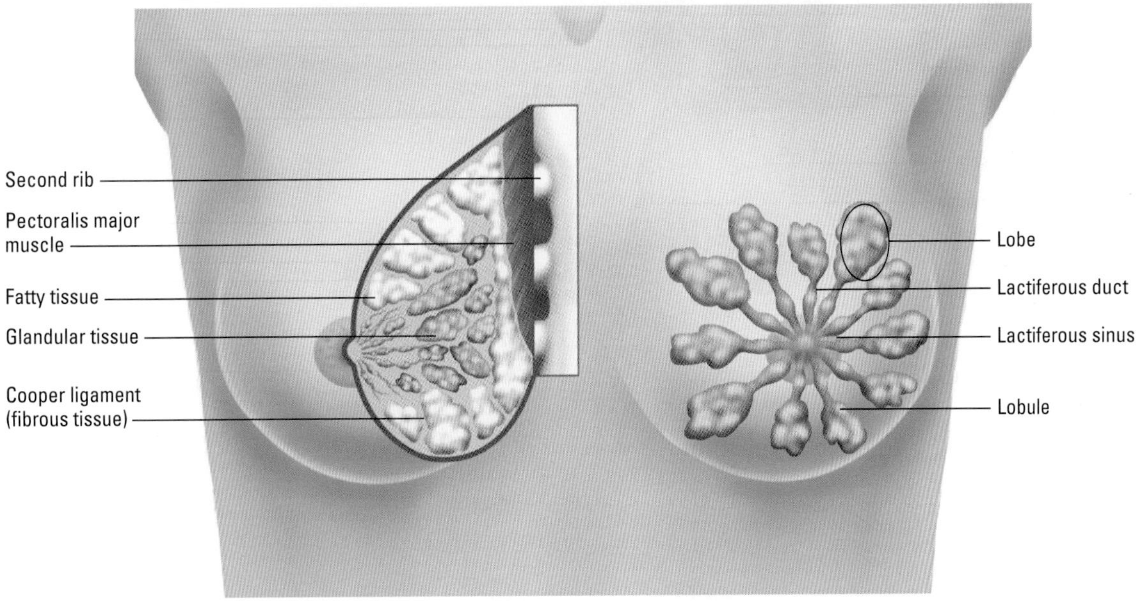
Second rib
Pectoralis major muscle
Fatty tissue
Glandular tissue
Cooper ligament (fibrous tissue)
Lobe
Lactiferous duct
Lactiferous sinus
Lobule

Lymph nodes

The breasts hold several lymph node chains, each serving different areas. The pectoral lymph nodes drain lymph fluid from most of the breast and anterior chest. The brachial nodes drain most of the arm. The subscapular nodes drain the posterior chest wall and part of the arm. The midaxillary nodes located near the ribs and the serratus anterior muscle high in the axilla are the central draining nodes for the pectoral, brachial, and subscapular nodes. In women, the internal mammary nodes drain the mammary lobes. The superficial lymphatic vessels drain the skin.

Lymph nodes of the breast and axillary region

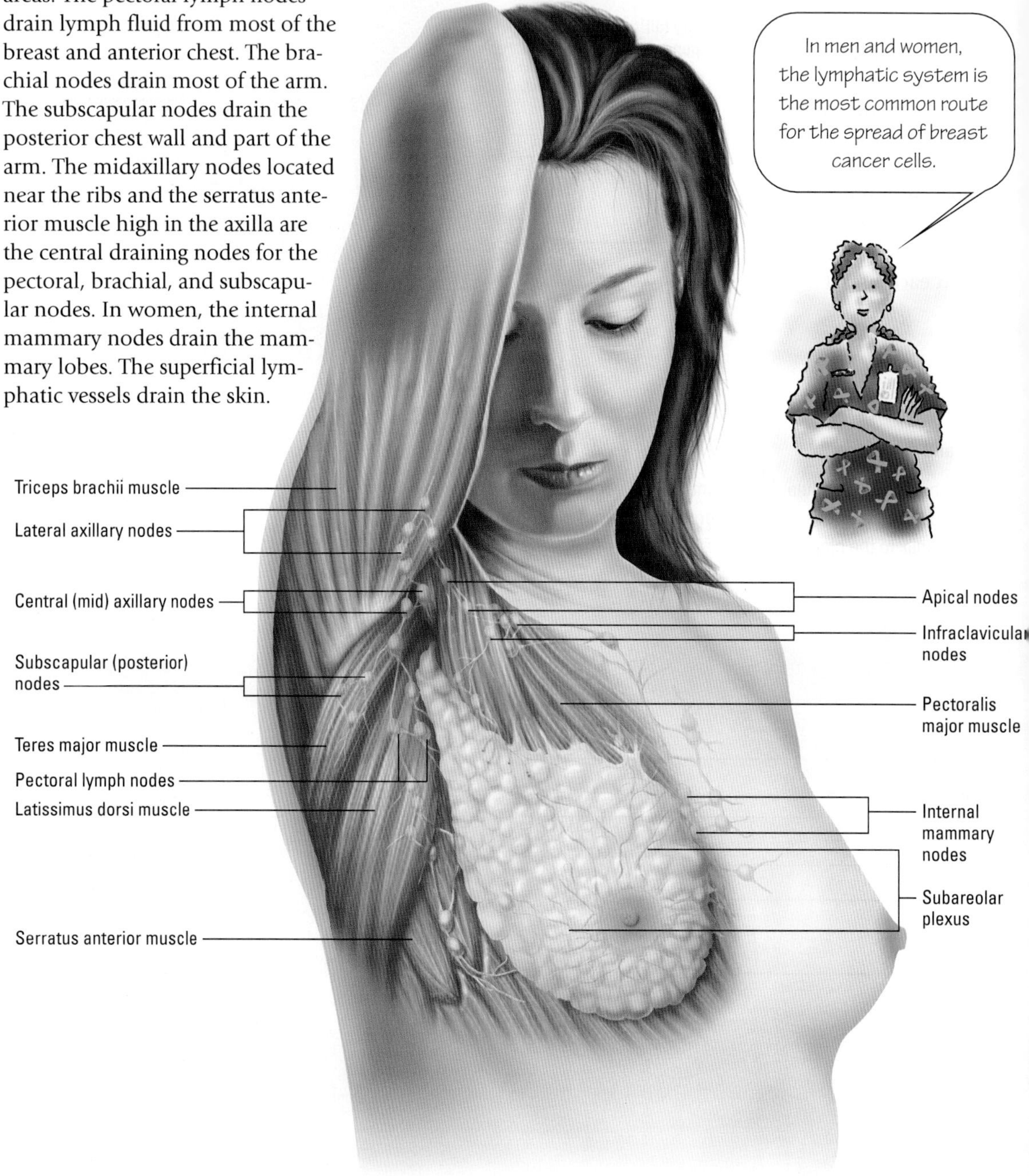
Triceps brachii muscle
Lateral axillary nodes
Central (mid) axillary nodes
Subscapular (posterior) nodes
Teres major muscle
Pectoral lymph nodes
Latissimus dorsi muscle
Serratus anterior muscle
Apical nodes
Infraclavicular nodes
Pectoralis major muscle
Internal mammary nodes
Subareolar plexus
In men and women, the lymphatic system is the most common route for the spread of breast cancer cells.

As time goes on

In females, the breasts start to change at puberty and continue changing during the reproductive years, pregnancy, and menopause.

Changes during puberty

Breast development is an early sign of puberty in girls and usually starts with the breast and nipple protruding as a single mound of flesh between ages 8 and 13. Development of breast tissue in girls younger than age 8 is abnormal.

Changes during the reproductive years

During the reproductive years, a woman's breasts may become full or tender in response to hormonal fluctuations during the menstrual cycle. During pregnancy, breast changes occur in response to hormones from the corpus luteum and the placenta.

Changes after menopause

After menopause, estrogen levels decrease, causing glandular tissue to atrophy and be replaced with fatty deposits.

Breast changes through the life span

Before age 8

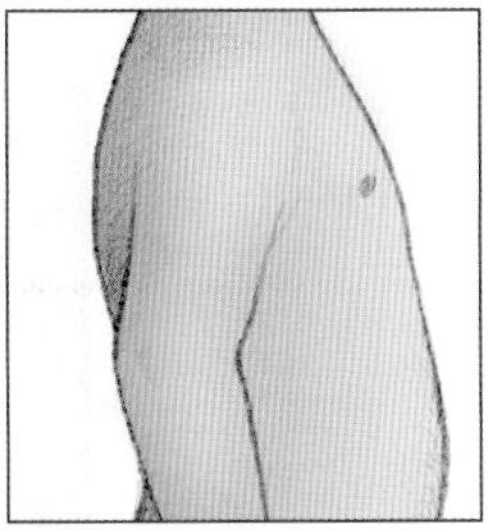

Between ages 8 and 13

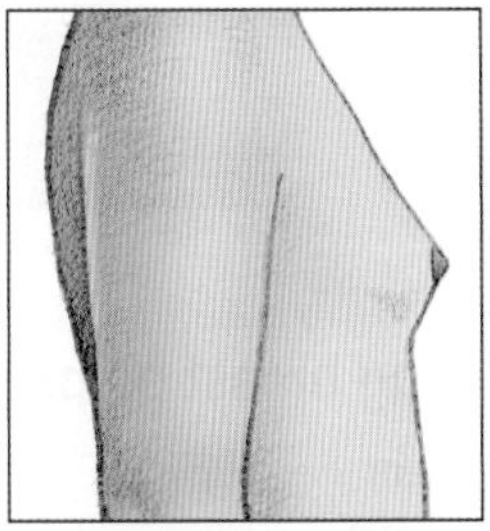

- The breast and nipple protrude as a single mound of flesh.

During adulthood (having never given birth)

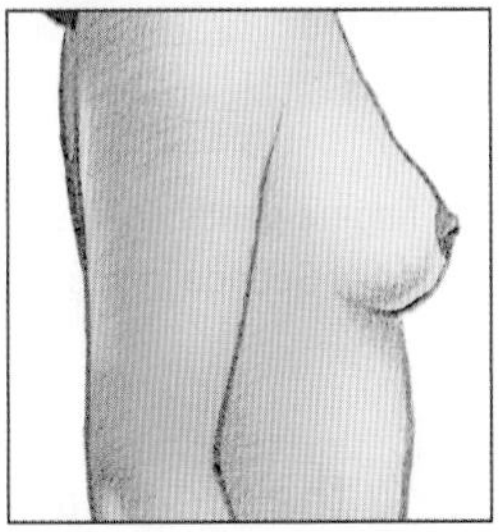

- Breasts may become full or tender in response to hormonal fluctuations during the menstrual cycle.

During pregnancy

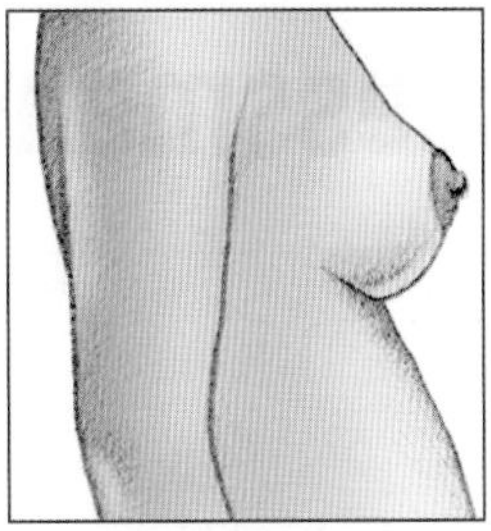

- The areola becomes deeply pigmented and increases in diameter.
- The nipple becomes darker, more prominent, and erect.
- The breasts enlarge because of the proliferation and hypertrophy of the alveolar cells and lactiferous ducts.
- As veins engorge, a venous pattern may become visible.
- Striae may appear as a result of stretching, and Montgomery tubercles may become prominent.

After pregnancy

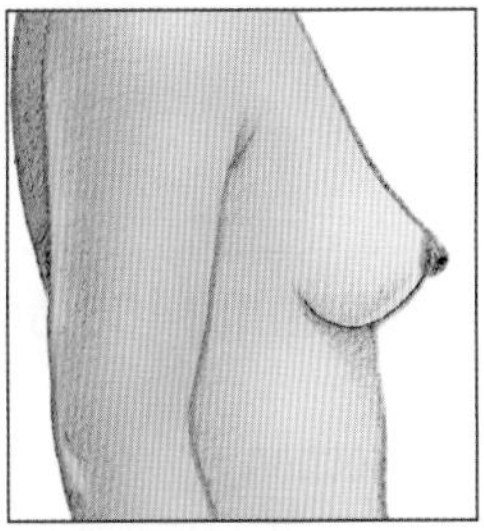

- During breast-feeding, a woman's breasts become full and tense and may feel firm and warm.
- After breast-feeding ceases, breast size decreases but usually doesn't return to the prepregnancy state.

After menopause

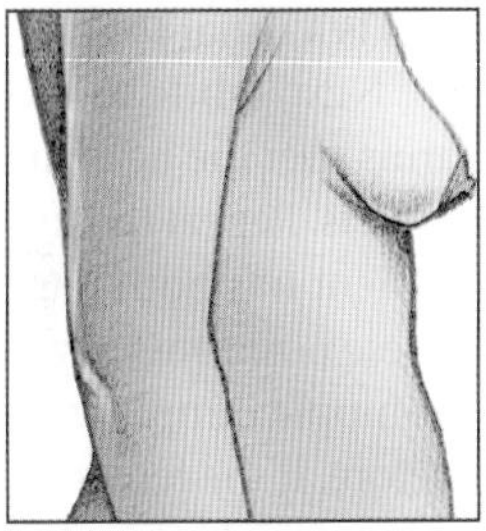

- The breasts become flabbier and smaller.
- As the ligaments relax, the breasts hang loosely from the chest.
- The nipples flatten, losing some of their erectile quality.
- The ducts around the nipples may feel like firm strings.

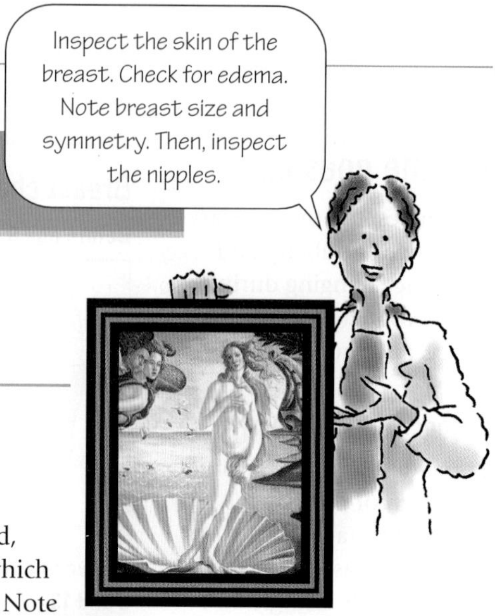
Inspect the skin of the breast. Check for edema. Note breast size and symmetry. Then, inspect the nipples.

Assessment

Examining the breasts

Inspection

Inspect the skin of the breast. It should be smooth, undimpled, and the same color as the rest of the skin. Check for edema, which can accompany lymphatic obstruction and may signal cancer. Note breast size, shape, and symmetry of the breast. Asymmetry may occur normally in some adult women, with the left breast usually larger than the right.

Inspect the nipples, noting their size and shape. If a nipple is inverted, dimpled, or creased, ask the patient when the abnormality was first noticed or if this is a usual finding for the patient.

Next, while the patient has both arms over the head, inspect the patient's breasts. Repeat the inspection while the patient has both hands on the hips. These positions may help you detect skin or nipple dimpling that wasn't obvious before. If the female patient has large or pendulous breasts, have her stand with her hands on the back of a chair and lean forward. This position helps reveal subtle breast or nipple asymmetry.

Palpation

Ask the patient to lie in a supine position, and place a small pillow under the shoulder on the side you're examining. Have the patient put the hand behind the head on the side you're examining. This spreads the breast evenly across the chest and makes finding nodules easier. If the breasts are small, the patient's arm can be left by the side.

Skill check

Performing breast palpation

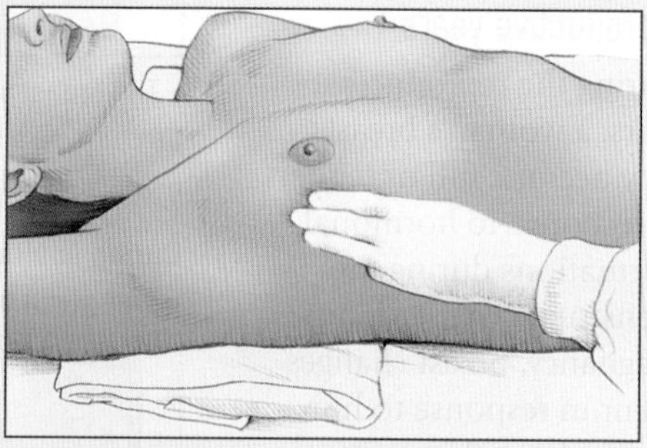

Ask the patient to place the arm above the head of the breast you are examining and then, use your three middle fingers to palpate the patient's breasts systematically. Rotate your fingers gently against the chest wall. Make sure you include the tail of Spence in your examination.

Examining the areola and nipple

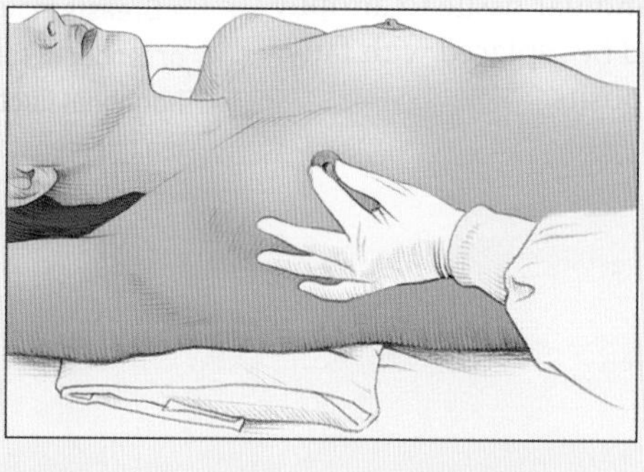

After palpating the breasts, palpate the areola and nipple. As the patients if they have had any unusual nipple discharge.

Breast palpation methods

Three methods may be used to palpate the breasts during a clinical examination: circular, wedged, or vertical strip. According to the American Cancer Society, the vertical strip method is the most effective method to ensure that the entire breast is palpated. Whatever method you use, be consistent and palpate the entire breast, including the periphery, tail of Spence, and the areola.

Circular

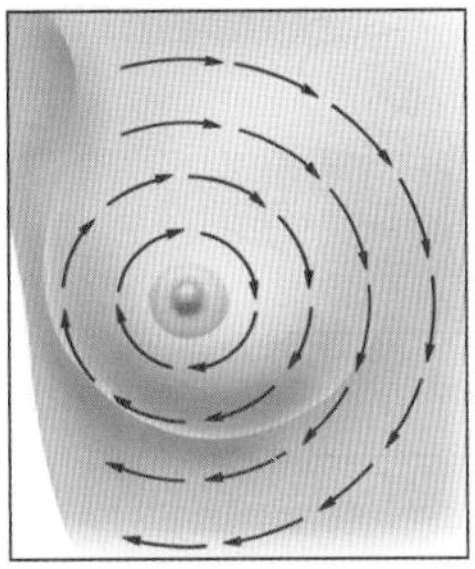

Wedged

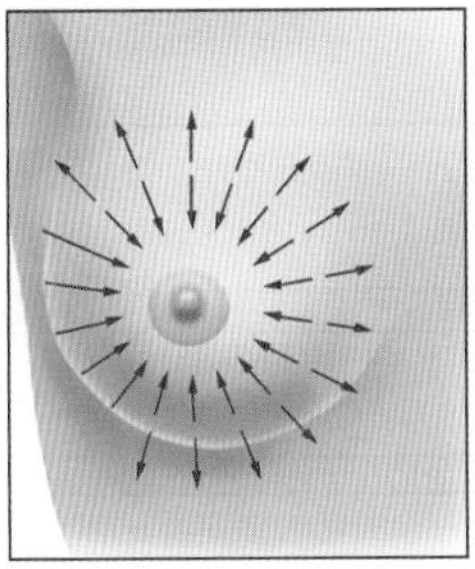

Vertical strip

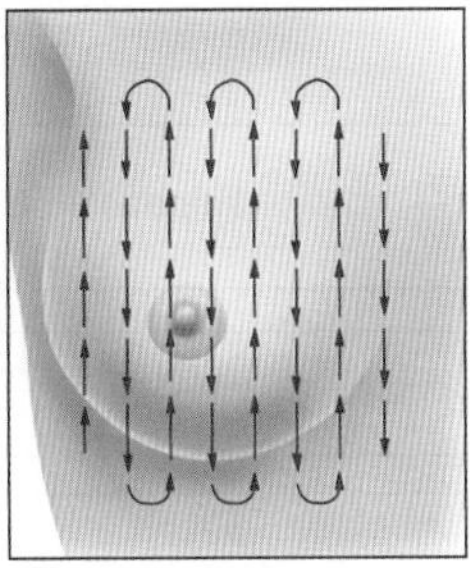

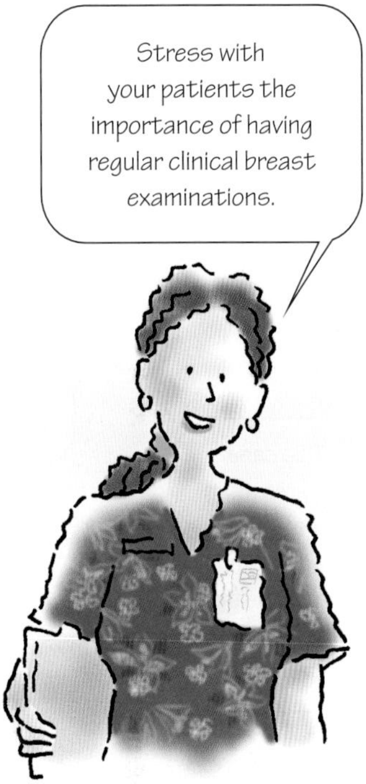
Stress with your patients the importance of having regular clinical breast examinations.

Identifying locations of breast lesions

Mentally divide the breast into four quadrants and a fifth segment, the tail of Spence. Describe your findings according to the appropriate quadrant or segment. You can also think of the breast as a clock, with the nipple in the center. Then specify locations according to the time (2 o'clock, for example). Either way, specify the location of a lesion or other findings by the distance in centimeters from the nipple.

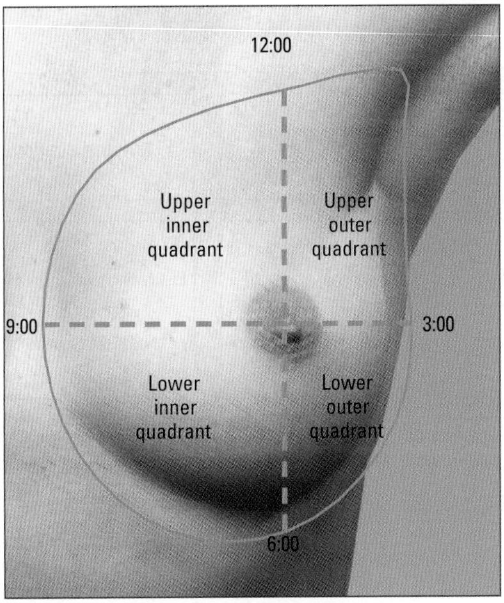
12:00
Upper inner quadrant
Upper outer quadrant
9:00
3:00
Lower inner quadrant
Lower outer quadrant
6:00

Documenting a breast lump

If you palpate a lump, record these characteristics:

- Size in centimeters
- Shape—round, discoid, regular, or irregular
- Consistency—soft, firm, or hard
- Mobility
- Degree of tenderness
- Location, using the quadrant or clock method.

Outside the norm

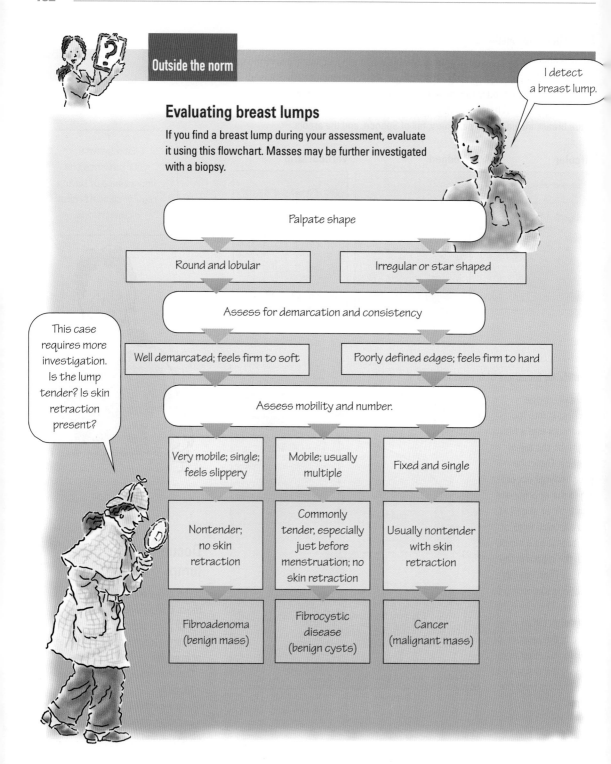
I detect
a breast lump.

Evaluating breast lumps

If you find a breast lump during your assessment, evaluate it using this flowchart. Masses may be further investigated with a biopsy.

Palpate shape

- Round and lobular
- Irregular or star shaped

Assess for demarcation and consistency

- Well demarcated; feels firm to soft
- Poorly defined edges; feels firm to hard

Assess mobility and number.

Very mobile; single; feels slippery	Mobile; usually multiple	Fixed and single
Nontender; no skin retraction	Commonly tender, especially just before menstruation; no skin retraction	Usually nontender with skin retraction
Fibroadenoma (benign mass)	Fibrocystic disease (benign cysts)	Cancer (malignant mass)

This case requires more investigation. Is the lump tender? Is skin retraction present?

Examining the axillae

Inspection

With the patient sitting or standing, inspect the skin of the axillae for rashes, infections, or unusual pigmentation.

Palpation

Ask the patient to relax the arm on the side you're examining. Support the elbow with one of your hands. Cup the fingers of your other hand, and reach high into the apex of the axilla. Place your fingers directly behind the pectoral muscles, pointing toward the midclavicle.

Assessing the axillary nodes

Palpate the central nodes by pressing your fingers downward and in toward the chest wall. You can usually palpate one or more of the nodes, which should be soft, small, and nontender. If you feel a hard, large, or tender lesion, try to palpate the other groups of lymph nodes for comparison.

Assessing the clavicular nodes

If the axillary nodes appear abnormal, assess the nodes in the clavicular area. To do this, have the patient relax the neck muscles by flexing the head slightly forward. Stand in front of the patient and hook your fingers over the clavicle beside the sternocleidomastoid muscle. Rotate your fingers deeply into this area to feel the supraclavicular nodes.

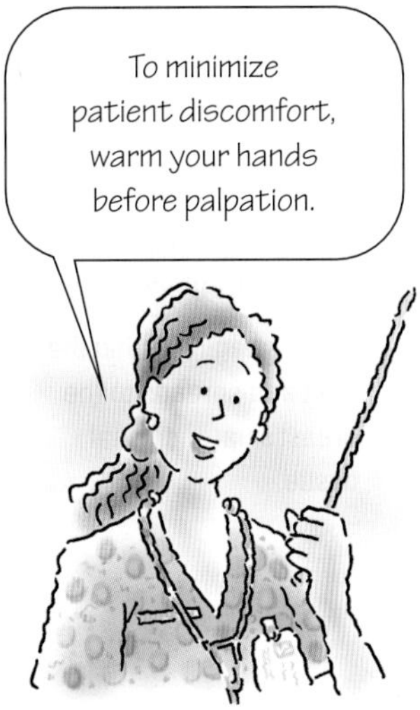
To minimize patient discomfort, warm your hands before palpation.

Skill check

Palpating the axilla

- Palpate the central nodes by pressing your fingers downward and in toward the chest wall, as shown.
- Palpate the pectoral and anterior nodes by grasping the anterior axillary fold between your thumb and fingers and palpating inside the borders of the pectoral muscles.
- Palpate the lateral nodes by pressing your fingers along the upper inner arm. Try to compress these nodes against the humerus.
- To palpate the subscapular or posterior nodes, stand behind the patient and press your fingers to feel the inside of the muscle of the posterior axillary fold.

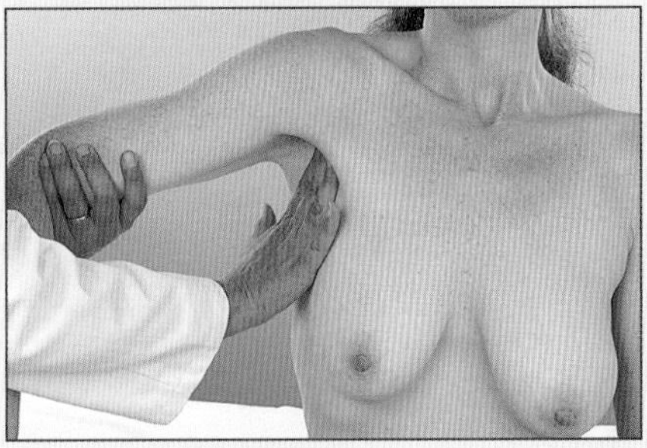

Abnormal findings

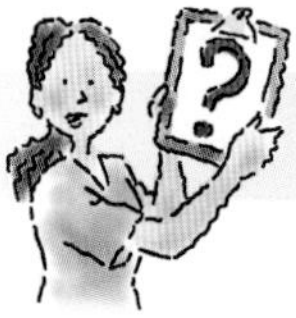

Outside the norm

Breast cancer mass

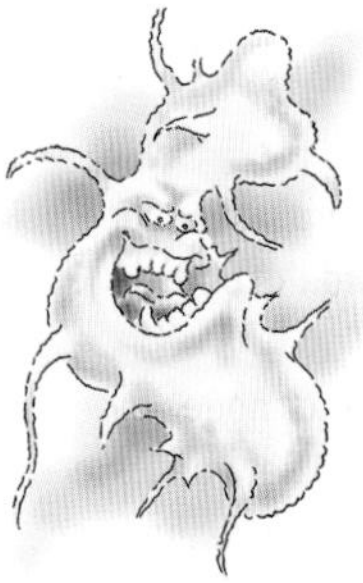

Breast cancer findings on palpation include an irregularly shaped mass with poorly defined edges. The mass is fixed, feels firm to hard, and is usually nontender. Evidence of skin retraction may be present.

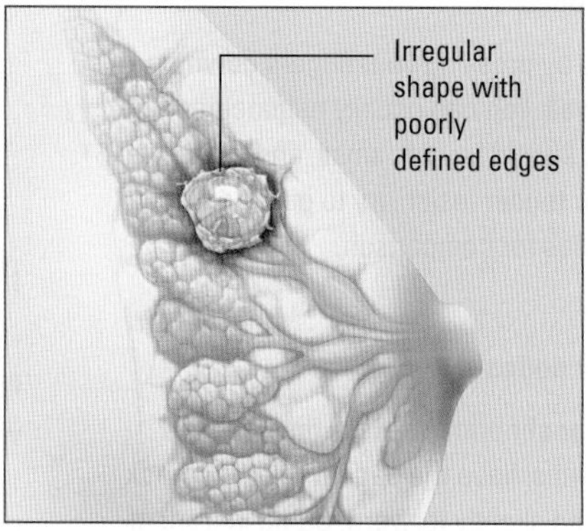
Irregular shape with poorly defined edges

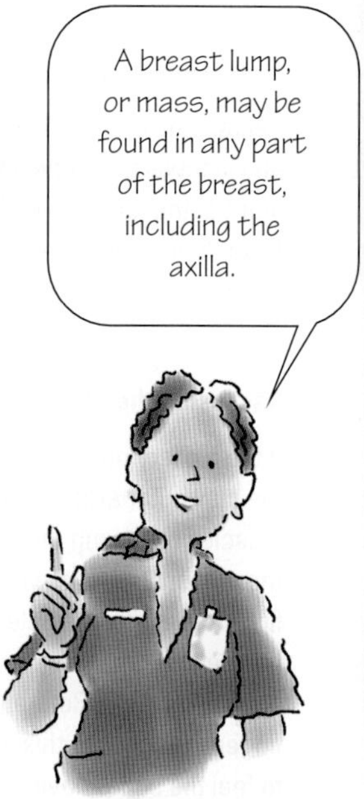
A breast lump, or mass, may be found in any part of the breast, including the axilla.

Ductal carcinoma in situ

Ductal carcinoma in situ is breast cancer in the earliest stage developing in the ducts.

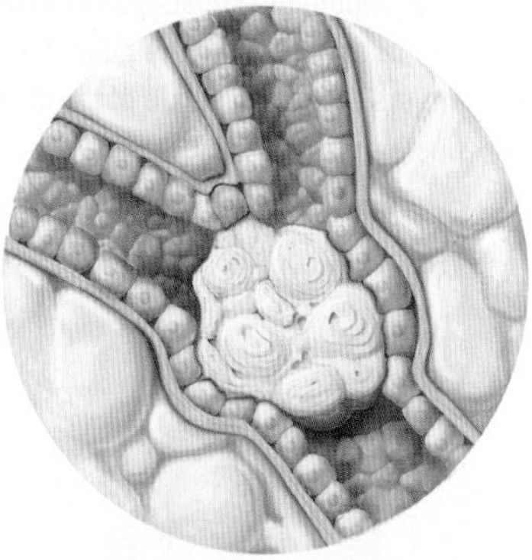

Infiltrating (invasive) ductal carcinoma

Cancer begins within the duct and spreads to the breast's parenchymal tissue.

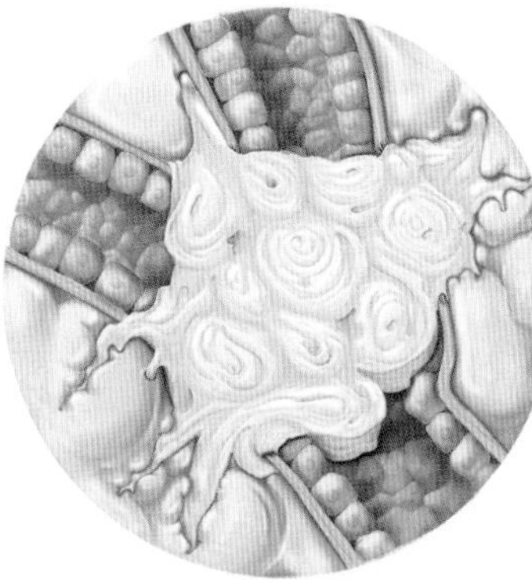

Dimpling

Breast dimpling—the puckering or retraction of skin on the breast—results from abnormal attachment of the skin to underlying tissue. It suggests an inflammatory or malignant mass beneath the skin surface and usually represents a late sign of breast cancer.

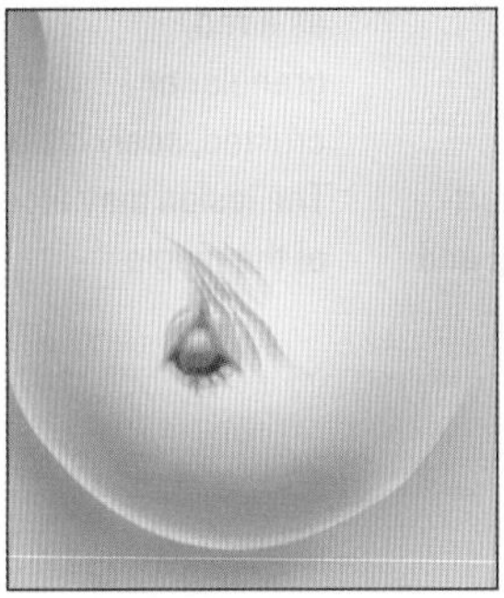

Fibrocystic changes

Fibrocystic changes (benign cysts) are round, elastic, mobile masses that are commonly tender on palpation, especially around menstruation. Multiple cysts may be present. Typically, there's no evidence of skin retraction.

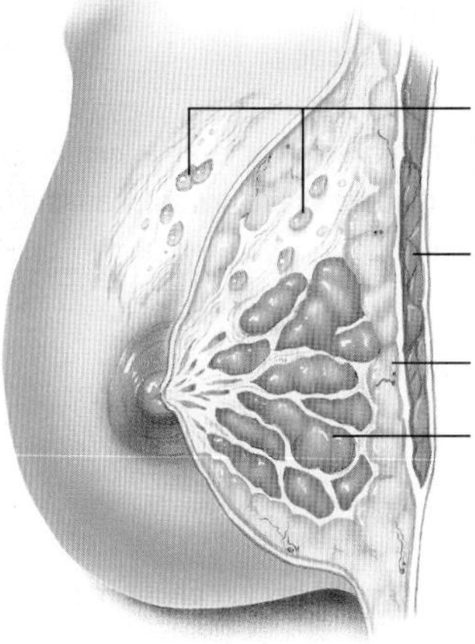
Dense fibrous tissue
Pectoralis muscle
Fat
Normal lobules

Peau d'orange

Usually a late sign of breast cancer, peau d'orange (orange peel skin) is the edematous thickening and pitting of breast skin. This sign can also occur with breast or axillary lymph node infection or Graves disease. Its striking orange peel appearance stems from lymphatic edema around deepened hair follicles.

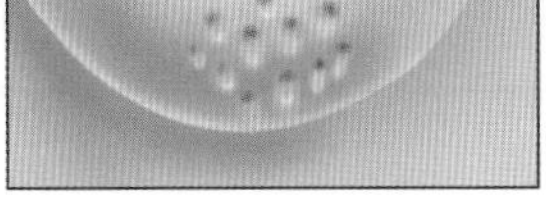

Fibroadenoma

A fibroadenoma is a benign, round, lobular, and well-demarcated mobile mass that feels slippery and firm to soft on palpation. It's usually nontender and causes no visible skin retraction.

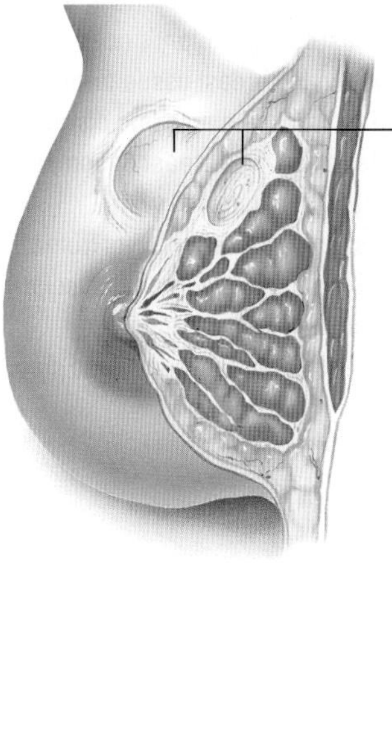
Rubbery, circumscribed, freely movable benign tumor

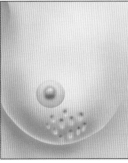

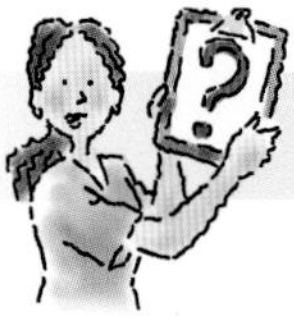

Outside the norm

Nipple retraction

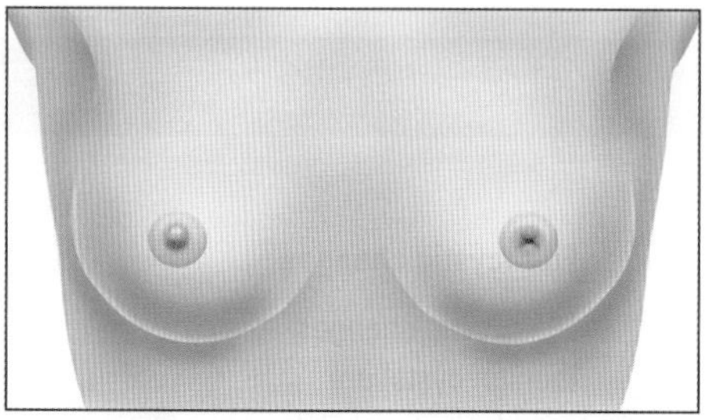

Nipple retraction, the inward displacement of the nipple below the level of surrounding breast tissue, that is not typical for the patient may indicate an inflammatory breast lesion or cancer. It results from scar tissue formation within a lesion or large mammary duct. As the scar tissue shortens, it pulls adjacent tissue inward, causing nipple deviation, flattening, and finally retraction.

Paget disease

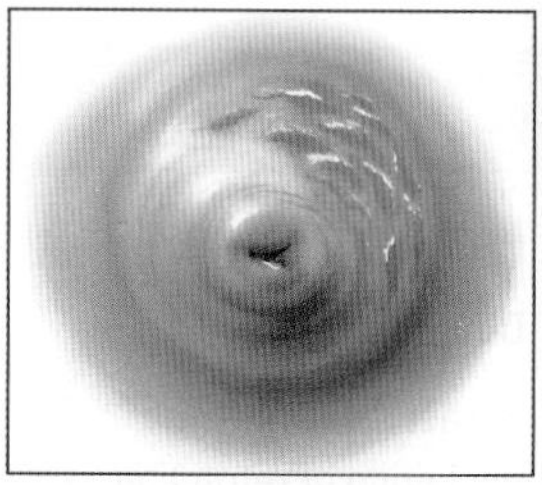

Paget disease is a rare form of breast cancer that usually starts as a red, granular or crusted, scaly lesion on the nipple or areola. The lesion may ulcerate and cause erosion of the nipple.

Mastitis and breast engorgement

Mastitis and breast engorgement are disorders that affect lactating females. Mastitis develops when a pathogen in the breast-feeding infant's nose or pharynx invades breast tissue through a fissured or cracked nipple and disrupts normal lactation. The breast becomes tender, hard, swollen, and warm.

Breast engorgement results from venous and lymphatic stasis and alveolar milk accumulation and causes painful breasts that feel heavy and may feel warm.

Mastitis

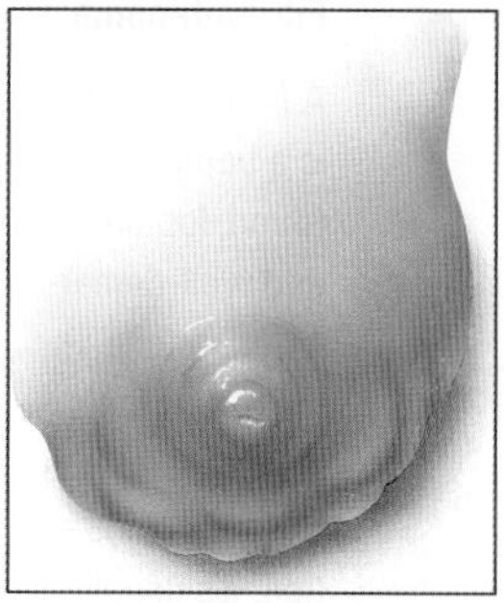

Engorgement

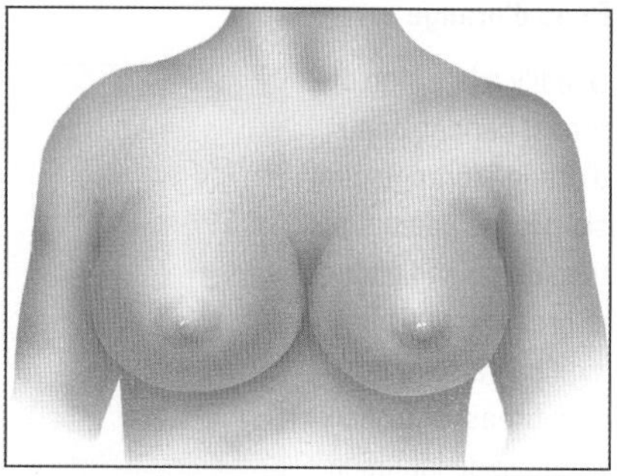

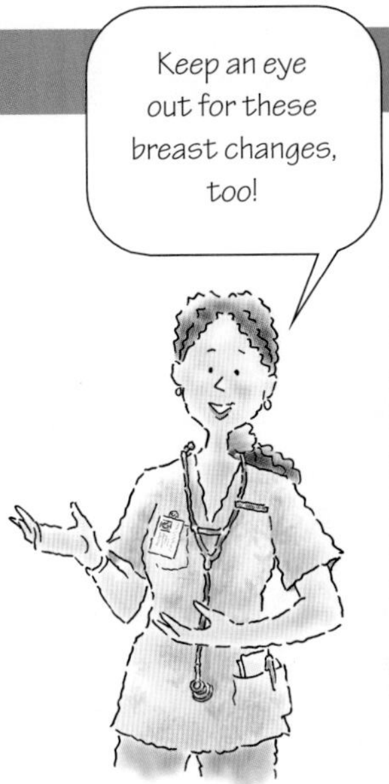
Keep an eye out for these breast changes, too!

Other breast abnormalities

Nipple discharge
Nipple discharge can occur spontaneously or can be elicited by nipple stimulation. It's characterized as intermittent or constant, as unilateral or bilateral, and by color, consistency, and composition. It can be a normal finding; however, nipple discharge can also signal serious underlying disease, particularly when accompanied by other breast changes. Significant causes include endocrine disorders, cancer, certain medications, and blocked lactiferous ducts.

Breast pain
Breast pain commonly results from benign breast disease, such as mastitis or fibrocystic changes. It may occur during rest or movement and may be aggravated by manipulation or palpation. Breast tenderness refers to pain elicited by physical contact.

Visible veins
Prominent veins in the breast may indicate cancer in some patients; however, they're considered normal in pregnant women because of engorgement.

Male breast concerns

Keep in mind that men also need clinical breast examinations and that the incidence of breast cancer in males is rising. Men with breast disorders may feel uneasy or embarrassed about being examined because they see their condition as being unmanly. Remember that a man needs a gentle, professional hand as much as a woman does.

Male breast cancer
Examine a man's breasts thoroughly during a complete physical assessment. Assess for the same changes you would in a woman. Breast cancer in men usually occurs in the areolar area.

Gynecomastia

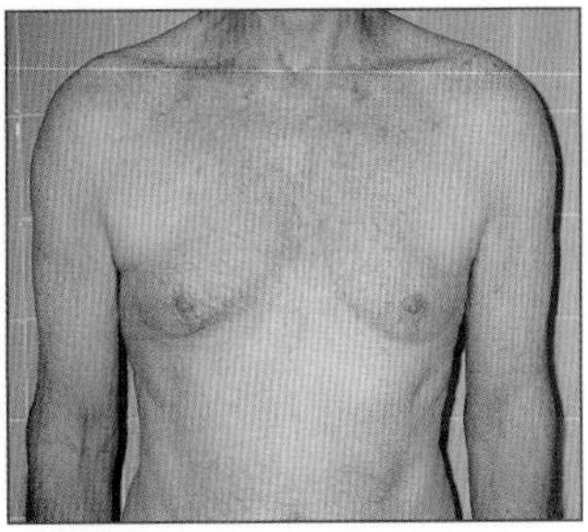

Gynecomastia (abnormal enlargement of the male breast) may be barely palpable and is usually bilateral. It can be caused by cirrhosis, leukemia, thyrotoxicosis, hormones, illicit drug use, certain medications, or alcohol consumption.

Understanding gynecomastia causes

Age-group	Description
Adolescent boys	• Temporary stimulation of breast tissue is caused by estrogen. • Adequate testosterone production usually ceases enlargement.
Elderly men	• Age-related hormonal alterations and certain medications can cause enlargement.

Q&A

Able to label?

Identify the skin structures indicated on this illustration.

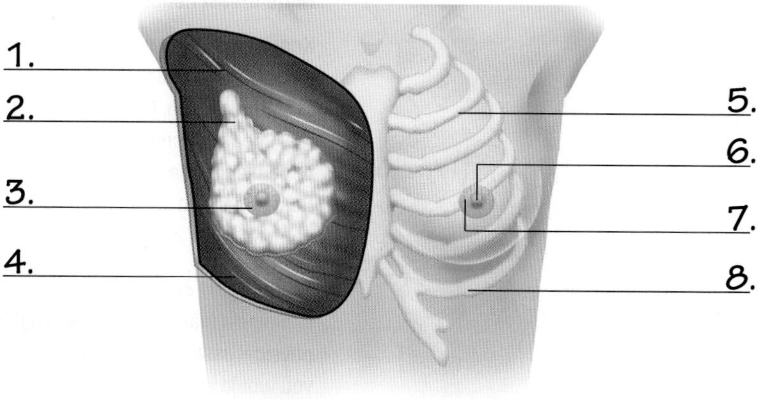
1.
2.
3.
4.
5.
6.
7.
8.

Matchmaker

Match the breast palpation technique shown with its correct name.

1. ____

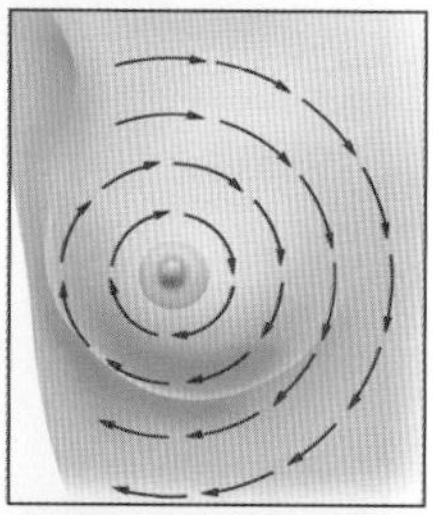

2. ____

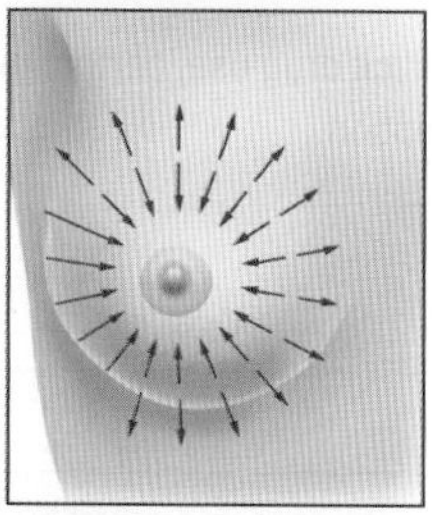

3. ____

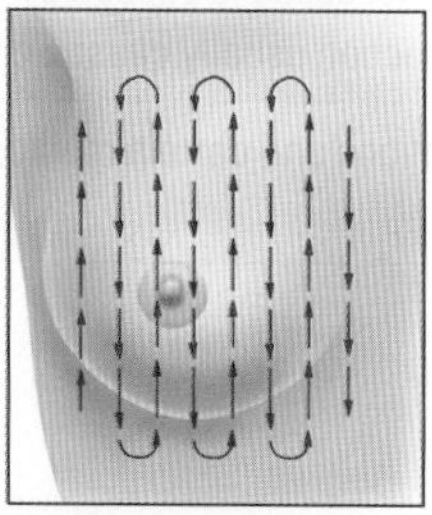

A. Wedged

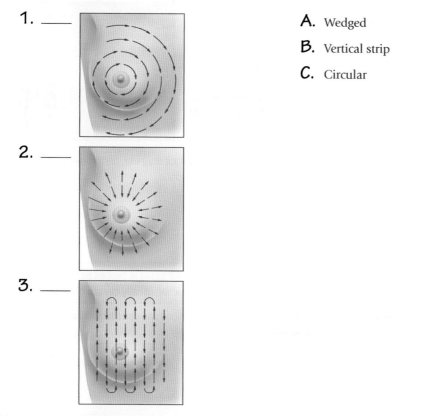

B. Vertical strip

C. Circular

Answers: Able to label? 1. Pectoralis major muscle, 2. Axillary tail of Spence, 3. Areola, 4. Serratus anterior muscle, 5. Second rib, 6. Nipple, 7. Montgomery tubercles, 8. Sixth rib; Matchmaker 1. C, 2. A, 3. B.

Selected References

American Cancer Society. (2015). *Breast awareness and self-exam*. Retrieved from http://www.cancer.org/cancer//breast-cancer/moreinformation/breastcancerearlydetection/breast-cancer-early-detection-acs-recs-bse

Hinkle, J. L., & Cheever, K. H. (2014). *Brunner and Suddarth's textbook of medical-surgical nursing* (13th ed.). Philadelphia, PA: Lippincott Williams & Wilkins.

Jensen, S. (2011). *Nursing health assessment: A best practice approach*. Philadelphia, PA: Lippincott Williams & Wilkins.

Taylor, C., Lillis, C., Lynn, P., & LeMone, P. (2015). *Fundamentals of nursing: The art and science of person-centered nursing care* (8th ed.). Philadelphia, PA: Lippincott Williams & Wilkins.

Weber, J. R., & Kelley, J. H. (2014). *Health assessment in nursing* (5th ed.). Philadelphia, PA: Lippincott Williams & Wilkins.

Chapter 8

Gastrointestinal system

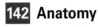

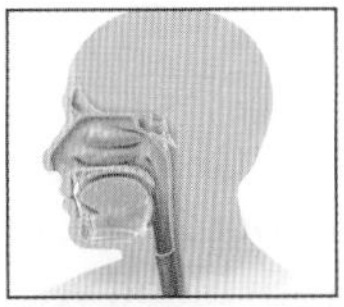
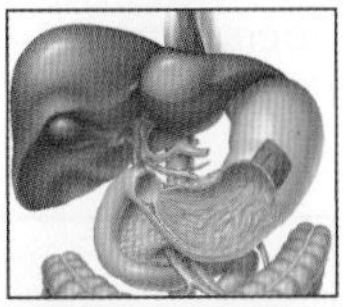
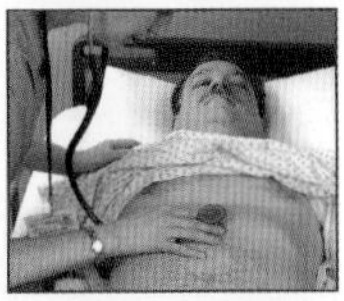
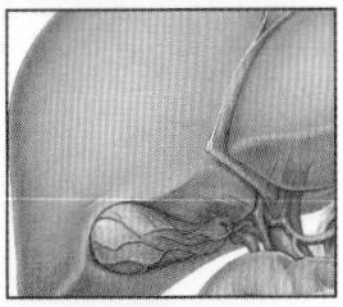
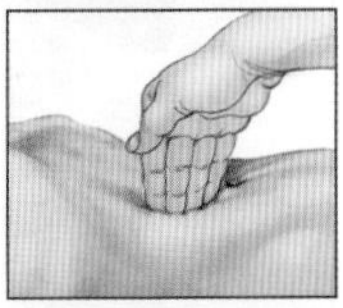
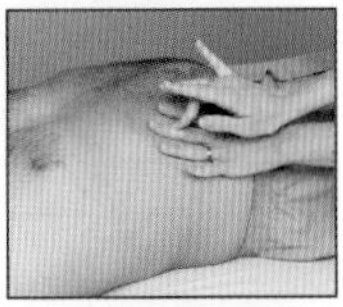
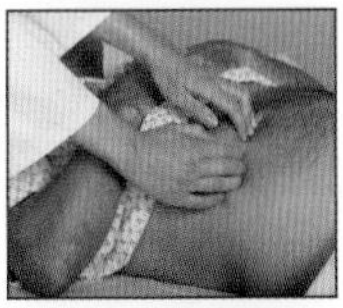
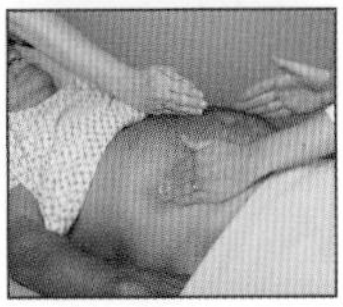
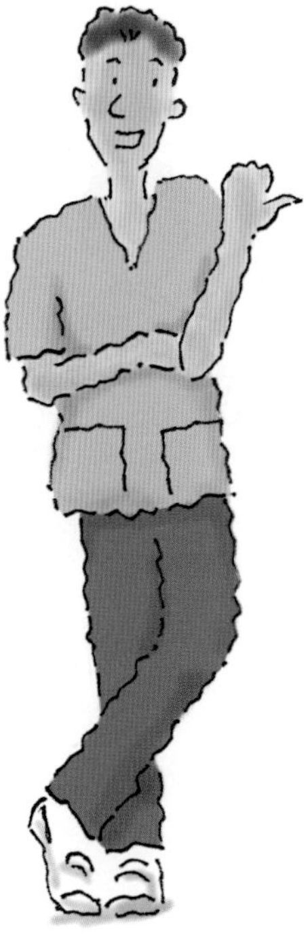

Anatomy

The GI tract is a hollow tube that begins at the mouth and ends at the anus. About 25′ (7.5 m) long, the GI tract consists of smooth muscle alternating with blood vessels and nerve tissue. Specialized circular and longitudinal fibers contract, causing peristalsis, which aids in propelling food through the GI tract.

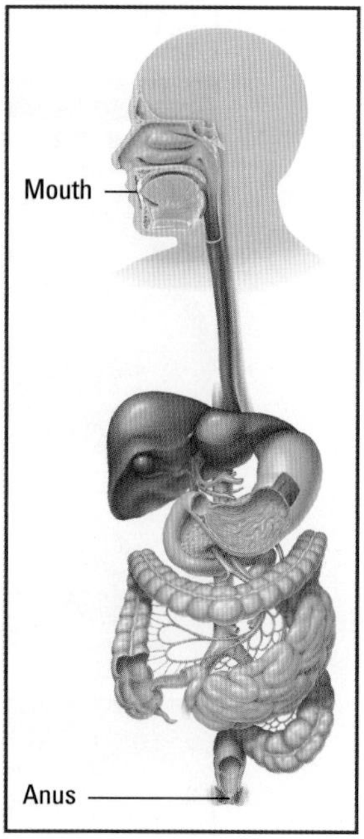
Mouth
Anus

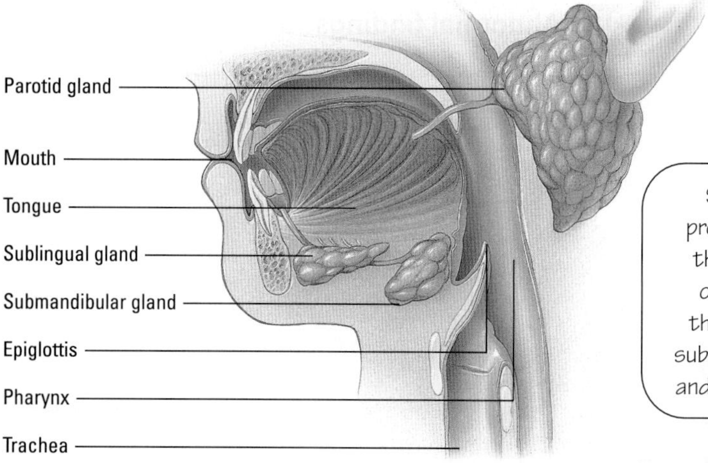
Parotid gland
Mouth
Tongue
Sublingual gland
Submandibular gland
Epiglottis
Pharynx
Trachea

Mouth
- Begins digestion through chewing, salivating, and swallowing

Tongue
- Provides sense of taste

Parotid, sublingual, and submandibular glands
- Produce saliva

Epiglottis
- Keeps food and fluid from being aspirated into the airway (trachea) by closing over the larynx when food is swallowed

Pharynx
- Consists of the nasopharynx, oropharynx, and laryngopharynx
- Allows the passage of food from the mouth to the esophagus
- Assists in swallowing
- Secretes mucus, which aids digestion

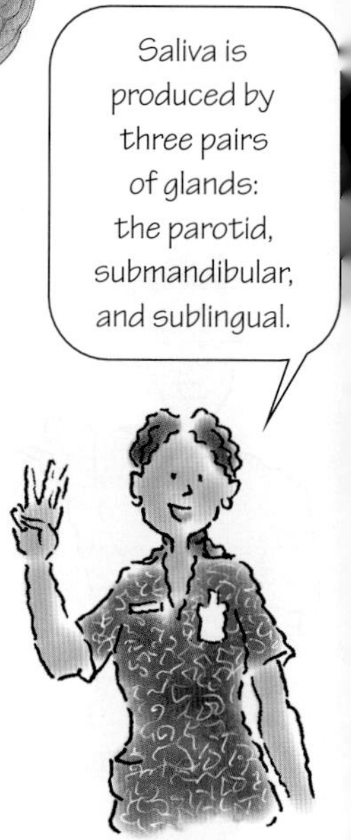
Saliva is produced by three pairs of glands: the parotid, submandibular, and sublingual.

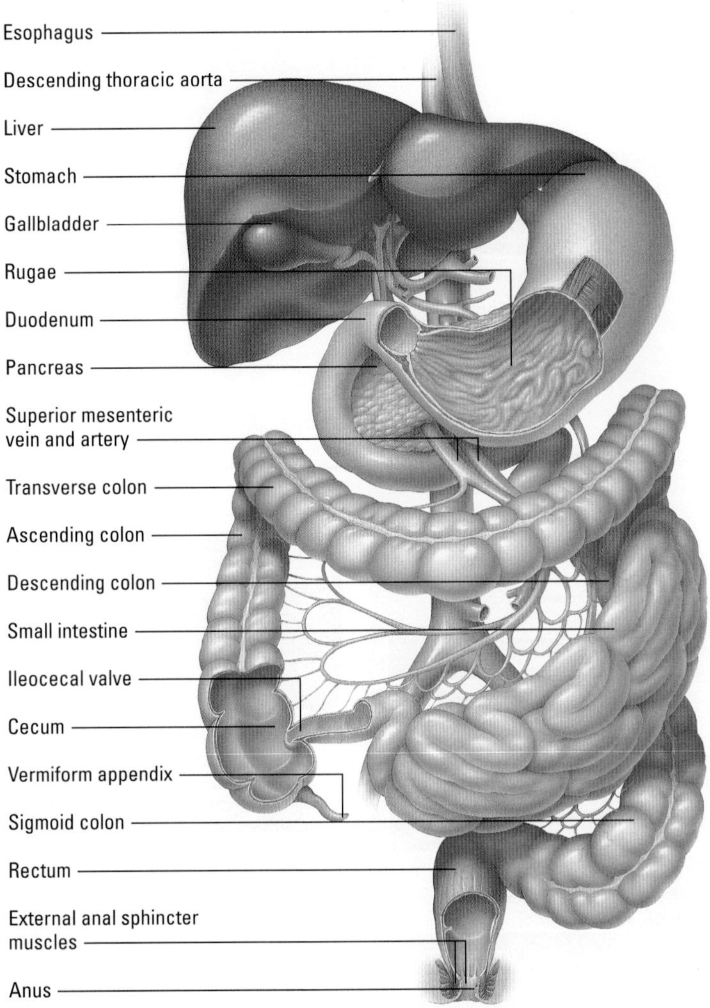
Esophagus
Descending thoracic aorta
Liver
Stomach
Gallbladder
Rugae
Duodenum
Pancreas
Superior mesenteric vein and artery
Transverse colon
Ascending colon
Descending colon
Small intestine
Ileocecal valve
Cecum
Vermiform appendix
Sigmoid colon
Rectum
External anal sphincter muscles
Anus

Esophagus

- Hollow, muscular tube that's approximately 10″ (25.5 cm) long
- Moves food from the pharynx to the stomach using peristalsis

Stomach

- Dilated, saclike structure that lies obliquely in the left upper quadrant
- Contains two important sphincters: the cardiac sphincter, which protects the entrance to the stomach, and the pyloric sphincter, which guards the exit
- Stores food and mixes it with gastric juices
- Passes chyme into the small intestine for further digestion and absorption

Rugae

- Accordion-like folds in the stomach lining
- Allow stomach to expand

Small intestine

- Consists of the duodenum, jejunum, and ileum
- Location of carbohydrate, fat, and protein breakdown
- Absorbs the end products of digestion

Vermiform appendix

- Finger-like projection that's attached to the cecum

Large intestine

- Consists of the cecum; ascending, transverse, descending, and sigmoid colons; rectum; and anus
- Absorbs excess water and electrolytes
- Stores food residue
- Eliminates waste products in the form of feces

Esophagogastric junction

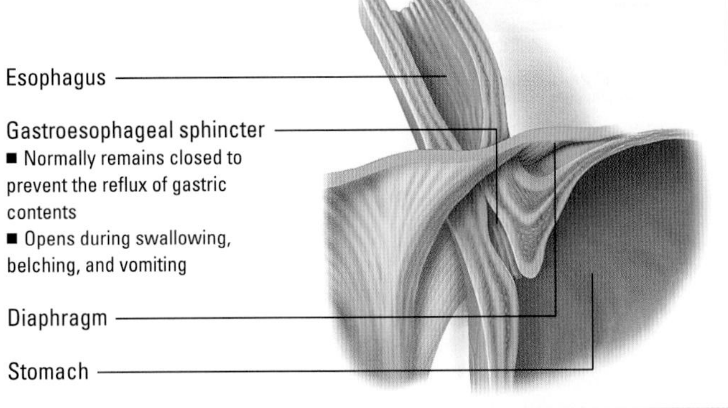
Esophagus
Gastroesophageal sphincter
■ Normally remains closed to prevent the reflux of gastric contents
■ Opens during swallowing, belching, and vomiting
Diaphragm
Stomach

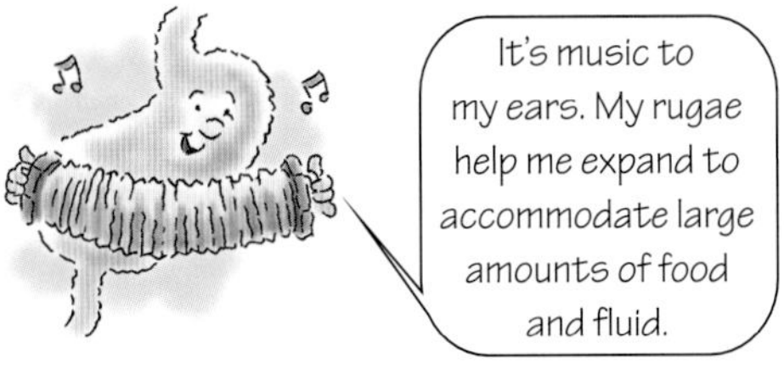
It's music to my ears. My rugae help me expand to accommodate large amounts of food and fluid.

A look at digestion

Digestion is the mechanical, chemical, and enzymatic process by which ingested food is broken down and converted into energy.

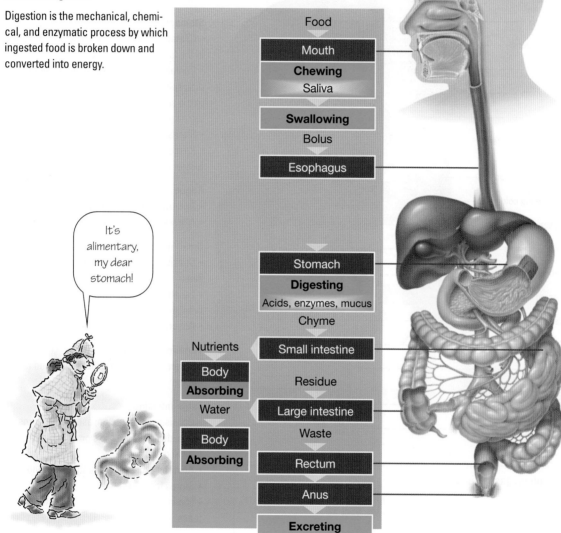

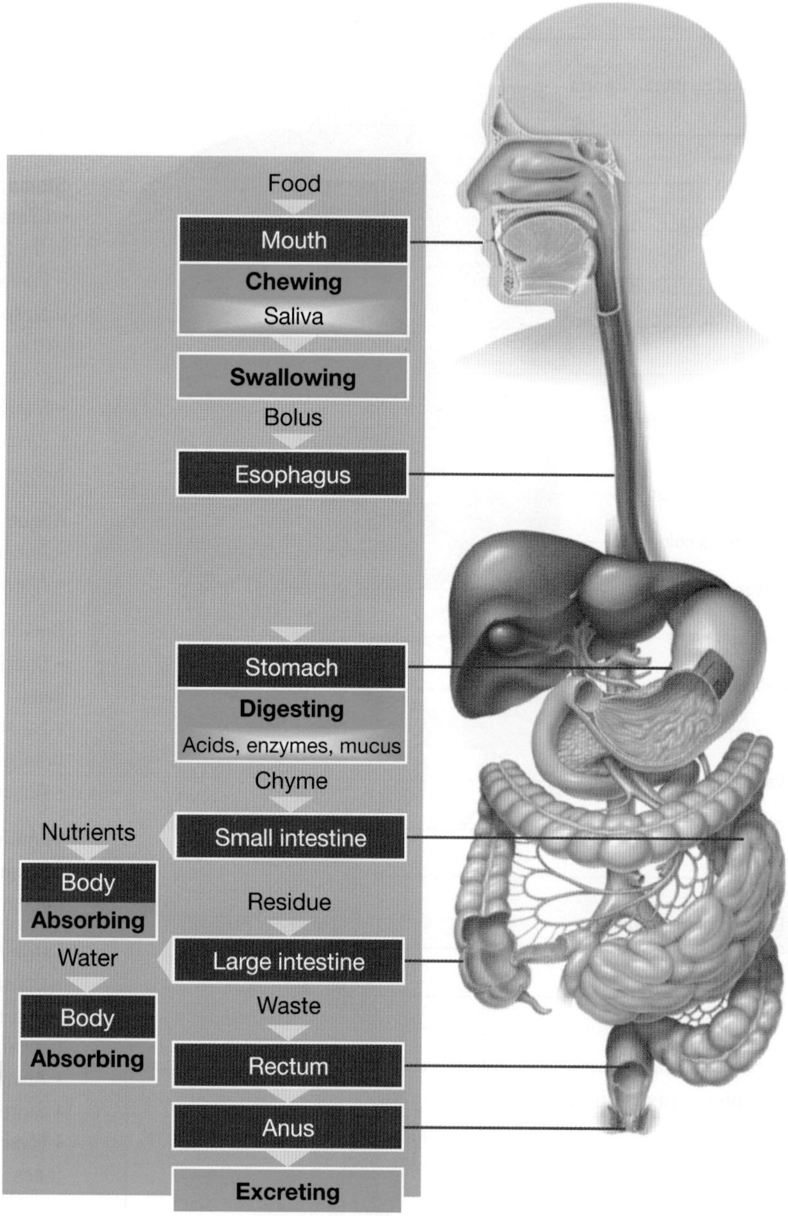
Food
Mouth
Chewing
Saliva
Swallowing
Bolus
Esophagus
Stomach
Digesting
Acids, enzymes, mucus
Chyme
Small intestine
Nutrients
Body
Absorbing
Residue
Large intestine
Water
Body
Absorbing
Waste
Rectum
Anus
Excreting

It's alimentary, my dear stomach!

Accessory GI organs and vessels

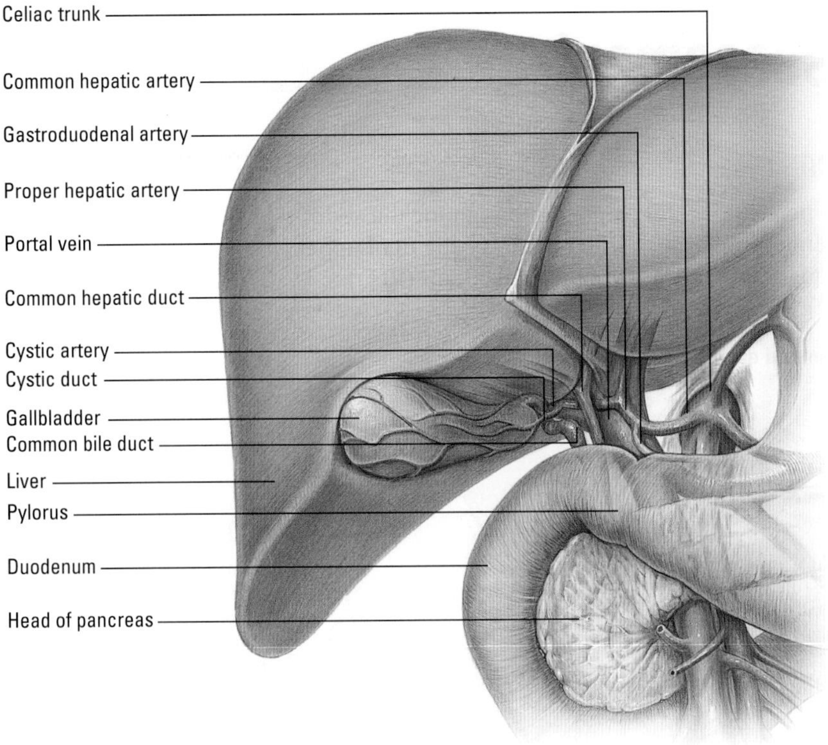

Celiac trunk
Common hepatic artery
Gastroduodenal artery
Proper hepatic artery
Portal vein
Common hepatic duct
Cystic artery
Cystic duct
Gallbladder
Common bile duct
Liver
Pylorus
Duodenum
Head of pancreas

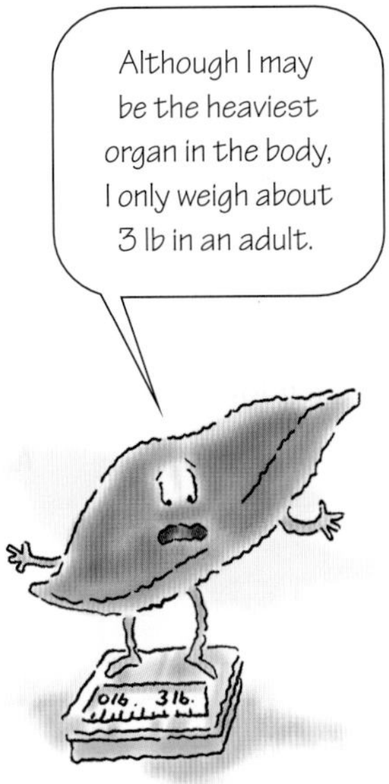

Although I may be the heaviest organ in the body, I only weigh about 3 lb in an adult.

Liver

- Metabolizes carbohydrates, fats, and proteins
- Detoxifies blood
- Converts ammonia to urea for excretion
- Synthesizes plasma proteins, nonessential amino acids, vitamins, and essential nutrients
- Secretes bile, a greenish fluid that helps digest fats and absorb fatty acids, cholesterol, and other lipids and gives stools their color

Gallbladder

- Stores bile from the liver until the bile empties into the duodenum

Bile ducts

- Hepatic ducts: drain bile from the liver
- Cystic duct: drains bile from the gallbladder
- Common bile duct: receives bile from the hepatic and cystic ducts and empties bile into the duodenum

Pancreas

- Measures 6″ to 8″ (15 to 20.5 cm) in length
- Consists of a head, body, and tail
- Releases insulin and glycogen into the bloodstream and produces enzymes that aid in digestion

Vessels

The abdominal aorta supplies blood to the GI tract. It enters the abdomen, separates into the common iliac arteries, and then branches into many arteries that extend the length of the GI tract. The gastric and splenic veins drain absorbed nutrients into the portal vein of the liver. After entering the liver, the venous blood circulates and then exits the liver through the hepatic vein, emptying into the inferior vena cava.

Assessment

Assessing the abdomen

Use inspection, auscultation, percussion, and palpation to examine the abdomen. Begin by mentally dividing the abdomen into four areas: the right upper quadrant (RUQ), left upper quadrant (LUQ), right lower quadrant (RLQ), and left lower quadrant (LLQ).

Abdominal quadrants and their structures

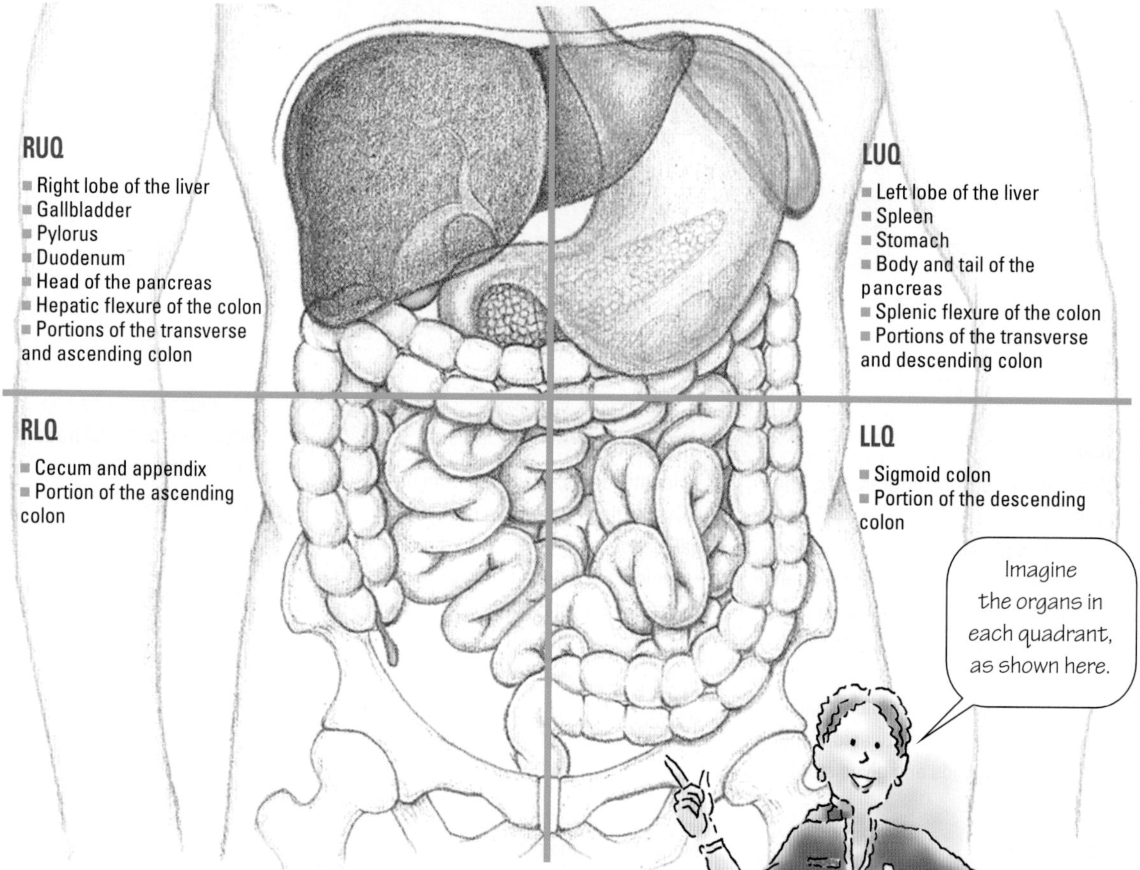
RUQ
Right lobe of the liver
Gallbladder
Pylorus
Duodenum
Head of the pancreas
Hepatic flexure of the colon
Portions of the transverse and ascending colon
LUQ
Left lobe of the liver
Spleen
Stomach
Body and tail of the pancreas
Splenic flexure of the colon
Portions of the transverse and descending colon
RLQ
Cecum and appendix
Portion of the ascending colon
LLQ
Sigmoid colon
Portion of the descending colon
Imagine the organs in each quadrant, as shown here.

Inspection

Observe the abdomen, checking for symmetry, bumps, bulges, or masses. Note the patient's abdominal shape and contour. Assess the umbilicus, which should be inverted and located in the abdominal midline.

Auscultation

Lightly place the diaphragm of your stethoscope in the RLQ, slightly below and to the right of the umbilicus. Auscultate in a clockwise fashion in each of the four quadrants. Note the character and quality of bowel sounds in each quadrant.

Skill check

Auscultating for vascular sounds

Auscultate the abdomen for vascular sounds with the bell of the stethoscope. Using firm pressure, listen over the aorta, as shown, as well as over the renal, iliac, and femoral arteries.

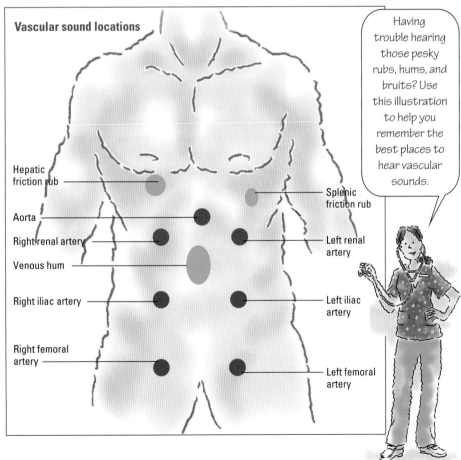

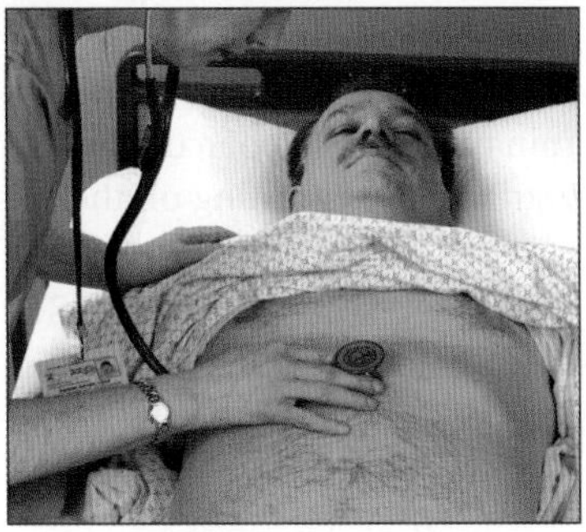

Vascular sound locations

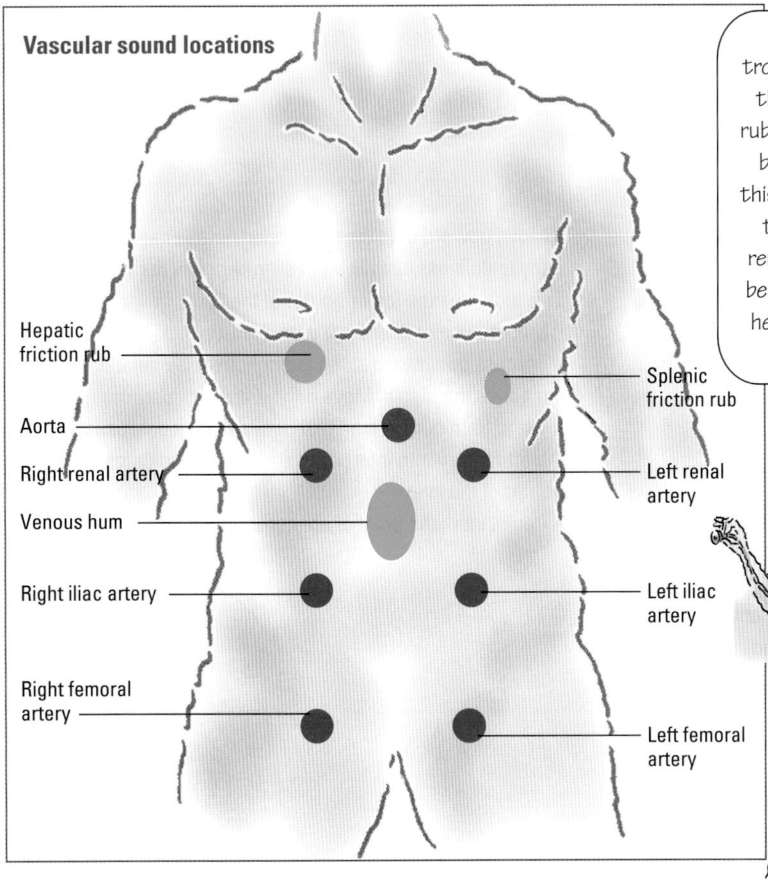
Hepatic friction rub
Splenic friction rub
Aorta
Right renal artery
Left renal artery
Venous hum
Right iliac artery
Left iliac artery
Right femoral artery
Left femoral artery

Having trouble hearing those pesky rubs, hums, and bruits? Use this illustration to help you remember the best places to hear vascular sounds.

What's all the bruit ha ha?

If the patient has hypertension or arterial stenosis, you may hear a bruit—a vascular sound similar to a heart murmur that is caused by turbulent blood flow through a narrowed artery. Occasionally, you may hear a bruit limited to systole in the epigastric region of a healthy person.

Percussion

Direct or indirect percussion is used to detect the size and location of abdominal organs and to detect air or fluid in the abdomen, stomach, or bowel. For direct percussion, strike your hand or finger directly against the patient's abdomen. For indirect percussion, use the middle finger of your dominant hand or a percussion hammer to strike a finger resting on the patient's abdomen. Begin percussion in the RLQ and proceed clockwise, covering all four quadrants. Note where percussed sounds change from tympany to dullness.

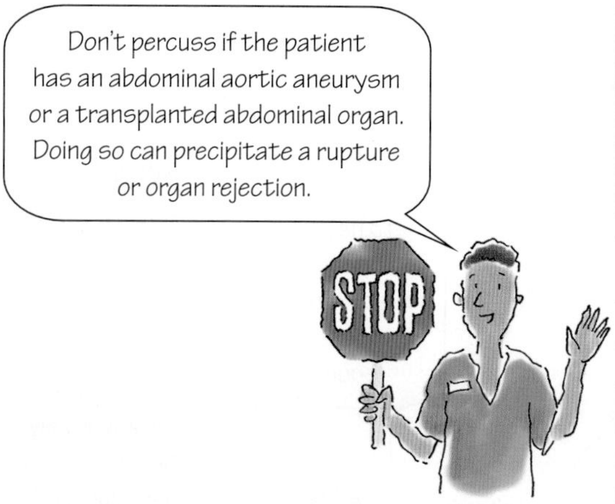
Don't percuss if the patient has an abdominal aortic aneurysm or a transplanted abdominal organ. Doing so can precipitate a rupture or organ rejection.
STOP

Drum and humdrum

Normally, two sounds can be heard during percussion of the abdomen: tympany and dullness. Tympany—a clear, hollow sound similar to a drum beating—occurs when you percuss over hollow organs such as an empty stomach or bowel. The degree of tympany depends on the amount of air present and gastric dilation.

When you percuss over solid organs, such as the liver, kidney, or feces-filled intestines, the sound changes to dullness.

Percussing and measuring the liver

Percussion of the liver can help you estimate its size.

Skill check

Percussing and measuring the liver

- Begin percussing the abdomen along the right midclavicular line, starting below the level of the umbilicus.

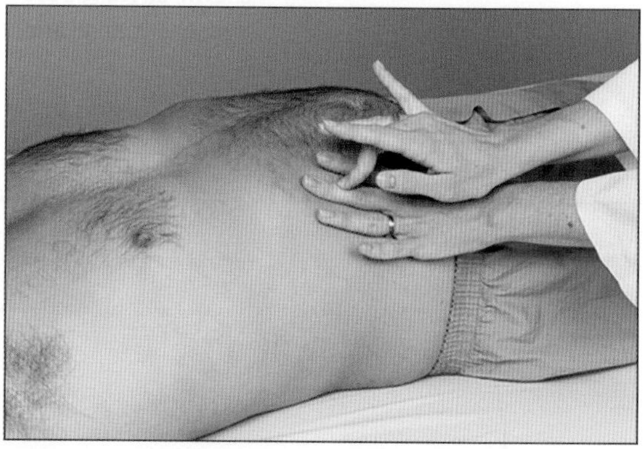

- Move upward until the percussion notes change from tympany to dullness, usually at or slightly below the costal margin. This indicates the lower border of the liver.
- Mark the point of change with a felt-tip pen.
- Percuss downward along the right midclavicular line, starting above the nipple. Move downward until percussion notes change from normal lung resonance to dullness, usually at the fifth to seventh intercostal space. This indicates the upper border of the liver.
- Again, mark the point of change with a felt-tip pen.

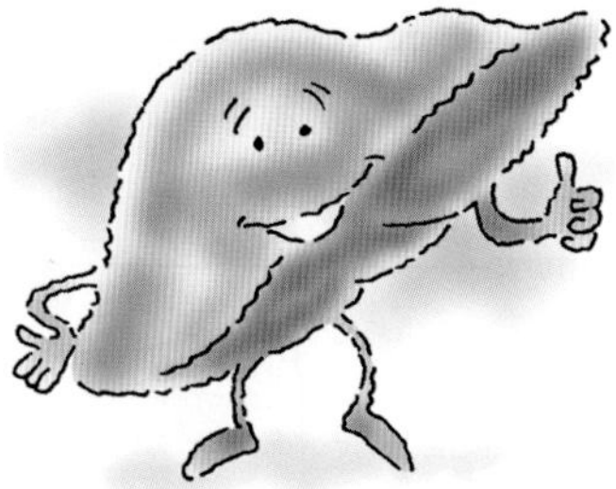

- Estimate the liver's size by measuring the distance between the two marks.
- In an adult, a normal liver span is 4 to 8 cm at the midsternal line and 6 to 12 cm at the right midclavicular line.

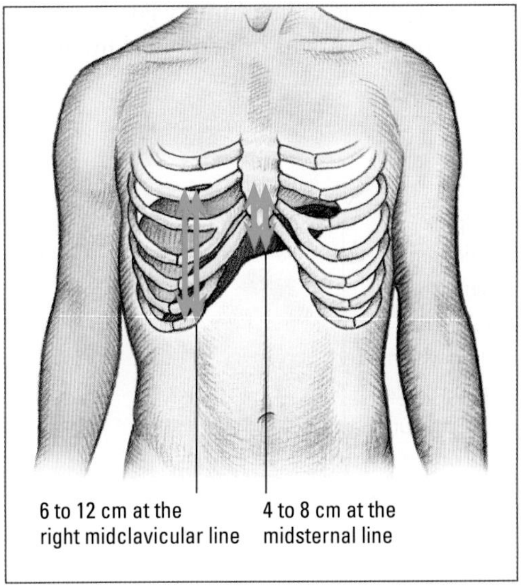
6 to 12 cm at the right midclavicular line
4 to 8 cm at the midsternal line

Percussing the spleen

The spleen is located at about the level of the 10th rib, in the left midaxillary line. Percussion may produce a small area of dullness, generally 7″ (17.8 cm) or less in adults. However, the spleen usually can't be percussed because tympany from the colon masks the dullness of the spleen.

Skill check

Percussing the spleen

- Percuss the lowest intercostal space in the left anterior axillary line; percussion notes should be tympanic.
- Ask the patient to take a deep breath, and then percuss this area again. If the spleen is normal in size, the area will remain tympanic. If the tympanic percussion note changes on inspiration to dullness, the spleen is probably enlarged.
- To estimate spleen size, outline the spleen's edges by percussing in several directions from areas of tympany to areas of dullness.

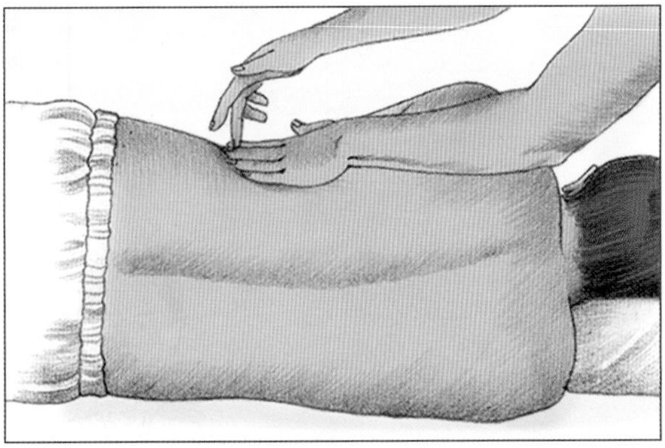

Palpation

To perform light palpation

- Put the fingers of one hand close together.
- Depress the skin about ½″ (1.5 cm) with the palmar surface of your fingers, and make gentle, rotating movements. Avoid short, quick jabs.

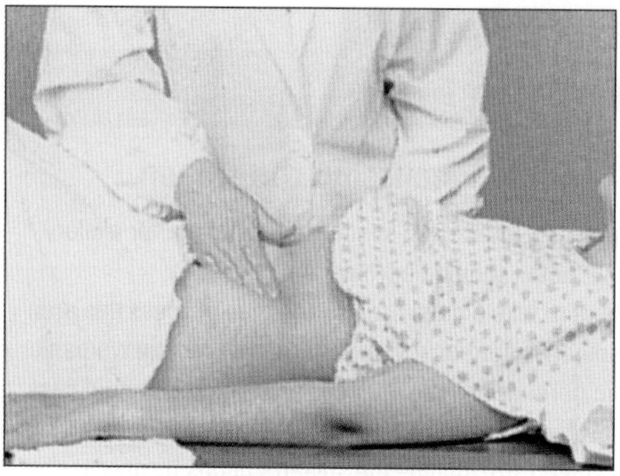

To perform deep palpation

- Push the abdomen down 2″ to 3″ (5 to 7.5 cm); in an obese patient, put one hand on top of the other and push.
- Palpate the entire abdomen in a clockwise direction, checking for tenderness, pulsations, organ enlargement, and masses.

The abdomen should be soft and nontender. As you palpate the four quadrants, note organs, masses, areas of fluid accumulation, and areas of tenderness or increased resistance. Determine whether resistance is due to the patient's being cold, tense, or ticklish, or if it's due to involuntary guarding or rigidity from muscle spasms or peritoneal inflammation.

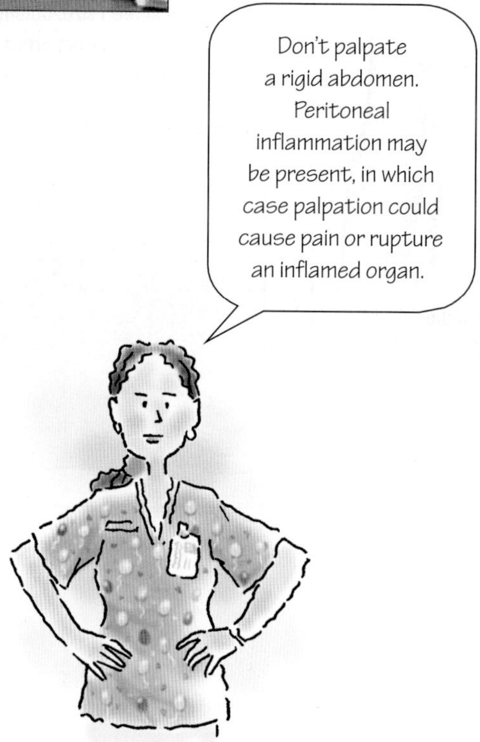
Don't palpate a rigid abdomen. Peritoneal inflammation may be present, in which case palpation could cause pain or rupture an inflamed organ.

Skill check

Palpating the liver

Palpate the patient's liver to check for enlargement and tenderness.

Method 1: Standard palpation

- Place the patient in the supine position. Standing at the patient's right side, place your left hand under the patient's back at the approximate location of the liver.
- Place your right hand slightly below the mark at the liver's upper border that you made during percussion. Point the fingers of your right hand toward the patient's head just under the right costal margin.
- As the patient inhales deeply, gently press in and up on the abdomen until the liver brushes under your right hand. The edge should be smooth, firm, and somewhat round. Note any tenderness.

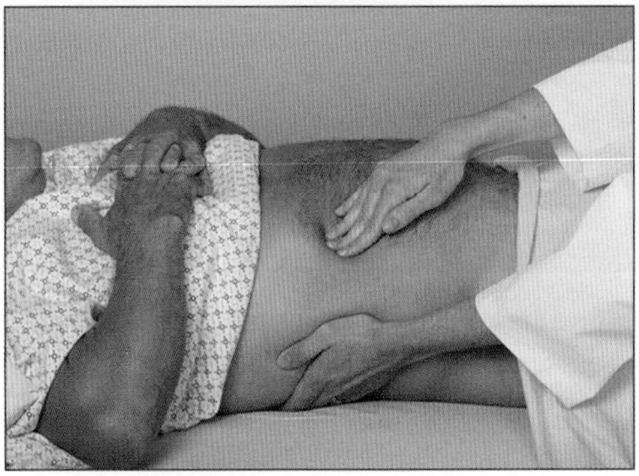

Method 2: Hooking the liver

- Stand next to the patient's right shoulder, facing the feet. Place your hands side by side, and hook your fingertips over the right costal margin, below the lower mark of dullness.
- Ask the patient to take a deep breath as you push your fingertips in and up. If the liver is palpable, you may feel its edge as it slides down in the abdomen as the patient breathes in.

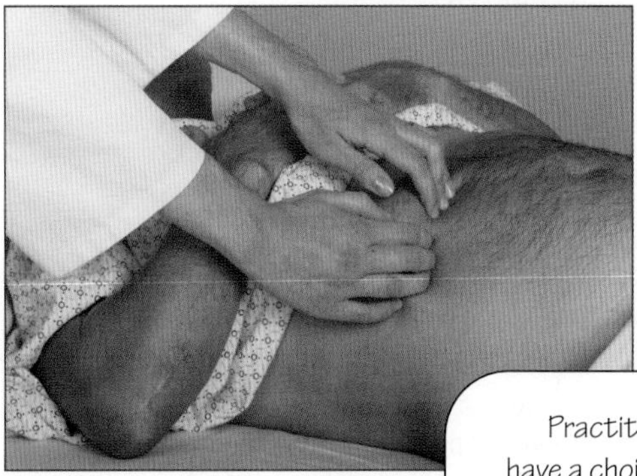

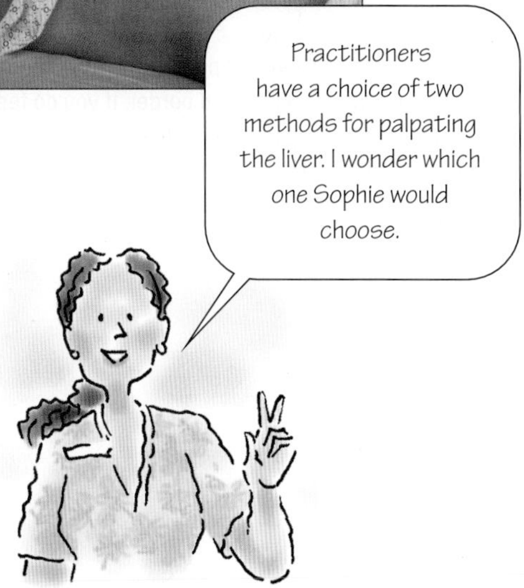
Practitioners have a choice of two methods for palpating the liver. I wonder which one Sophie would choose.

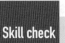

Skill check

Palpating the spleen

Palpate the spleen to detect tenderness and enlargement. Splenic tenderness may result from infections, which are common in a patient with an immunodeficiency disorder.

- With the patient in a supine position and you at the right side, reach across the patient and support the posterior lower left rib cage with your left hand.
- Place your right hand below the left costal margin and press inward.

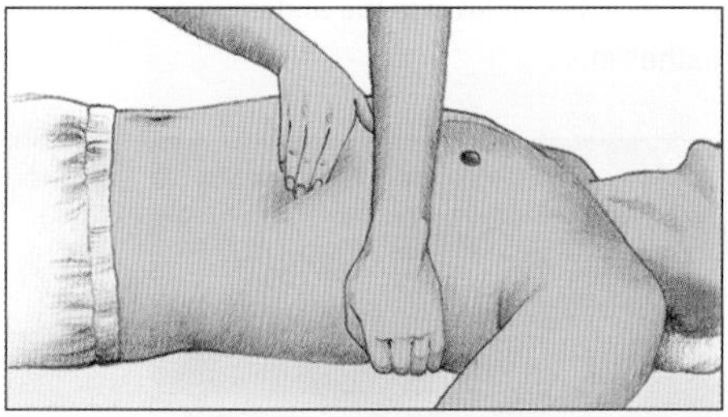

- Instruct the patient to take a deep breath. The spleen normally shouldn't descend on deep inspiration below the 9th or 10th intercostal space in the posterior midaxillary line.
- Normally, the spleen isn't palpable. If the spleen is enlarged, you'll feel its rigid border. If you do feel the spleen, stop palpating immediately because an enlarged spleen can easily rupture.

Special assessment techniques

Check for ascites, a large accumulation of fluid in the peritoneal cavity caused by advanced liver disease, heart failure, pancreatitis, or cancer.

Skill check

Checking for ascites

- Have an assistant place the ulnar edge of one hand firmly on the patient's abdomen at its midline.
- As you stand facing the patient's head, place the palm of your left hand against the patient's right flank, as shown below.

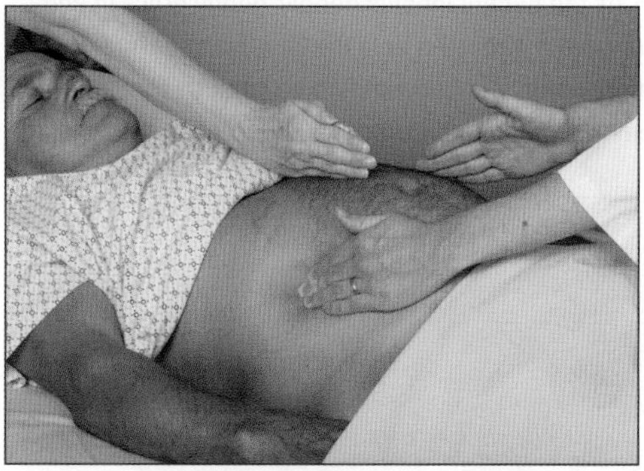

- Give the left abdomen a firm tap with your right hand. If ascites is present, you may see and feel a "fluid wave" ripple across the abdomen.
- If you detect ascites, use a tape measure to measure the fullest part of the abdomen. Mark this point on the patient's abdomen with a felt-tip pen so you'll be sure to measure it consistently. This measurement is important, especially if fluid removal or paracentesis is performed. If the patient is hospitalized, perform this measurement at the same time each day.

Then inspect and palpate the abdominal aorta.

Skill check

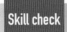

Assessing the abdominal aorta

- Inspect the abdomen for aortic pulsations, which may indicate an aortic aneurysm. Don't palpate a suspected aortic aneurysm because of the risk of rupture.
- If no visible pulsatile mass is visible, palpate the upper abdomen to the left of the midline for the aortic pulsation, as shown. Normally, the aortic pulsation is regular and moderately strong.
- In patients older than age 50, assess the width of the aorta by pressing firmly into the upper abdomen with one hand on each side of the aorta. The width of the normal aorta should be less than 1¼″ (3 cm).

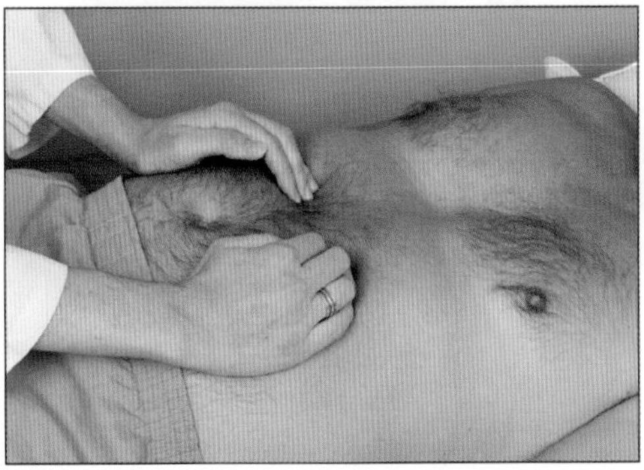

Perform the test for rebound tenderness and iliopsoas and obturator sign when you suspect peritoneal inflammation. Perform these assessment techniques at the end of your abdominal examination.

Eliciting rebound tenderness in children

Eliciting rebound tenderness in young children who can't verbalize how they feel may be difficult. Be alert for such clues as an anguished facial expression, a grimace, or intensified crying.

When attempting to assess this symptom, use techniques that elicit minimal tenderness. For example, have the child hop or jump to allow tissue to rebound gently while you watch closely for signs of pain. With this technique, the child won't associate the exacerbation of pain with your actions, and you may gain the child's cooperation.

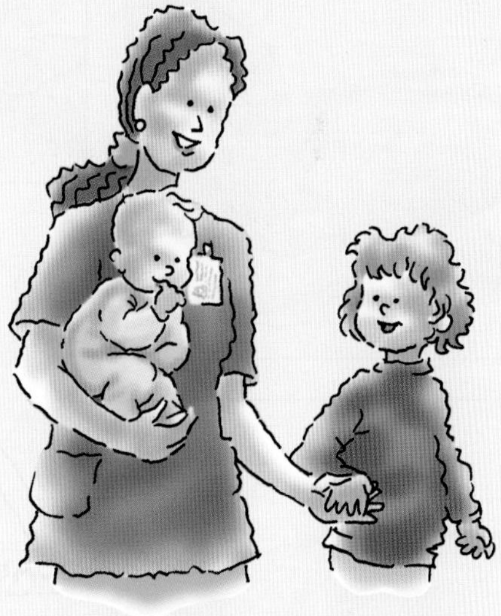

Skill check

Eliciting abdominal pain

Rebound tenderness and the iliopsoas and obturator signs can indicate such conditions as appendicitis and peritonitis.

Rebound tenderness

- Help the patient into a supine position with knees flexed to relax the abdominal muscles.
- Place your hands gently on the right lower quadrant at McBurney point (located about midway between the umbilicus and the anterior superior iliac spine).
- Slowly and deeply dip your fingers into the area; then release the pressure in a quick, smooth motion.
- Pain on release—rebound tenderness—is a positive sign. The pain may radiate to the umbilicus.

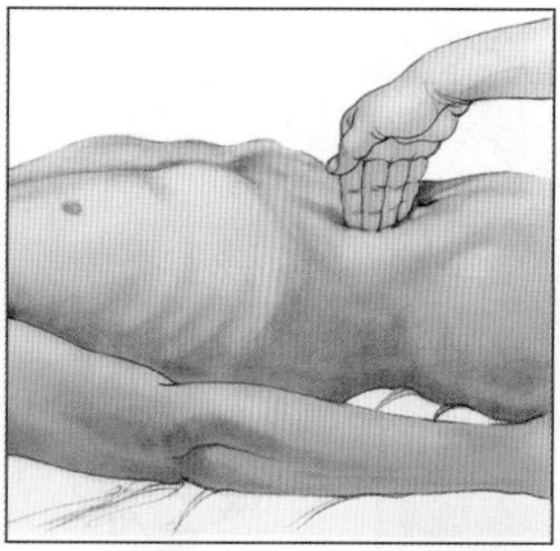

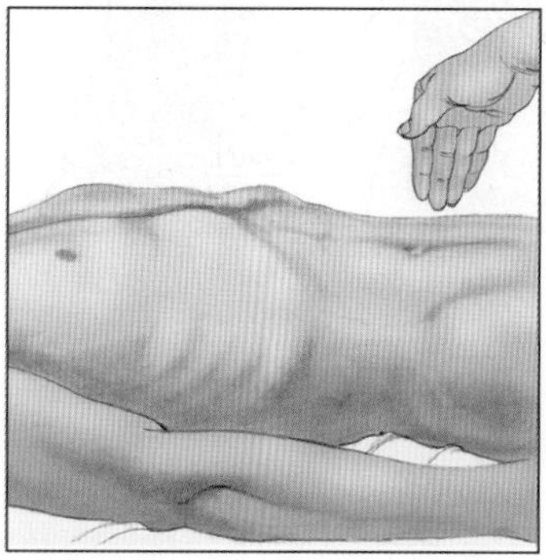

Iliopsoas sign

- Help the patient into a supine position with legs straight.
- Instruct the patient to raise the right leg upward as you exert slight downward pressure with your hand on the right thigh.
- Repeat the maneuver with the left leg.
- When testing either leg, increased abdominal pain is a positive result, indicating irritation of the psoas muscle.

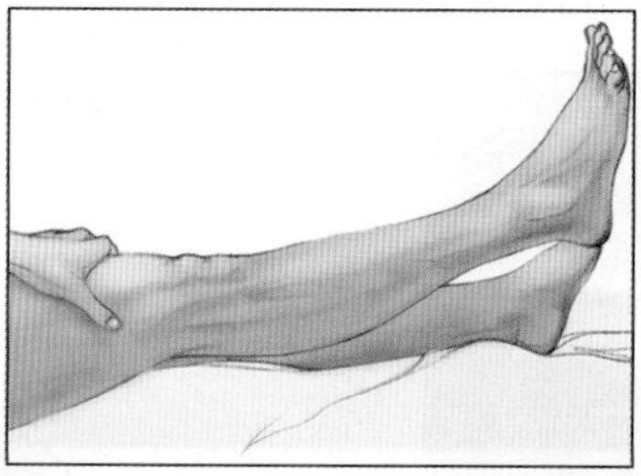

Obturator sign

- Help the patient into a supine position with the right leg flexed 90 degrees at the hip and knee.
- Hold the leg just above the knee and at the ankle; then rotate the leg laterally and medially.
- Pain in the hypogastric region is a positive sign, indicating irritation of the obturator muscle.

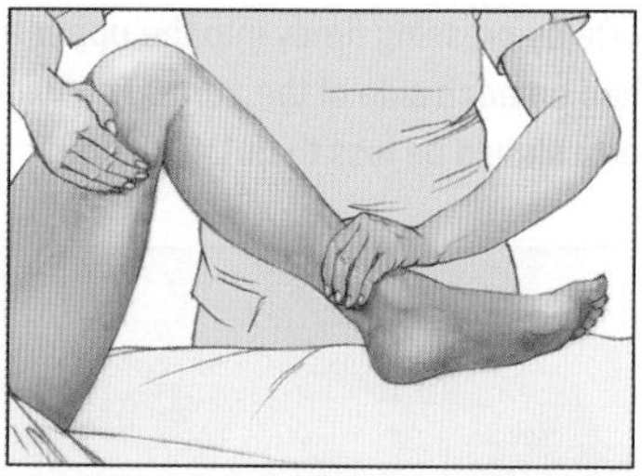

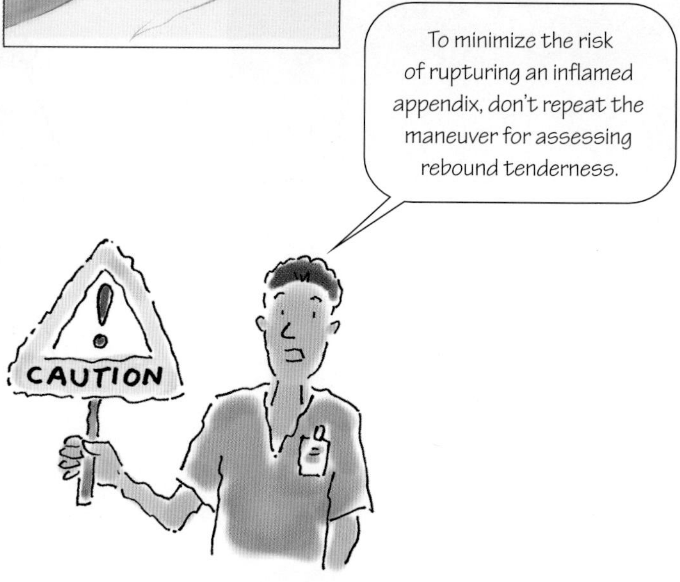
To minimize the risk of rupturing an inflamed appendix, don't repeat the maneuver for assessing rebound tenderness.
CAUTION

Examining the rectum and anus

If your patient is age 40 or older, perform a rectal examination as part of your GI assessment. Be sure to explain the procedure to the patient before you begin.

Inspection

Put on gloves and spread the buttocks to expose the anus and surrounding tissue. The skin in the perianal area is normally somewhat darker than that of the surrounding area. Check for fissures, lesions, scars, inflammation, discharge, rectal prolapse, skin tags, and external hemorrhoids. Then ask the patient to strain as if he or she is having a bowel movement. This action may reveal internal hemorrhoids, polyps, or fissures.

Palpation

Apply a water-soluble lubricant to your gloved index finger. Tell the patient to relax and warn the patient about a feeling of pressure during the exam. Ask the patient to bear down. As the sphincter opens, gently insert your finger into the rectum, toward the umbilicus. To palpate as much of the rectal wall as possible, rotate your finger clockwise and then counterclockwise. The rectal walls should feel soft and smooth, without masses, fecal impaction, or tenderness.

Remove your finger from the rectum, and inspect the glove for stool, blood, and mucus. Test fecal matter adhering to the glove for occult blood using a guaiac test.

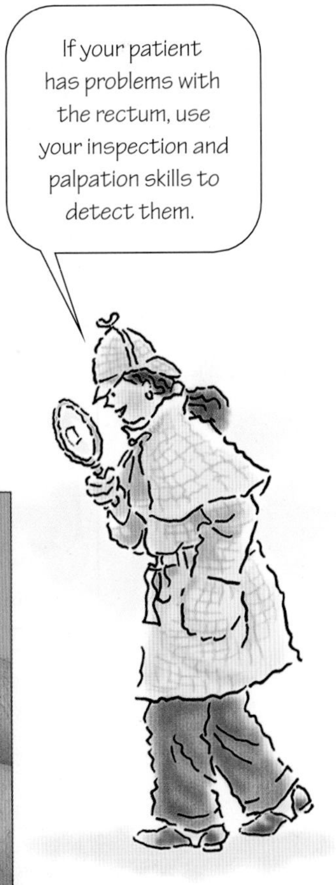
If your patient has problems with the rectum, use your inspection and palpation skills to detect them.

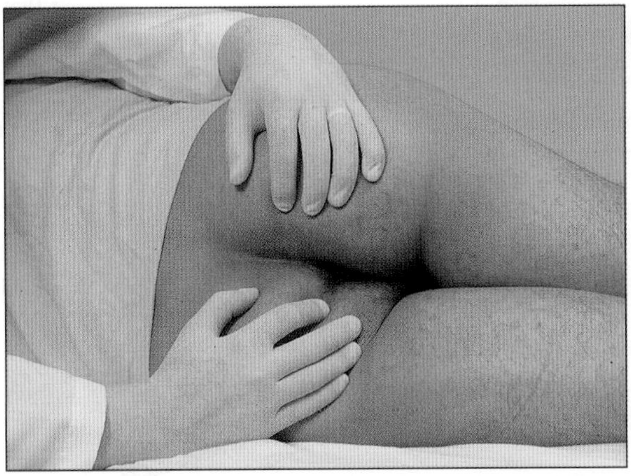

Abnormal findings

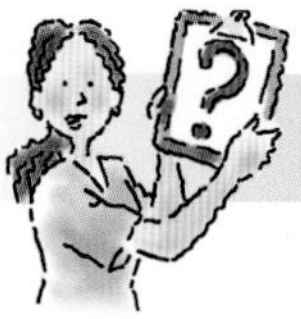

Outside the norm

Abdominal distention

Distention may result from gas, a tumor, or a colon filled with feces. It may also be caused by an incisional hernia, which may protrude when the patient lifts the head and shoulders.

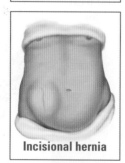

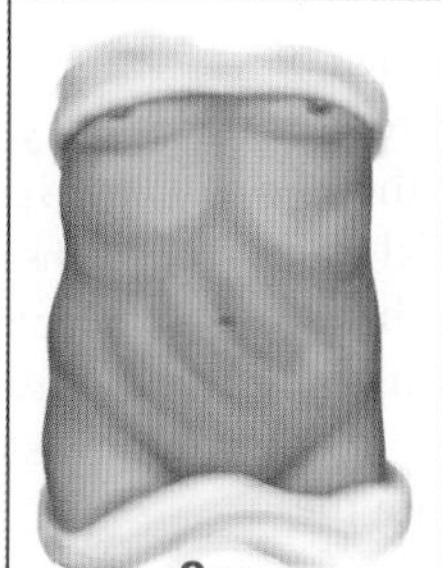

Gas

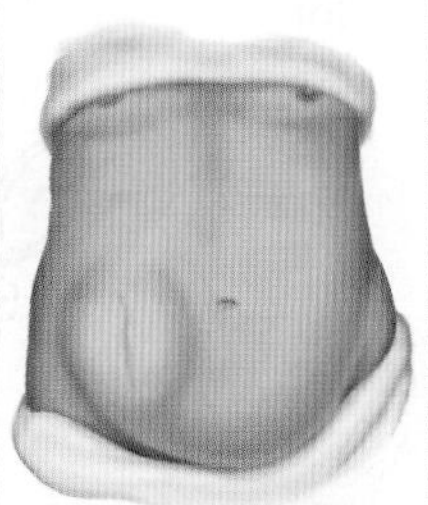

Incisional hernia

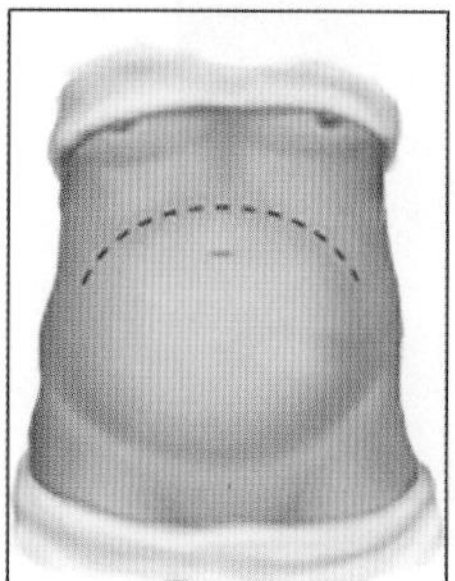

Tumor

Abdominal pain

Abdominal pain may indicate ulcers, intestinal obstruction, appendicitis, cholecystitis, peritonitis, or other inflammatory disorders. For example, a duodenal ulcer can cause gnawing abdominal pain in the midepigastrium 1½ to 3 hours after the patient has eaten.

If your patient complains of abdominal pain, ask the patient to describe the pain and when it started. As shown in the table below, the type of pain is a clue to its possible cause.

Type of abdominal pain	Possible cause
Burning	• Peptic ulcer • Gastroesophageal reflux disease
Cramping	• Biliary colic • Irritable bowel syndrome • Diarrhea • Constipation • Flatulence
Severe cramping	• Appendicitis • Crohn disease • Diverticulitis
Stabbing	• Pancreatitis • Cholecystitis

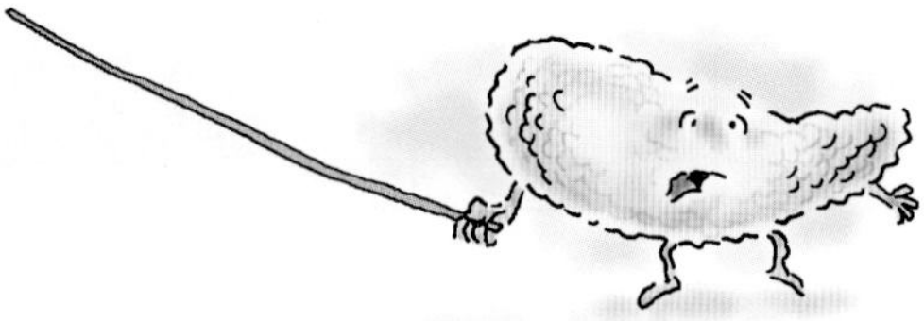

Abdominal pain origins

Affected organ	Visceral pain	Parietal pain	Referred pain
Stomach	Midepigastrium	Midepigastrium and left upper quadrant	Shoulders
Small intestine	Periumbilical area	Over affected site	Midback (rare)
Appendix	Periumbilical area	Right lower quadrant	Right lower quadrant
Proximal colon	Periumbilical area and right flank for ascending colon	Over affected site	Right lower quadrant and back (rare)
Distal colon	Hypogastrium and left flank for descending colon	Over affected site	Left lower quadrant and back (rare)
Gallbladder	Midepigastrium	Right upper quadrant	Right subscapular area
Ureters	Costovertebral angle	Over affected site	Groin; scrotum in men, labia in women (rare)
Pancreas	Midepigastrium and left upper quadrant	Midepigastrium and left upper quadrant	Back and left shoulder
Ovaries, fallopian tubes, and uterus	Hypogastrium and groin	Over affected site	Inner thighs

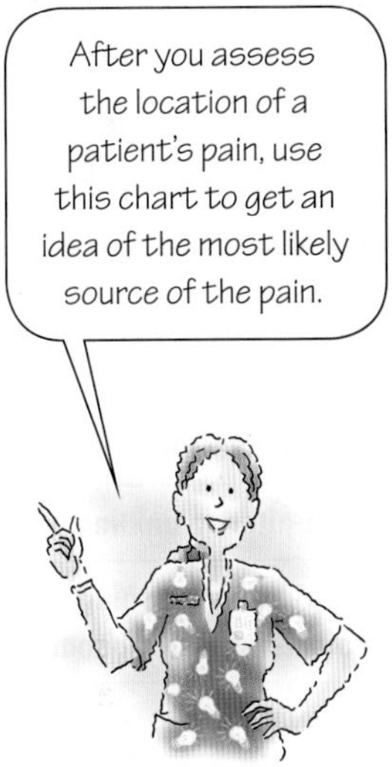
After you assess the location of a patient's pain, use this chart to get an idea of the most likely source of the pain.

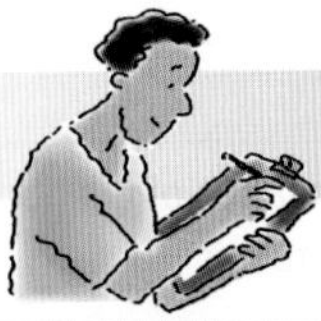

Take note

Documenting abdominal pain

2/19/2010	1345	Admitted to emergency department at 1330 c/o burning LUQ abdominal pain rated as 5 on 0 to 10 scale. Episode of vomiting x 1, approx. 200 ml of coffee-ground emesis. LUQ tenderness on palpation, no distention, no abdominal bruits. Bowels sounds heard in all four quadrants. Skin cool and dry, color pale, lips and nail beds pink. I.V. started in left hand with #16 gauge Angiocath and 1,000 ml D_5NSS infusing at 125 ml/hour. Lab work drawn. Patient's provider in room at 1335, and CT scan of the abdomen scheduled for 1400.
		Antoinette Stewart, RN

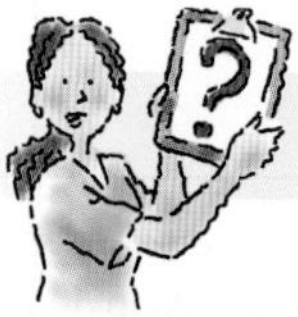

Outside the norm

Abnormal abdominal sounds

Sound and description	Location	Possible cause
Abnormal bowel sounds		
Hyperactive sounds (unrelated to hunger)	Any quadrant	Diarrhea, laxative use, or early intestinal obstruction
Hypoactive, then absent sounds	Any quadrant	Paralytic ileus or peritonitis
High-pitched tinkling sounds	Any quadrant	Intestinal fluid and air under tension in a dilated bowel
High-pitched rushing sounds coinciding with abdominal cramps	Any quadrant	Intestinal obstruction (life threatening)
Systolic bruits		
Vascular blowing sounds resembling cardiac murmurs	Over abdominal aorta	Partial arterial obstruction or turbulent blood flow
	Over renal artery	Renal artery stenosis
	Over iliac artery	Iliac artery stenosis
Venous hum		
Continuous, medium-pitched tone created by blood flow in a large engorged vascular organ such as the liver	Epigastric and umbilical regions	Increased collateral circulation between portal and systemic venous systems, such as in cirrhosis
Friction rub		
Harsh, grating sound like two pieces of sandpaper rubbing together	Over liver and spleen	Inflammation of the peritoneal surface of liver, such as from a tumor

Skin color changes

Areas of abdominal redness may indicate inflammation. Dilated, tortuous, visible abdominal veins may indicate inferior vena cava obstruction. Other changes include jaundice, icteric sclera, spider angiomas, Cullen sign, and Grey Turner sign.

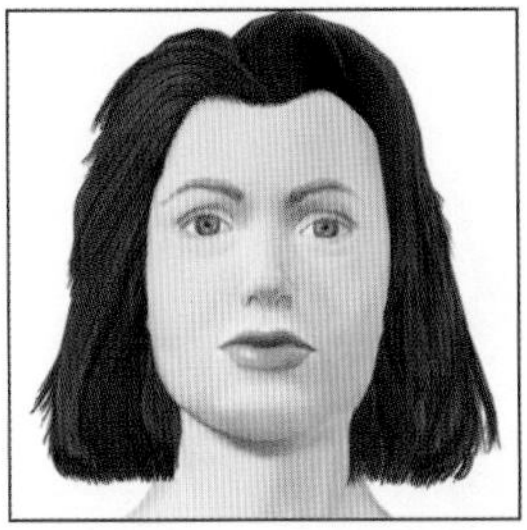

Jaundice
Yellowing of the skin indicates liver or biliary tract disease.

Spider angiomas
Cutaneous spider angiomas—areas of dilated capillaries or arterioles—may signal liver disease.

Cullen sign
Cullen sign, a bluish periumbilical discoloration, signals intra-abdominal hemorrhage. It may be seen in acute hemorrhagic pancreatitis, with massive hemorrhage after trauma.

Usually, Cullen sign appears gradually. Blood travels from a retroperitoneal organ or structure to the periumbilical area, where it diffuses through subcutaneous tissue. The extent of discoloration depends on the extent of bleeding. This sign may be difficult to detect in a dark-skinned person.

Grey Turner sign
Grey Turner sign (also known as *Turner sign*) is a bruiselike skin discoloration of the flank area. This sign typically appears 6 to 24 hours after the onset of retroperitoneal hemorrhage associated with acute pancreatitis.

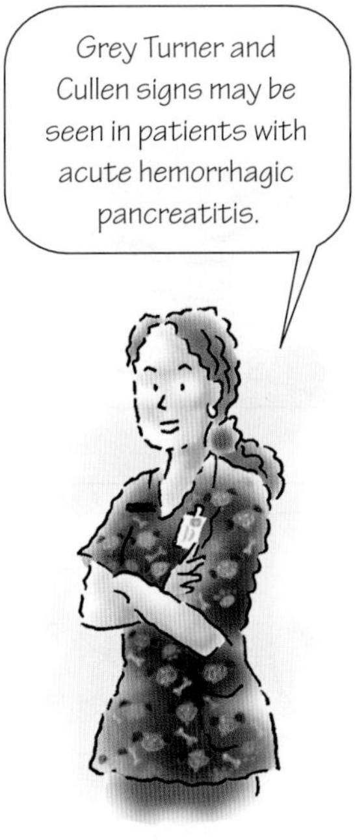
Grey Turner and Cullen signs may be seen in patients with acute hemorrhagic pancreatitis.

Other common GI abnormalities

Bloody stools
The passage of bloody stools, also known as *hematochezia,* usually indicates GI bleeding. It may also result from colorectal cancer, colitis, Crohn disease, or an anal fissure or hemorrhoids.

Constipation
Constipation can be caused by immobility, a sedentary lifestyle, and side effects of medications. The patient may complain of a dull ache in the abdomen, low back pain, rectal pressure, and a full abdominal feeling. A patient with complete intestinal obstruction will not pass flatus or stools and will not have bowel sounds below the obstruction. Constipation occurs more commonly in older patients.

Diarrhea
Diarrhea may be caused by toxins, medications, or a GI condition such as Crohn disease. Cramping, abdominal tenderness, anorexia, and hyperactive bowel sounds may accompany diarrhea. Bloody diarrhea may be a sign of ulcerative colitis or Crohn disease.

Dysphagia
Dysphagia, or difficulty swallowing, may be accompanied by weight loss. It can be caused by an obstruction, achalasia of the lower esophagogastric junction, or a neurologic disease, such as stroke or Parkinson disease. Dysphagia can lead to aspiration and pneumonia.

Nausea and vomiting
Usually occurring together, nausea and vomiting can be caused by existing illnesses, such as myocardial infarction, gastric and peritoneal irritation, appendicitis, bowel obstruction, cholecystitis, acute pancreatitis, bulimia nervosa, and neurologic disturbances, or by some medications.

Hepatomegaly
Hepatomegaly (enlargement of the liver) is commonly associated with hepatitis and other liver diseases.

Splenomegaly
Splenomegaly is enlargement of the spleen. Conditions that cause splenomegaly include mononucleosis, trauma, and illnesses that destroy red blood cells, such as sickle cell anemia and some cancers.

Q&A

Color my world

In the illustration shown, color the liver brown, the stomach pink, and the gallbladder green.

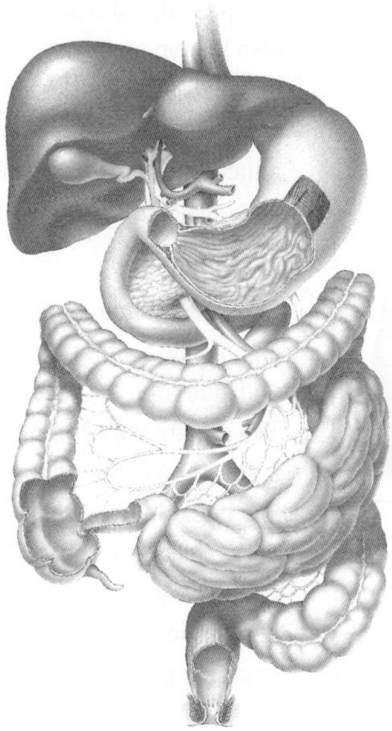

Matchmaker

Match each of the assessment techniques listed with the image that shows the best way to perform it.

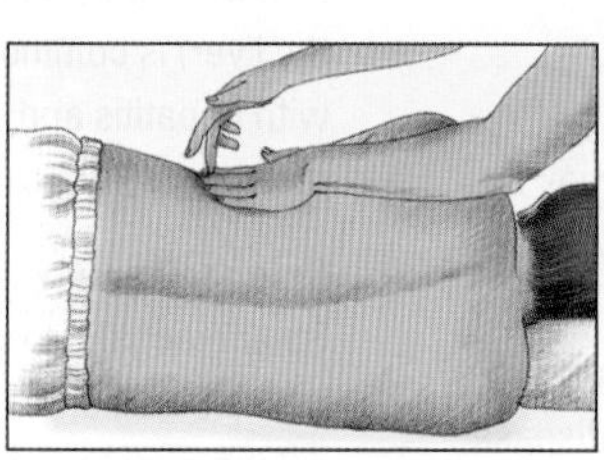

1. ______

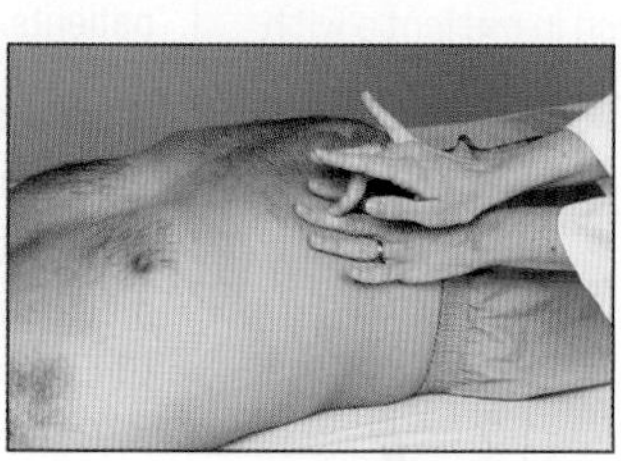

2. ______

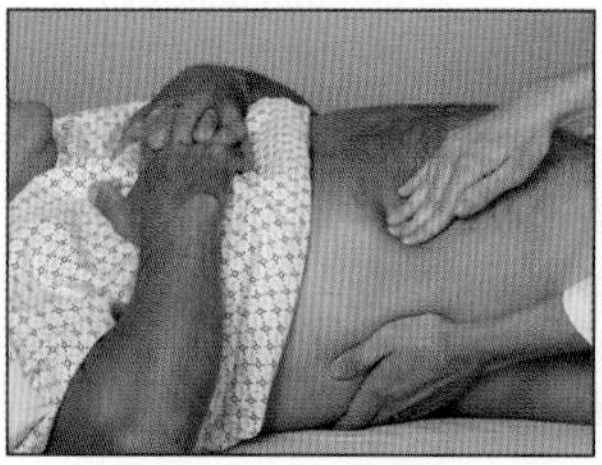

3. ______

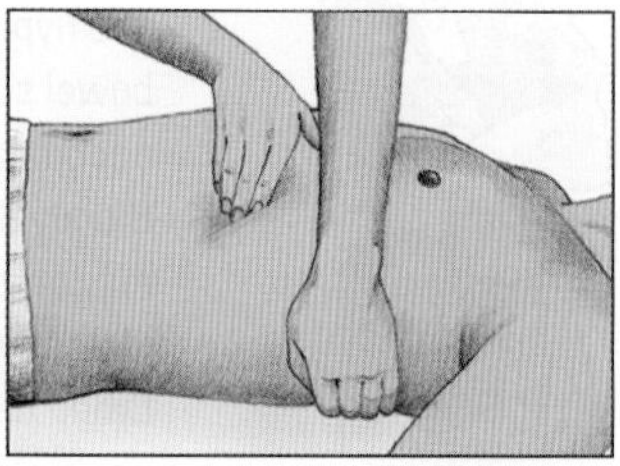

4. ______

A. Liver percussion

B. Liver palpation

C. Spleen percussion

D. Spleen palpation

Answers: Color my world See page 143; Matchmaker 1. C, 2. A, 3. B, 4. D.

Selected References

Bickley, L. (2012). *Bates guide to physical examination and history taking* (7th ed.). Philadelphia, PA: Lippincott Williams & Wilkins.

Buckius, M., McGrath, B., Monk, J., Grim, M., Bell, T., & Ahuja, B. (2012). Changing epidemiology of acute appendicitis in the United States: Study period 1993–2008. *Journal of Surgical Research, 175*(2), 185–190.

Gans, S., Pols, M., Stoker, J., & Boermeester, M. (2015). Guideline for the diagnostic pathway in patients with acute abdominal pain. *Digestive Surgery, 32*(1), 23–31.

McGibbon, A., Grant, C., Peltekian, K., & Belduyzen van Zanten, S. (2007). An evidence-based manual for abdominal paracentesis. *Digestive Diseases and Sciences, 52*(12), 3307–3315.

Penner, R., Fishman, M., & Majumdae, S. (2015). Evaluation of the adult with abdominal pain. Retrieved from http://www.uptodate.com/contents/evaluation-of-the-adult-with-abdominal-pain

Chapter 9

Musculoskeletal system

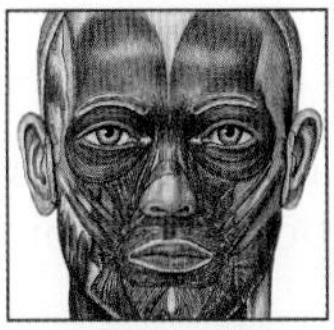

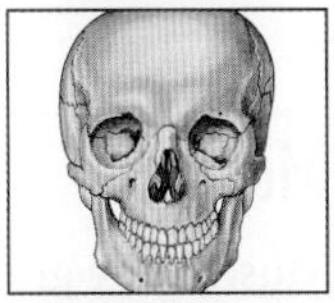

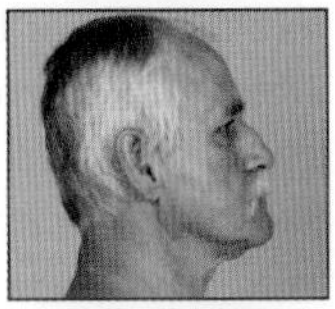

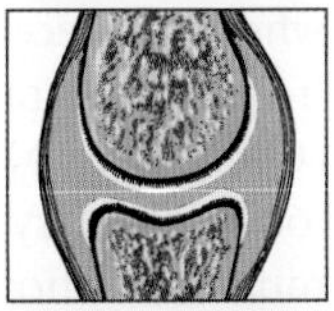

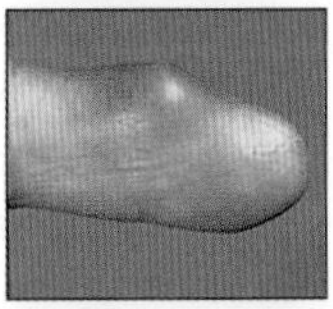

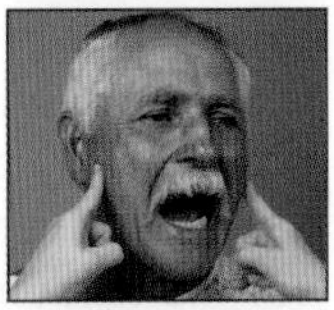

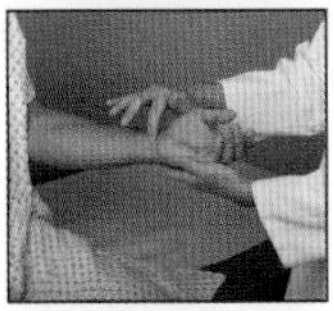

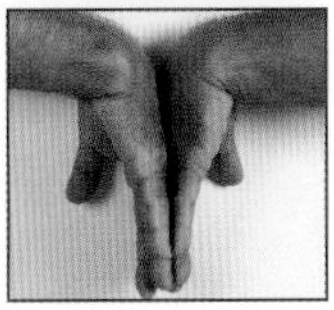

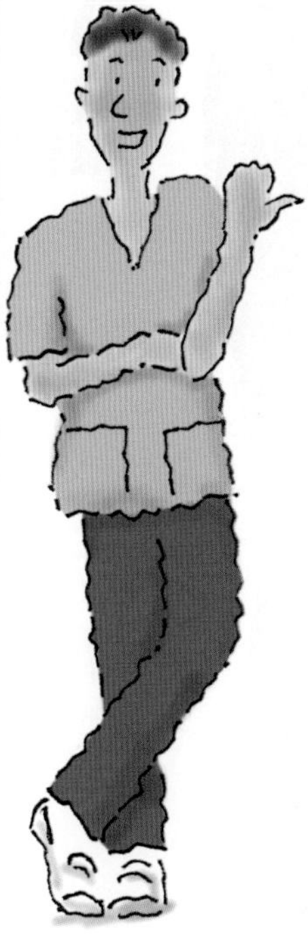

Anatomy

The three main parts of the musculoskeletal system are the muscles, bones, and joints.

Muscles

Muscles are groups of contractile cells or fibers that affect movement of an organ or another part of the body. Skeletal muscles contract and produce skeletal movement when they receive a stimulus from the central nervous system (CNS). The CNS is responsible for involuntary and voluntary muscle function.

Tendons are tough fibrous portions of muscle that attach the muscles to bone.

Bursae are sacs filled with friction-reducing synovial fluid that are located in areas of high friction such as the knee. Bursae allow adjacent muscles or muscles and tendons to glide smoothly over each other during movement.

Thanks to the bursae, there's less friction between us.
BURSAE

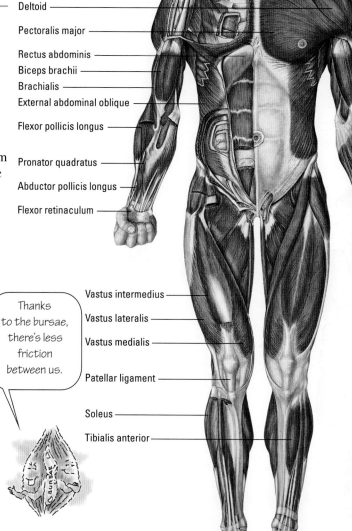

Major muscles of the body

Anterior view

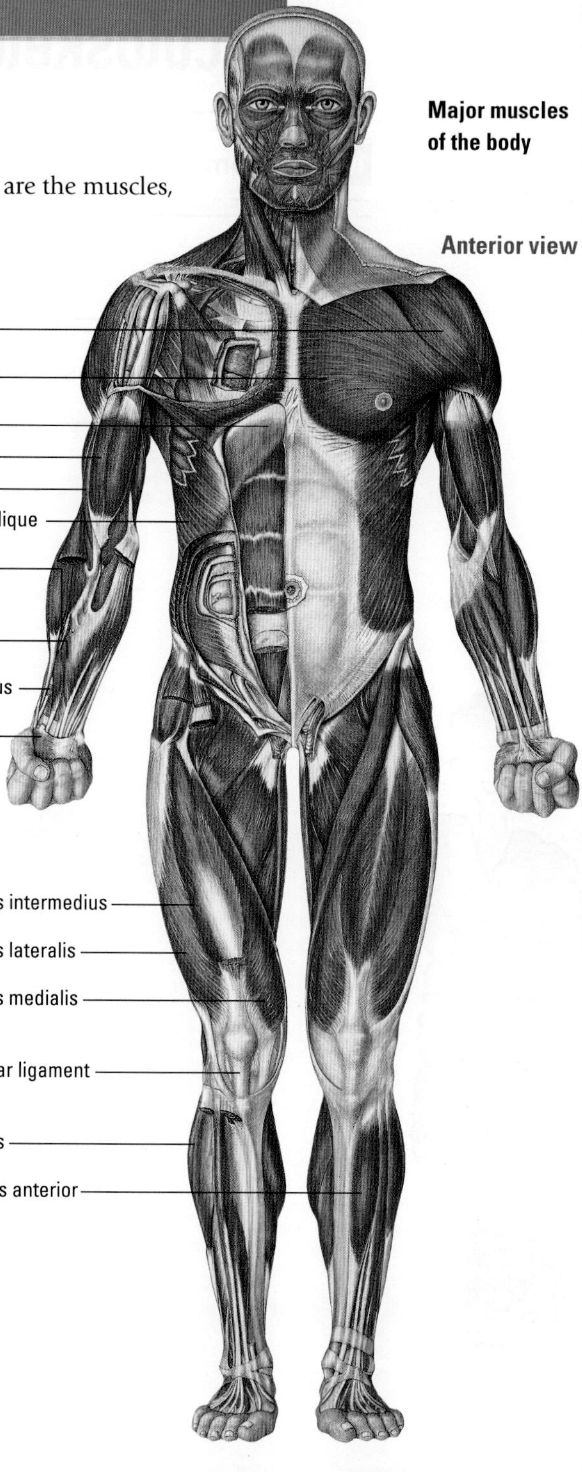
Deltoid
Pectoralis major
Rectus abdominis
Biceps brachii
Brachialis
External abdominal oblique
Flexor pollicis longus
Pronator quadratus
Abductor pollicis longus
Flexor retinaculum
Vastus intermedius
Vastus lateralis
Vastus medialis
Patellar ligament
Soleus
Tibialis anterior

Posterior view

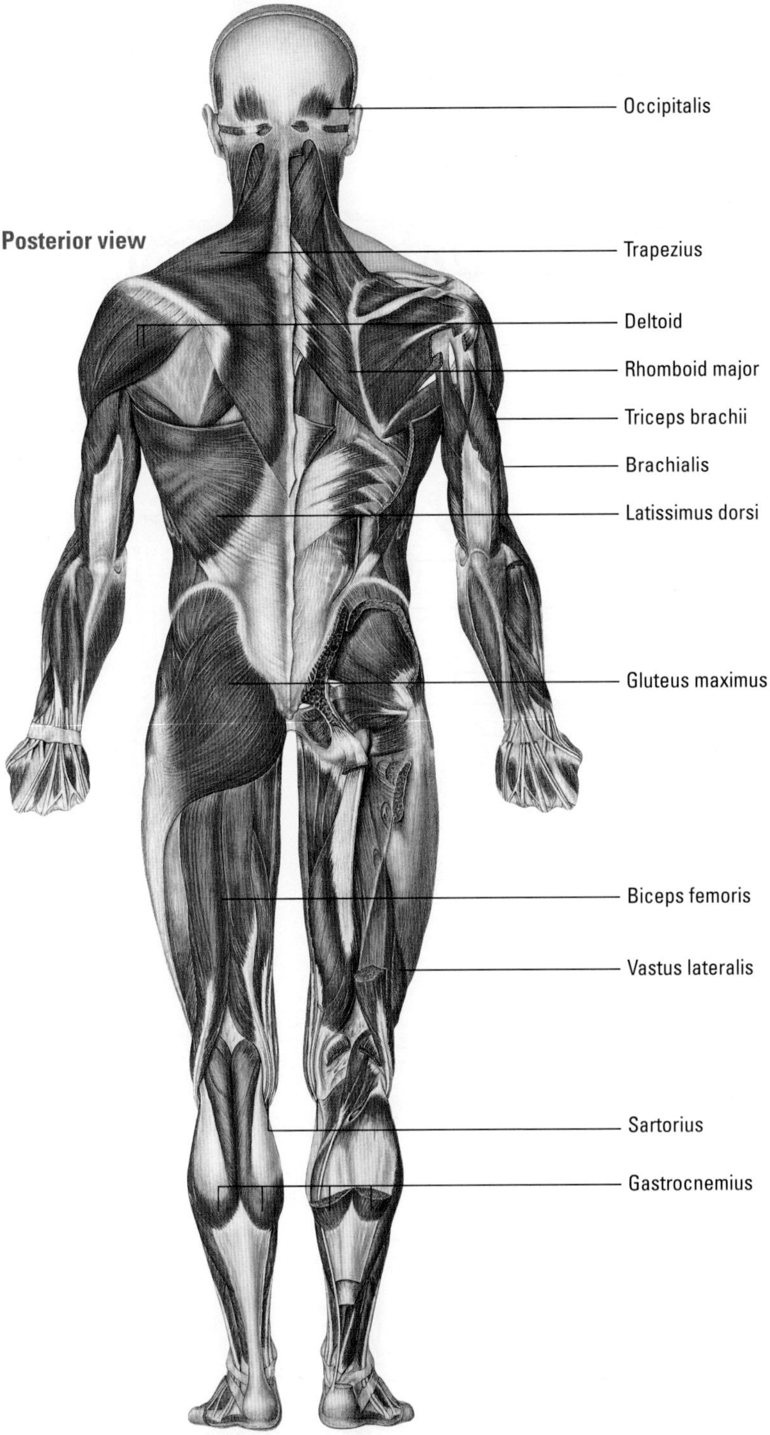
Occipitalis
Trapezius
Deltoid
Rhomboid major
Triceps brachii
Brachialis
Latissimus dorsi
Gluteus maximus
Biceps femoris
Vastus lateralis
Sartorius
Gastrocnemius

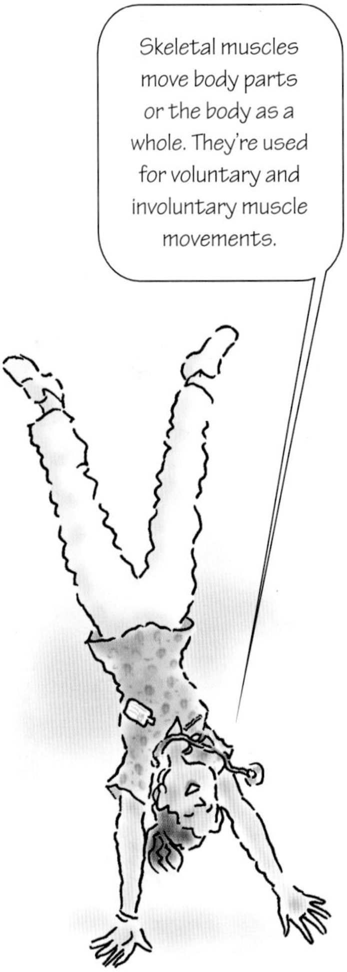
Skeletal muscles move body parts or the body as a whole. They're used for voluntary and involuntary muscle movements.

Bones

The 206 bones of the skeleton form the body's framework, supporting and protecting organs and tissues. The bones also serve as storage sites for minerals such as calcium, and they contain bone marrow, which produces red blood cells.

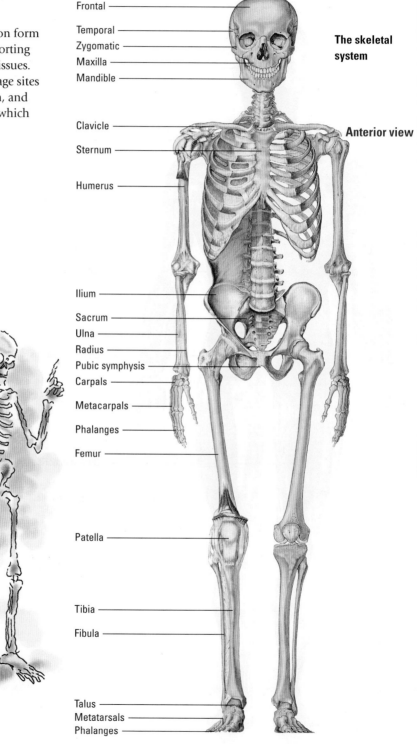

The skeletal system

Anterior view

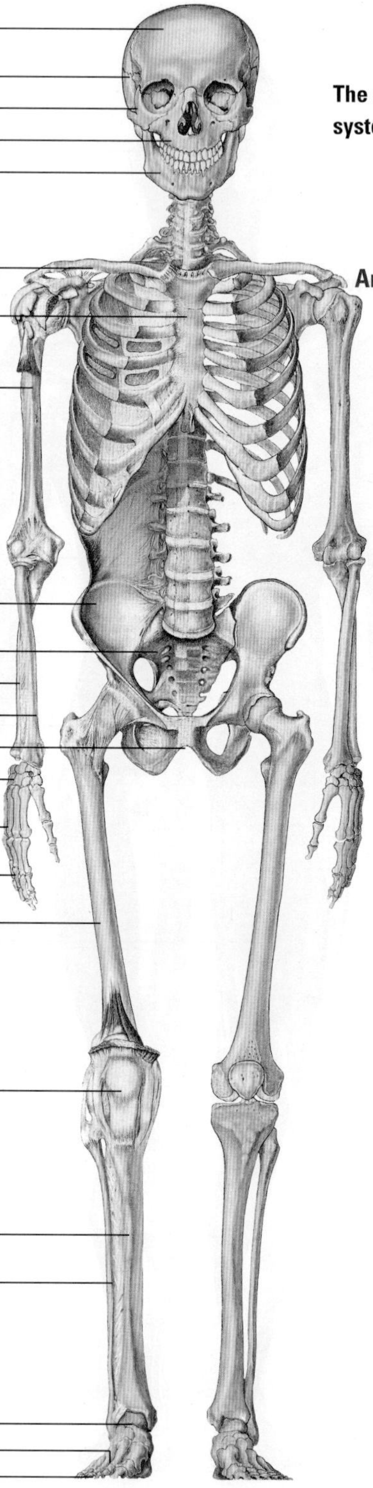
Frontal
Temporal
Zygomatic
Maxilla
Mandible
Clavicle
Sternum
Humerus
Ilium
Sacrum
Ulna
Radius
Pubic symphysis
Carpals
Metacarpals
Phalanges
Femur
Patella
Tibia
Fibula
Talus
Metatarsals
Phalanges

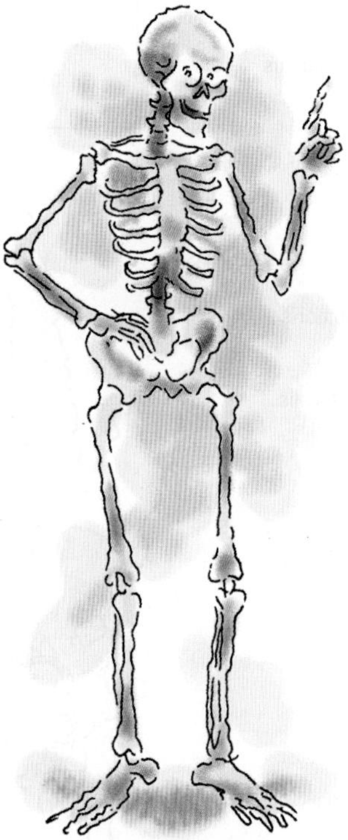

Posterior view

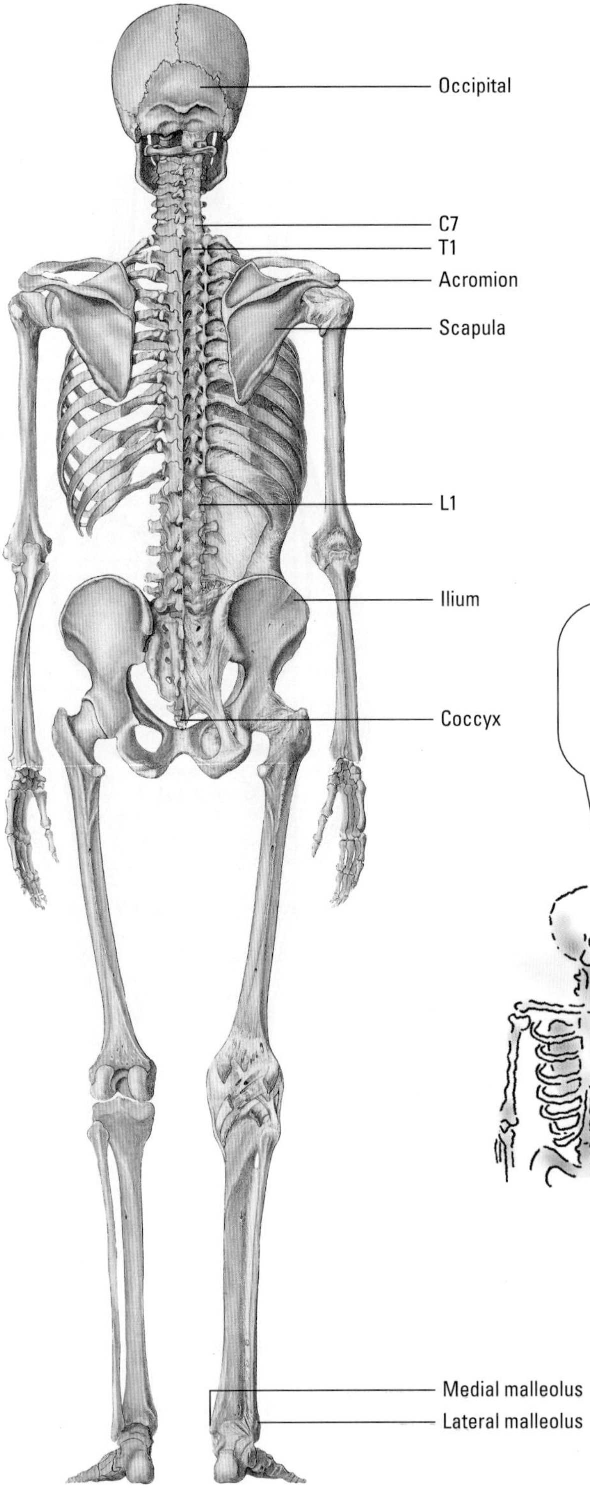
Occipital
C7
T1
Acromion
Scapula
L1
Ilium
Coccyx
Medial malleolus
Lateral malleolus

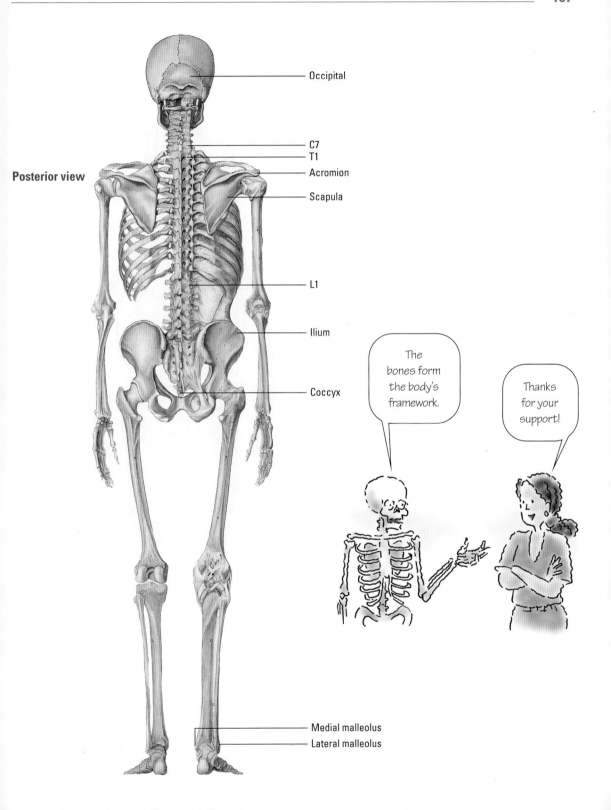
The bones form the body's framework.
Thanks for your support!

Joints

The junction of two or more bones is called a *joint*. Joints stabilize the bones and allow a specific type of movement. The two types of joints are nonsynovial and synovial.

Nonsynovial

In nonsynovial joints, the bones are connected by fibrous tissue, or cartilage. The bones may be immovable, like the sutures in the skull, or slightly movable, like the vertebrae.

Synovial

Synovial joints move freely; the bones are separate from each other and meet in a cavity filled with synovial fluid, a lubricant. These joints are surrounded by a fibrous capsule that stabilizes the joint structures and surrounds the joint's ligaments—the tough, fibrous bands that join one bone to another.

A look at a synovial joint

Normally, bones fit together. Cartilage—a smooth, fibrous tissue—cushions the end of each bone, and synovial fluid fills the joint space. This fluid lubricates the joint and eases movement, much as the brake fluid functions in a car.

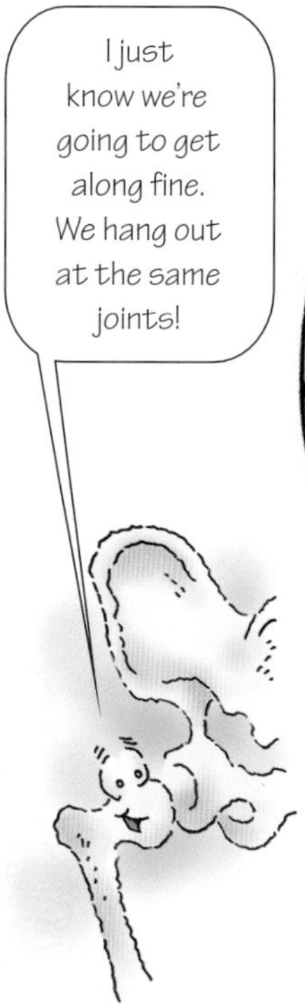
I just know we're going to get along fine. We hang out at the same joints!

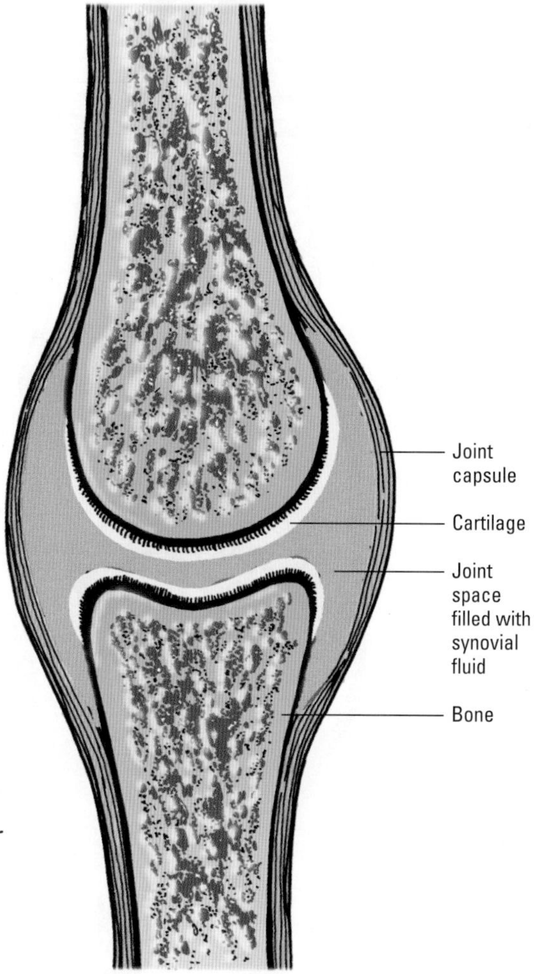
Joint capsule
Cartilage
Joint space filled with synovial fluid
Bone

Popular joints

Ball-and-socket joints

- Located in the shoulders and hips
- Allow flexion, extension, adduction, and abduction
- Rotate in their sockets
- Are assessed by their degree of internal and external rotation

Hinge joints

- Include the knee and elbow
- Move in flexion and extension

Types of joint motion

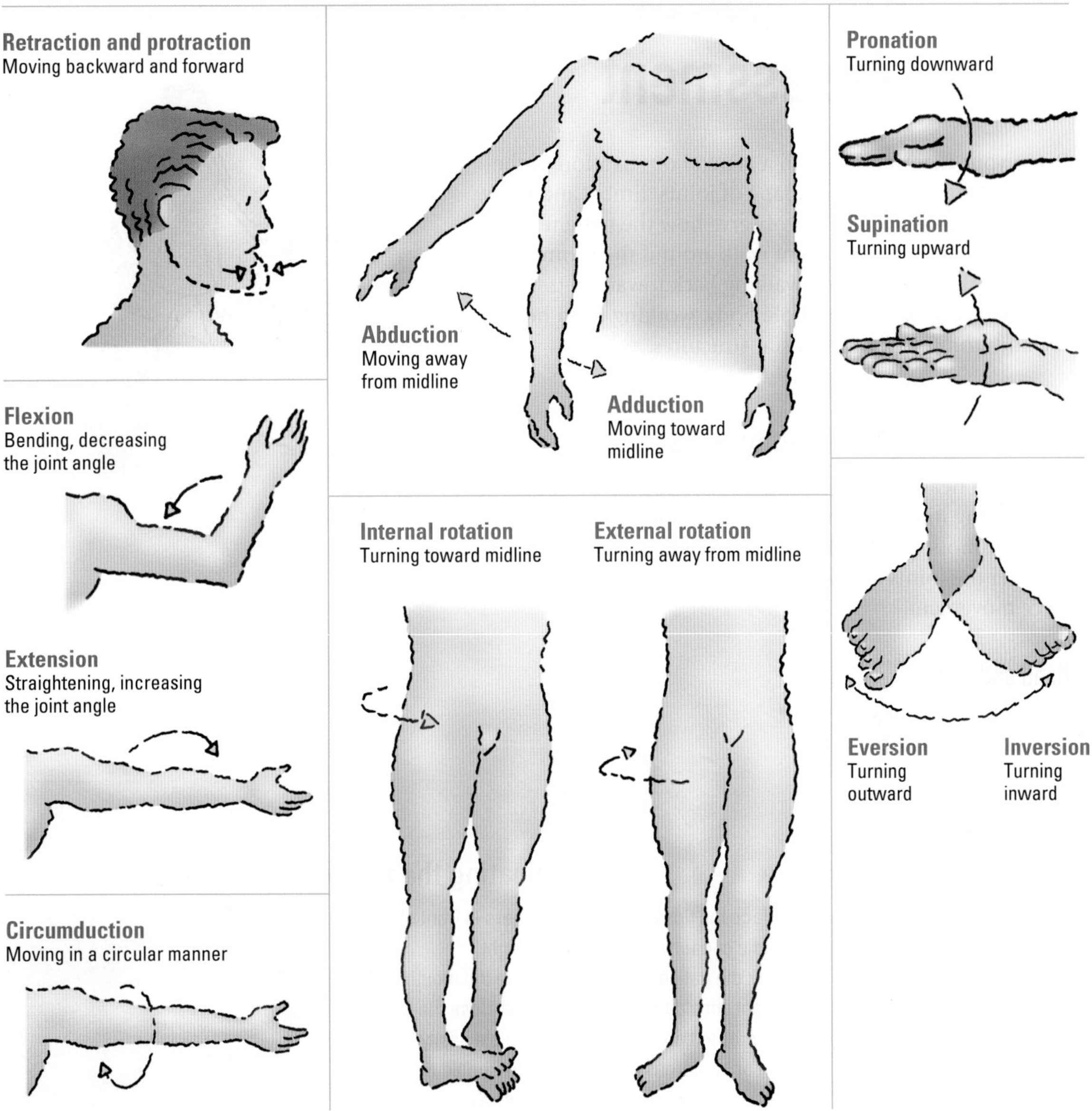
Retraction and protraction
Moving backward and forward
Abduction
Moving away from midline
Adduction
Moving toward midline
Pronation
Turning downward
Supination
Turning upward
Flexion
Bending, decreasing the joint angle
Internal rotation
Turning toward midline
External rotation
Turning away from midline
Extension
Straightening, increasing the joint angle
Eversion
Turning outward
Inversion
Turning inward
Circumduction
Moving in a circular manner

Assessment

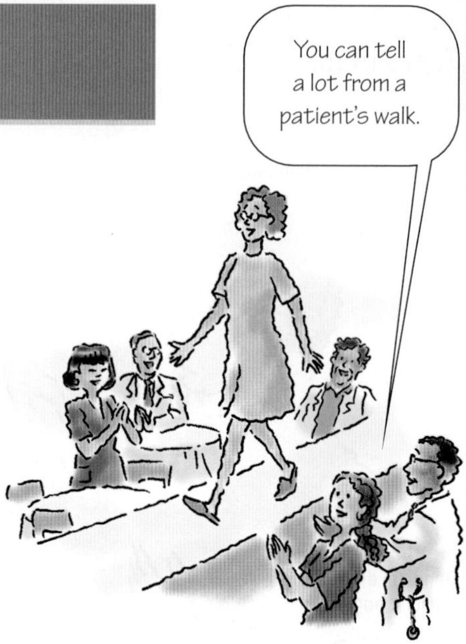
You can tell a lot from a patient's walk.

Begin your examination with a general observation of the patient. Note the size and shape of joints, limbs, and body regions. Whenever possible, observe how the patient stands and moves. Watch the patient walk around the room: to the door, turning around, and walking back toward you. Then systematically assess the whole body, working from head to toe and from proximal to distal structures.

Assessing the bones and joints

Perform a head-to-toe evaluation of your patient's bones and joints using inspection and palpation. Then perform passive range-of-motion (ROM) exercises to help you determine whether the joints are healthy. Remember, you should never force movement.

Head and jaw

Inspect the patient's face for swelling, symmetry, and evidence of trauma. The mandible should be in the midline, not shifted to the right or left. Then evaluate ROM in the temporomandibular joint.

Skill check

Evaluating the temporomandibular joint

- Place the tips of your index fingers in front of the middle of each ear, as shown at right.
- Ask the patient to open and close the mouth. The patient should be able to open and close the jaw and protract and retract the mandible easily, without pain or tenderness. Your fingertips should drop into the depressed areas over the joints as the patient's mouth opens.
- If you hear or palpate a click as the patient's mouth opens, suspect an improperly aligned jaw. Swelling of the area, crepitus, or pain may occur.

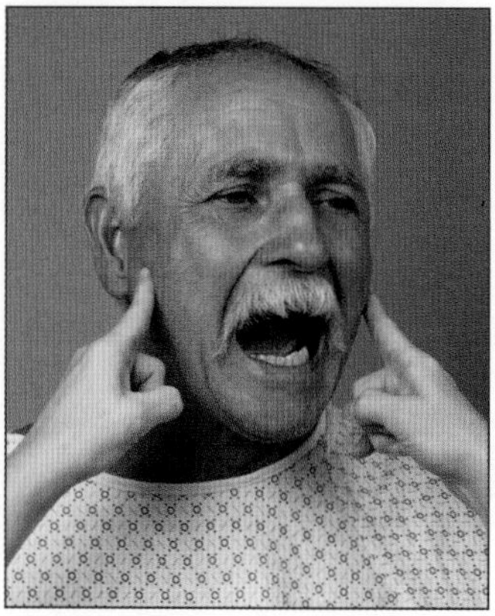

Neck

Inspect the front, back, and sides of the patient's neck, noting muscle asymmetry or masses. Then palpate the spinous processes of the cervical vertebrae and the areas above each clavicle (supraclavicular fossae) for tenderness, swelling, or nodules. To palpate the neck area:

- Stand facing the patient with your hands placed lightly on the sides of the neck.
- Ask the patient to turn the head from side to side, flex the neck forward, and then extend it backward.
- Feel for any lumps or tender areas.
- As the patient moves the neck, listen and palpate for crepitus, an abnormal grating sound. Note that this sound is different from the occasional crack that can be heard from joints.

After inspecting and palpating, check ROM in the neck.

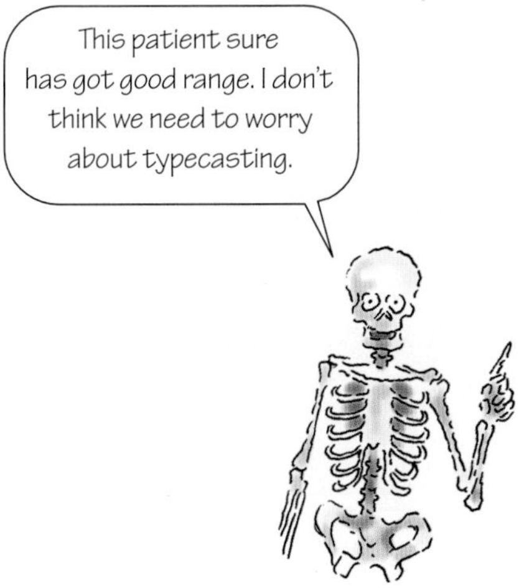
This patient sure has got good range. I don't think we need to worry about typecasting.

Skill check

Assessing neck range of motion

- Ask the patient to try touching right ear to right shoulder and left ear to left shoulder. The usual range of motion is 40 degrees on each side.

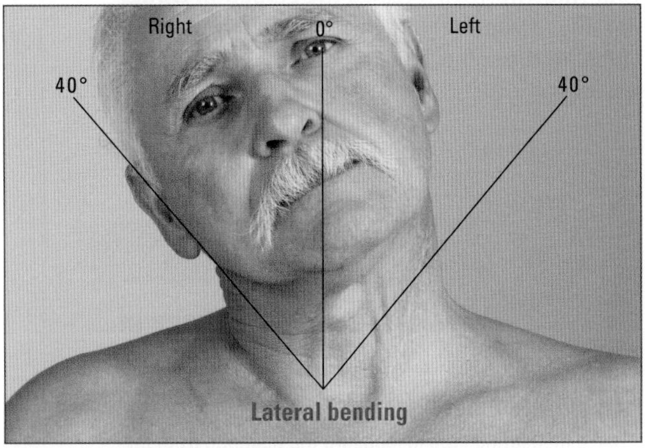
Right
0°
Left
40°
40°
Lateral bending

- Ask the patient to touch chin to chest and then to point the chin up toward the ceiling. While doing this, the patient's neck should flex forward 45 degrees and extend backward 55 degrees.

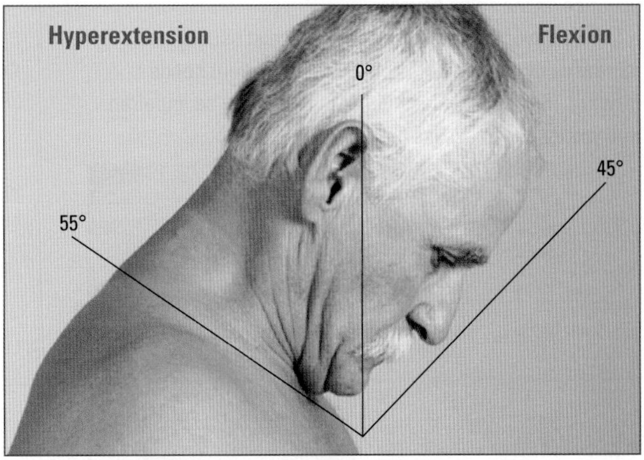
Hyperextension
Flexion
0°
45°
55°

- To assess rotation, watch while the patient moves the head side to side without moving the trunk of the body. During this movement, the chin should remain parallel to the shoulders.
- Finally, ask the patient to move the head in a circle—normal rotation is 70 degrees.

Spine

Assess spinal position and curvature and the range of spinal movement. Then palpate the spinal processes and the areas lateral to the spine. Have the patient bend at the waist and let the arms hang loosely at the sides. Palpate the spine with your fingertips. Then repeat the palpation using the side of your hand, lightly striking the areas lateral to the spine. Note tenderness, swelling, or spasm.

Skill check

Assessing the range of spinal movement

- Ask the patient to straighten up.
- Use a measuring tape to measure the distance from the nape of the neck to the waist.
- Ask the patient to bend forward at the waist.
- Continue to hold the tape at the patient's neck, letting it slip through your fingers slightly to accommodate the increased distance as the spine flexes.
- The length of the spine from neck to waist usually increases by at least 2″ (5 cm) when the patient bends forward. If it doesn't, the patient's mobility may be impaired, and you'll need to assess this further.

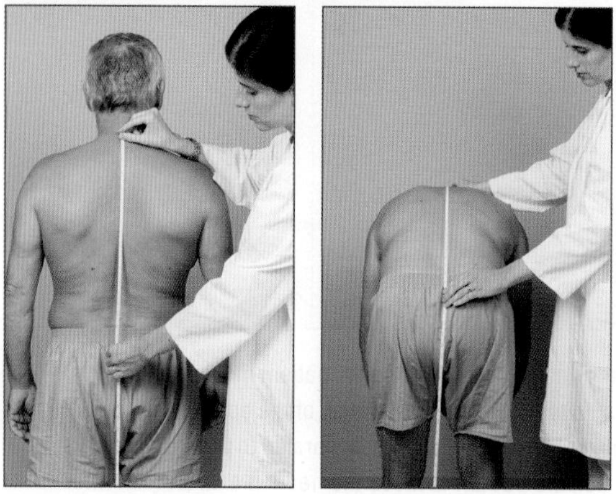

Normal position of spine

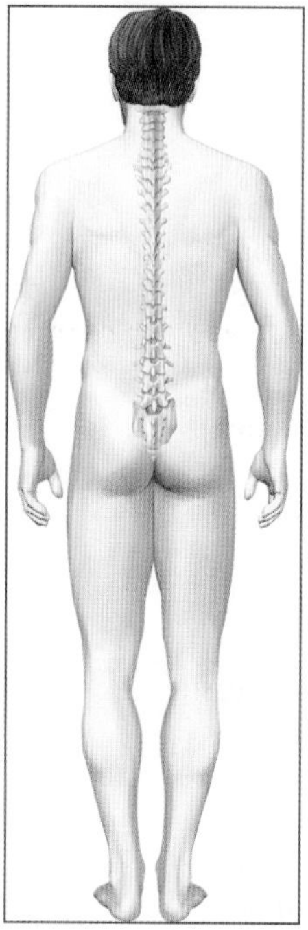

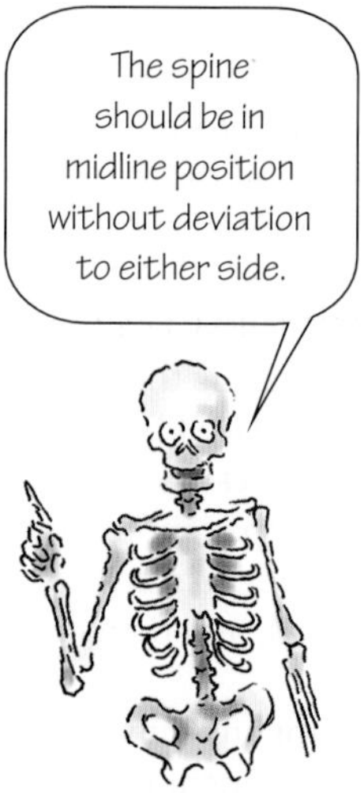
The spine should be in midline position without deviation to either side.

Normal curvature of spine

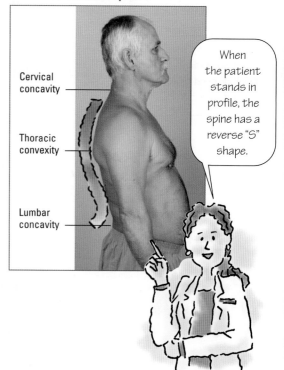

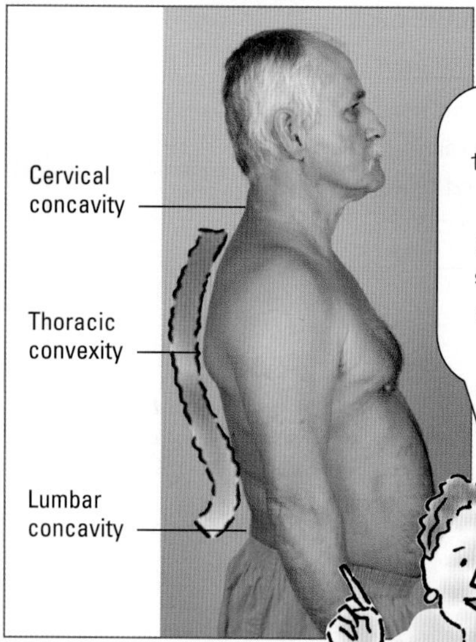
Cervical concavity
Thoracic convexity
Lumbar concavity

When the patient stands in profile, the spine has a reverse "S" shape.

Shoulders and elbows

With the patient sitting or standing, observe the shoulders, noting asymmetry, muscle atrophy, or deformity. Palpate the shoulders with the palmar surfaces of your fingers to locate bony landmarks; note crepitus or tenderness. Using your entire hand, palpate the shoulder muscles for firmness and symmetry. Also palpate the elbow and the ulna for subcutaneous nodules that occur with rheumatoid arthritis. Assess ROM.

Skill check

Assessing shoulder and elbow range of motion

Shoulder flexion and extension

- To assess flexion, ask the patient to move each arm anteriorly from the side to over the head, as if reaching for the sky. Full flexion is 180 degrees.
- To assess extension, have the patient move, with the arms, from the neutral position posteriorly as far as possible. Normal extension ranges from 30 to 50 degrees.

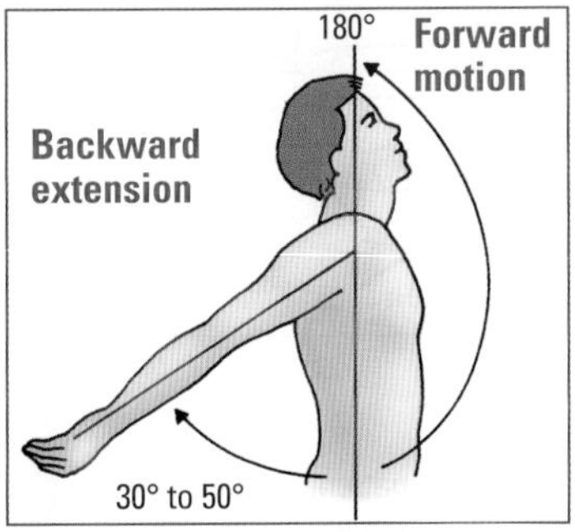
180°
Forward motion
Backward extension
30° to 50°

Shoulder external and internal rotation

- Have the patient abduct each arm with the elbow bent.
- Ask the patient to place each hand first behind the head and then behind the small of the back. Normal external and internal rotation is 90 degrees.

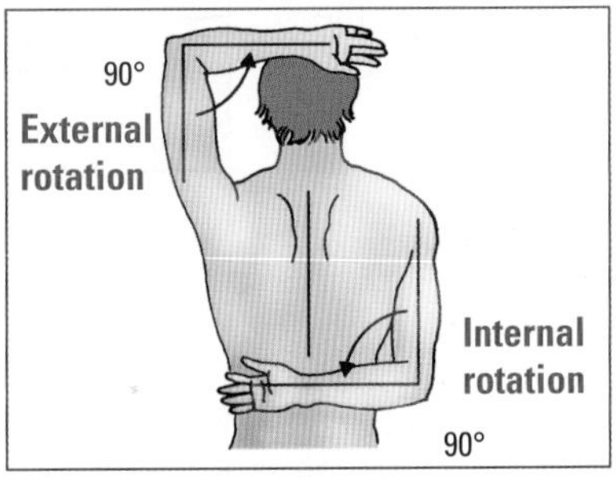
90°
External rotation
Internal rotation
90°

Shoulder abduction and adduction

- To assess abduction, ask the patient to move the arm from the neutral position laterally as far as possible. Normal range of motion (ROM) is 180 degrees.
- To assess adduction, have the patient move the arm from the neutral position across the front of the body as far as possible. Normal ROM is 50 degrees.

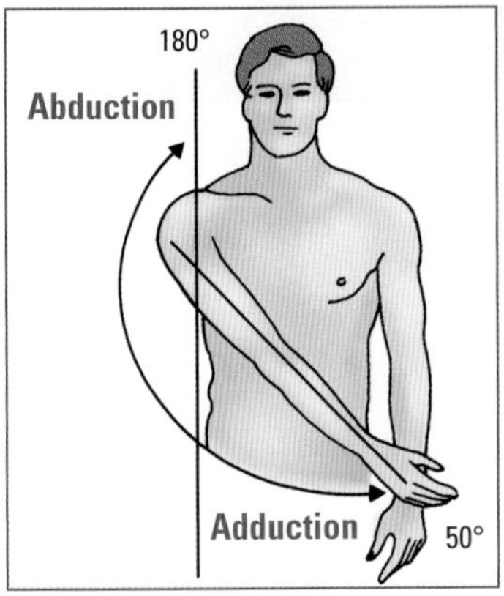
180°
Abduction
Adduction
50°

Elbow flexion and extension

- Have the patient rest with arms at the sides.
- Ask the patient to flex each elbow and then extend it. Normal ROM is 90 degrees for both flexion and extension.

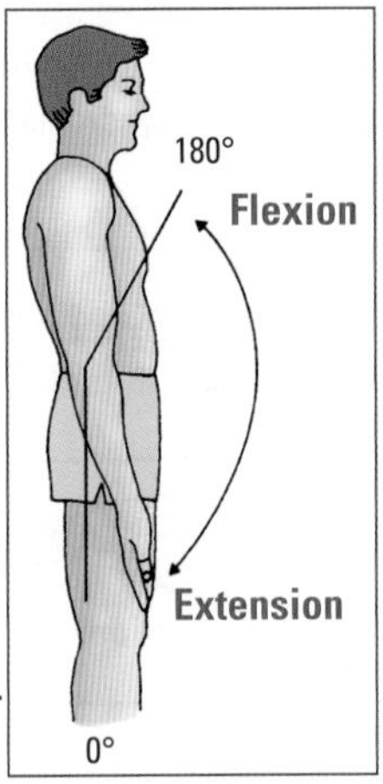
180°
Flexion
Extension
0°

Elbow pronation and supination

- Have the patient place the side of each hand on a flat surface with the thumb on top.
- Ask the patient to rotate palm down for pronation and upward for supination. The normal angle of elbow rotation is 90 degrees in each direction.

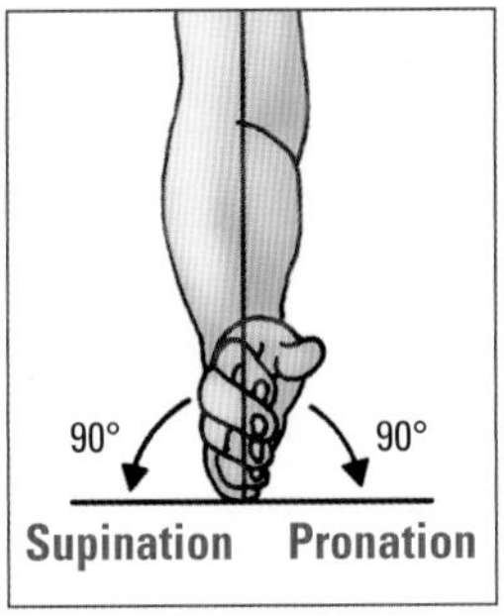
90°
90°
Supination
Pronation

Wrists, hands, and fingers

Inspect the wrists and hands for contour, and compare them for symmetry. Also check for nodules, redness, swelling, deformities, and webbing between fingers.

Use your thumb and index finger to palpate both wrists and each finger joint. Note any tenderness, nodules, or bogginess. Then assess ROM of the wrists and fingers.

Skill check

Assessing wrist range of motion

Radial and ulnar deviation

- Ask the patient to rotate each wrist by moving the entire hand—first laterally and then medially—as if waxing a car.
- Normal range of motion is 55 degrees laterally (ulnar deviation) and 20 degrees medially (radial deviation).

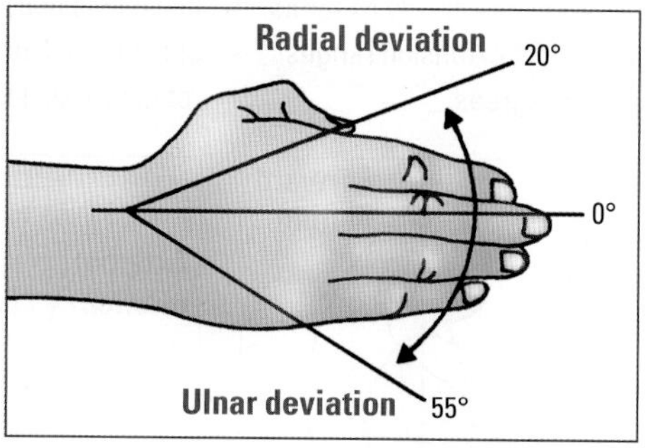
Radial deviation
20°
0°
Ulnar deviation
55°

Extension and flexion

- Observe the wrist while the patient extends the fingers up toward the ceiling and down toward the floor, as if flapping the hand. The patient should be able to extend the wrist 70 degrees and flex it 90 degrees.
- If these movements cause pain or numbness, the patient may have carpal tunnel syndrome. Further assessment is needed.

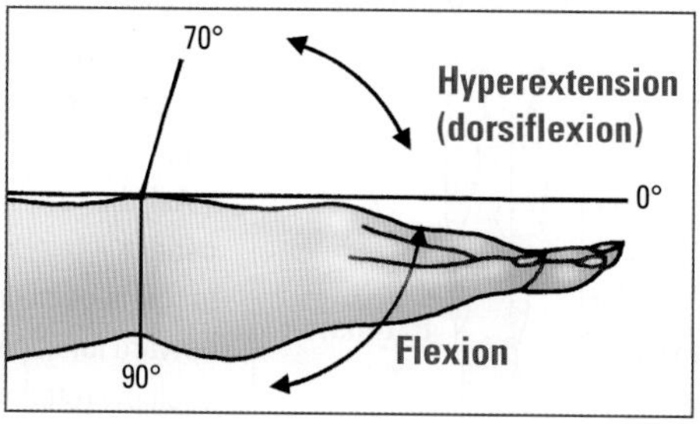
70°
Hyperextension
(dorsiflexion)
0°
Flexion
90°

Testing for carpal tunnel syndrome

Tinel sign

- Lightly percuss the transverse carpal ligament over the median nerve where the patient's palm and wrist meet.
- If this action produces numbness and tingling shooting into the palm and finger, the patient has Tinel sign and may have carpal tunnel syndrome.

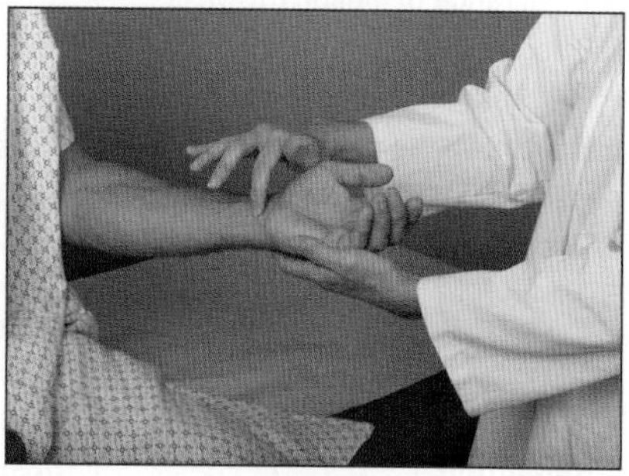

Assessing finger range of motion

Phalen maneuver

- Have the patient put the backs of the hands together and flex the wrists downward at a 90-degree angle.
- Pain or numbness in the hand or fingers during this maneuver indicates a positive Phalen sign. The more severe the carpal tunnel syndrome, the more rapidly the symptoms develop.

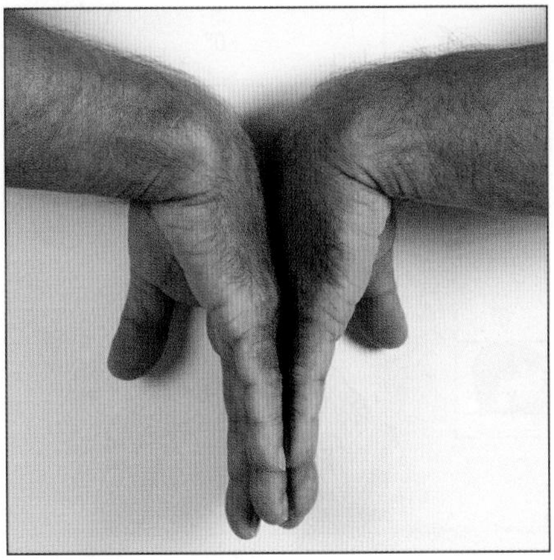

Extension and flexion

- Ask the patient to keep the wrist still and move only the fingers—first up toward the ceiling and then down toward the floor.
- Have the patient make a fist with the thumb remaining straight.
- Normal hyperextension is 30 degrees; normal flexion, 90 degrees.
- Ask the patient to touch the thumb to the little finger of the same hand. The patient should be able to fold or flex the thumb across the palm of the hand so that it touches or points toward the base of the little finger.
- To assess flexion of all of the fingers, ask the patient to form a fist.

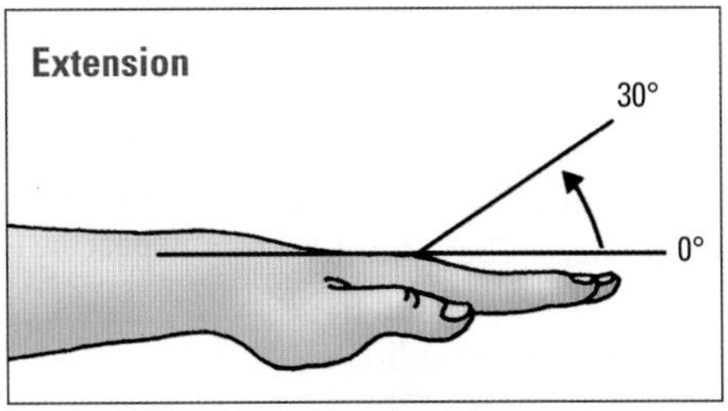
Extension
30°
0°

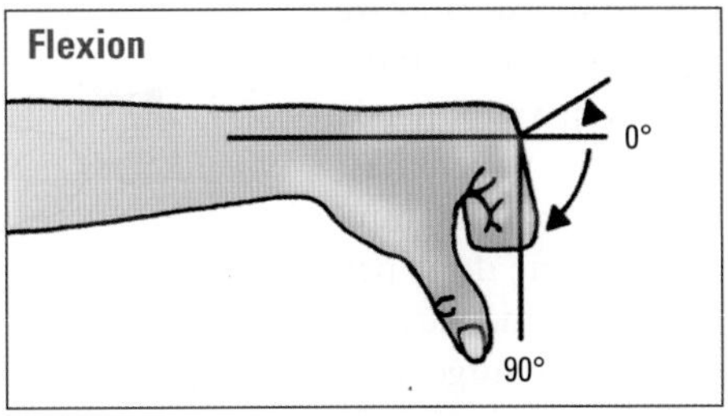
Flexion
0°
90°

Abduction and adduction

- To test abduction, have the patient spread the fingers apart.
- To test adduction, have the patient draw the fingers back together.

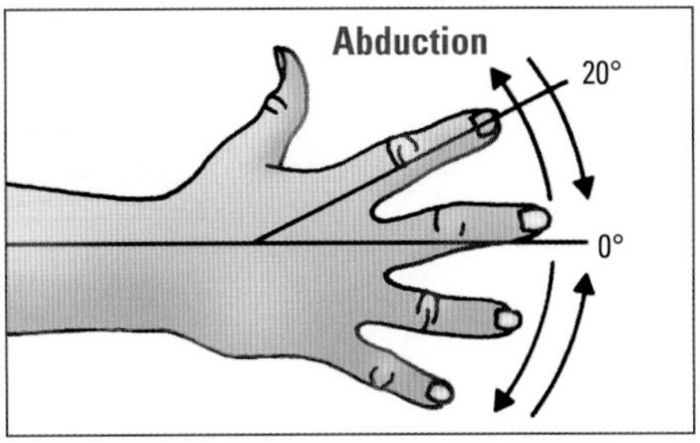
Abduction
20°
0°

Hips and knees

Inspect the hip area for contour and symmetry. Inspect the position of the knees, noting whether the patient is bowlegged, with knees that point out, or knock-kneed, with knees that turn in.

Palpate each hip over the iliac crest and trochanteric area for tenderness or instability. Palpate both knees. They should feel smooth, and the tissues should feel solid.

Assess ROM in the hip. These exercises are typically done with the patient in a supine position. If the patient has undergone a total hip replacement, don't perform these maneuvers without the surgeon's permission; motion can dislocate the prosthesis. Next, assess ROM in the knee.

Skill check

Assessing hip range of motion

Flexion

- Have the patient lie on the back.
- Have the patient bend one knee and pull it toward the abdomen and chest as far as possible.
- As the patient flexes the knee, the opposite hip and thigh should remain flat.
- Repeat the test on the opposite side.

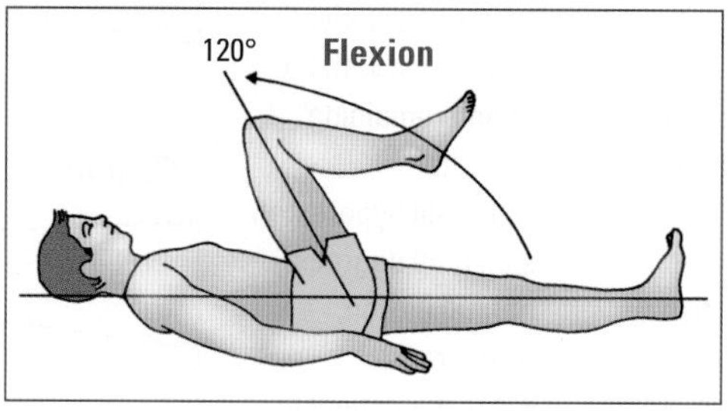
120°
Flexion

Extension

- Have the patient lie in a prone position (facedown).
- Gently extend the thigh upward.
- Repeat the test on the other thigh.

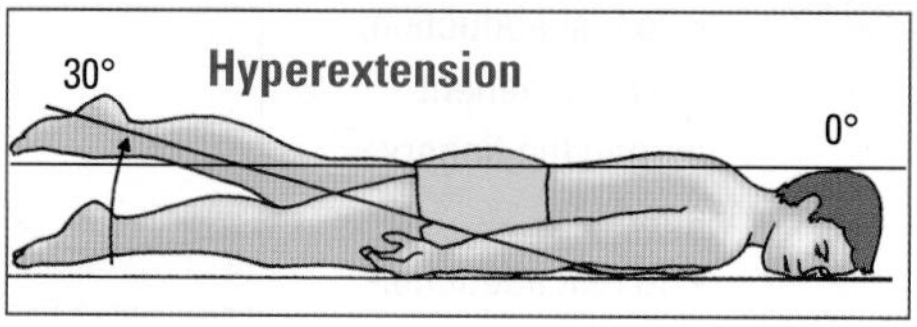
30°
Hyperextension
0°

Internal and external rotation

- Ask the patient to bend one knee while turning the leg inward.
- Then ask the patient to turn the leg outward.
- Normal ROM for internal rotation is 40 degrees and for external rotation, 45 degrees.

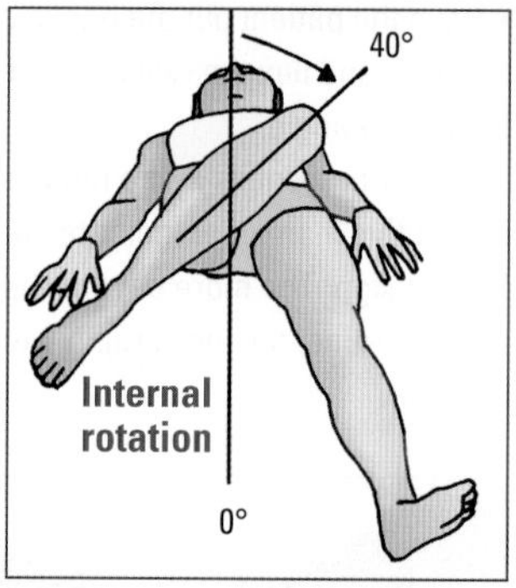
40°
Internal rotation
0°

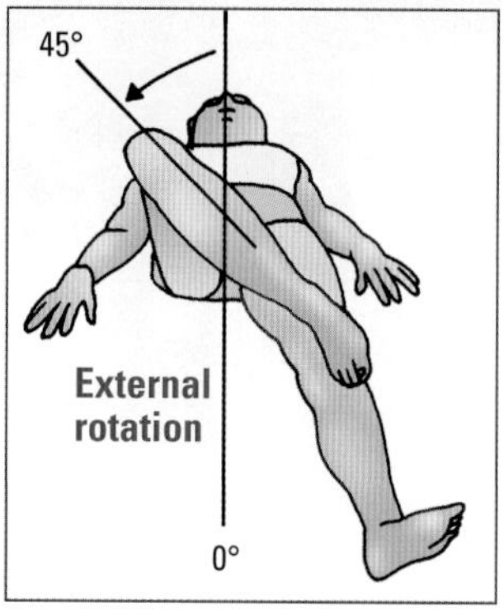
45°
External rotation
0°

Abduction and adduction

- Stand alongside the patient and press down on the superior iliac spine of the opposite hip with one hand to stabilize the pelvis.
- With your other hand, hold the patient's leg by the ankle and gently abduct the hip until you feel the iliac spine move. That movement indicates the limit of hip abduction.
- While still stabilizing the pelvis, move the ankle medially across the patient's body to assess hip adduction.
- Repeat on the other side.
- Normal range of motion (ROM) is about 45 degrees for abduction and 30 degrees for adduction.

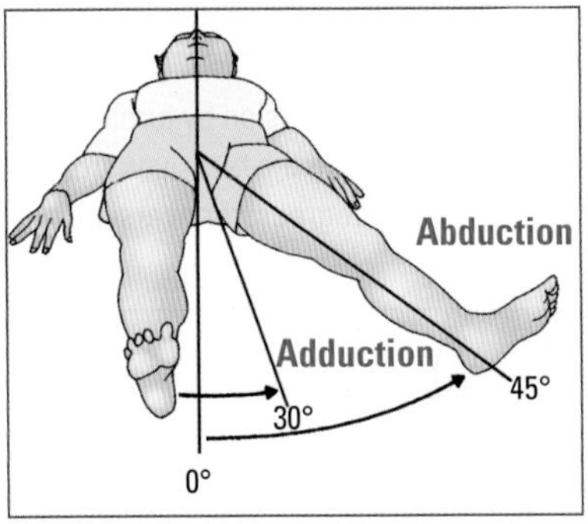
Abduction
Adduction
30°
45°
0°

Assessing knee range of motion

- If this is done while the patient is standing, it can be done by asking for the patient to bend the knee heel to buttocks, as shown. Normal range of motion for flexion is 120 to 130 degrees.
- If the patient is lying down, ask for the patient to draw a knee up toward the chest. The calf should touch the back of the thigh.
- Knee extension returns the knee to a neutral position of 0 degrees; however, some knees may normally be hyperextended 15 degrees.
- If the patient can't extend the leg fully or if the knee pops audibly and painfully, consider the response abnormal. Pronounced crepitus may signal a degenerative disease of the knee. Sudden buckling may indicate a ligament injury.

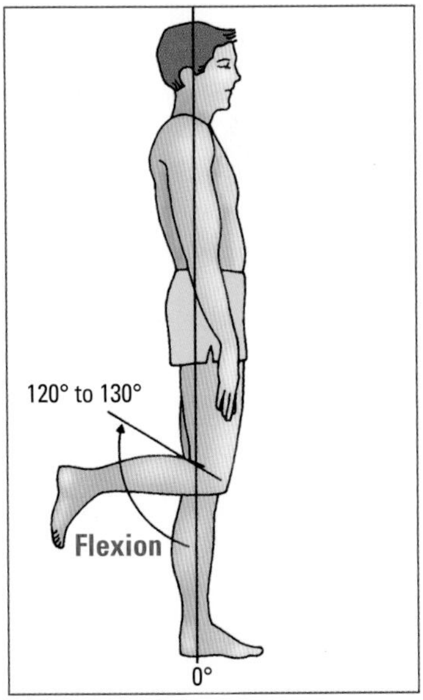
120° to 130°
Flexion
0°

Assessing for bulge sign

The bulge sign indicates excess fluid in the joint. To assess the patient for this sign, ask the patient to lie down and palpate the knee. Then give the medial side of the knee two to four firm strokes, as shown, to displace excess fluid.

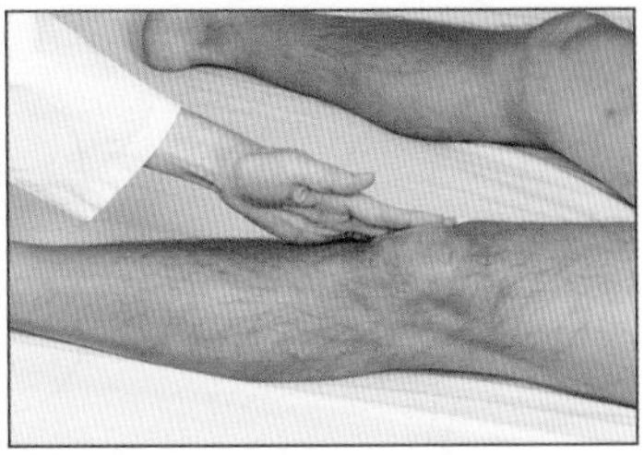

Lateral check

Next, tap the lateral aspect of the knee while checking for a fluid wave on the medial aspect.

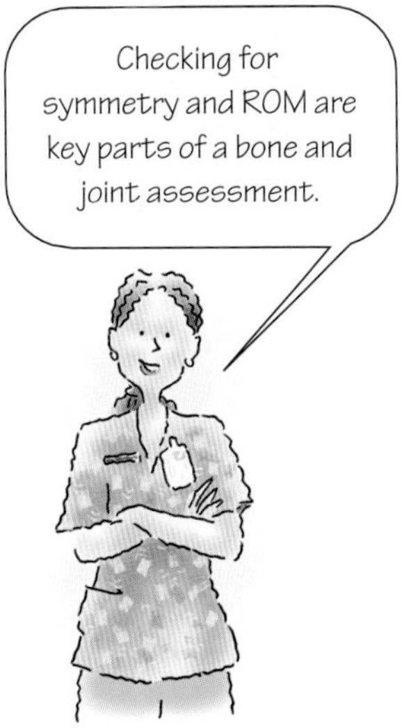
Checking for symmetry and ROM are key parts of a bone and joint assessment.

Ankles and feet

Inspect the ankles and feet for swelling, redness, nodules, and other deformities. Check the arch of the foot and look for toe deformities. Also note calluses, bunions, corns, ingrown toenails, plantar warts, trophic ulcers, hair loss, or unusual pigmentation.

Use your fingertips to palpate the bony and muscular structures of the ankles and feet. Palpate each toe joint by compressing it with your thumb and fingers. Then assess ROM.

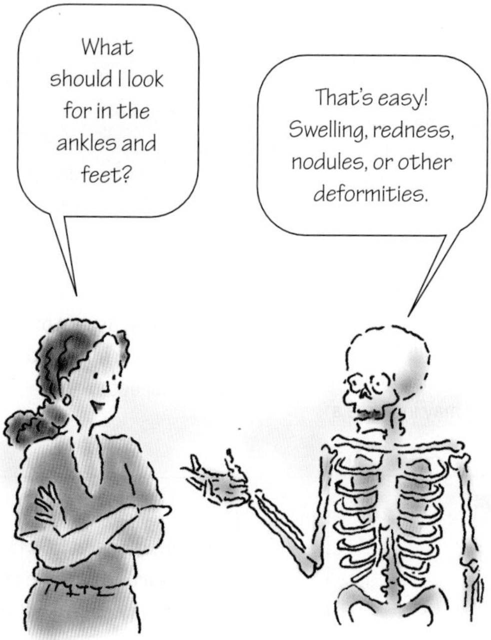
What should I look for in the ankles and feet?
That's easy! Swelling, redness, nodules, or other deformities.

Skill check

Assessing ankle and foot range of motion

- Have the patient sit in a chair or on the side of a bed.
- Test plantar flexion of the ankle by asking the patient to point the toes toward the floor.
- Test dorsiflexion by having the patient point toes toward the ceiling.
- Normal range of motion (ROM) for plantar flexion is about 45 degrees; for dorsiflexion, 20 degrees.

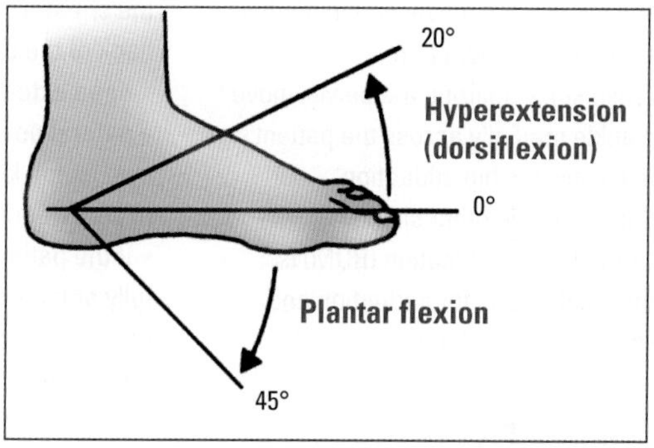
20°
Hyperextension (dorsiflexion)
0°
Plantar flexion
45°

- Ask the patient to demonstrate inversion by turning the feet inward, and eversion by turning the feet outward. Normal ROM for inversion is 30 degrees; for eversion, 20 degrees.

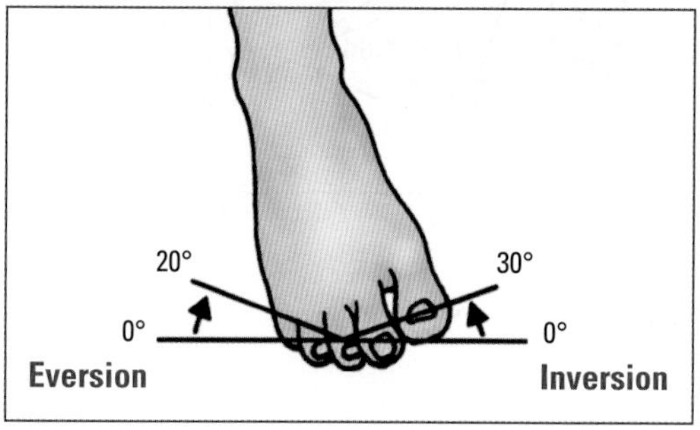
20°
30°
0°
0°
Eversion
Inversion

- To assess the metatarsophalangeal joints, ask the patient to first flex the toes and then straighten them.

Assessing the muscles

Inspect all major muscle groups. Check for symmetry. If a muscle appears atrophied or hypertrophied, measure it by wrapping a tape measure around the largest circumference of the muscle on each side of the body and comparing the two numbers. Note contracture and abnormal movements, such as spasms, tics, tremors, and fasciculation.

Muscle tone

Muscle tone describes muscular resistance to passive stretching. To test the patient's arm muscle tone, move the shoulder through passive ROM exercises. You should feel a slight resistance. Then let the arm drop. It should fall easily to the side.

Test leg muscle tone by putting the patient's hip through passive ROM exercises and then letting the leg fall to the examination table or bed. Like the arm, the leg should fall easily. Abnormal findings include muscle rigidity and flaccidity.

Muscle strength

Observe the patient's gait and movements to form an idea of general muscle strength. Grade muscle strength on a scale of 0 to 5. Document the results as a fraction, with the score as the numerator and maximum strength as the denominator. Then test specific muscle groups.

Grading muscle strength

Grade muscle strength on a scale of 0 to 5, as follows:

5/5 **Normal:** Patient moves joint through full range of motion (ROM) and against gravity with full resistance.

4/5 **Good:** Patient completes ROM against gravity with moderate resistance.

3/5 **Fair:** Patient completes ROM against gravity only.

2/5 **Poor:** Patient completes full ROM with gravity eliminated (passive motion).

1/5 **Trace:** Patient's attempt at muscle contraction is palpable but without joint movement.

0/5 **Zero:** No evidence of muscle contraction.

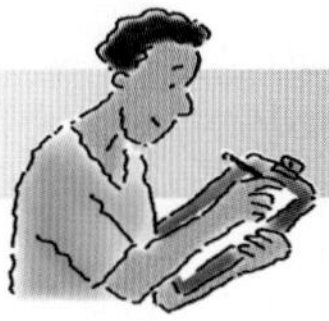

Take note

Documenting muscle strength

3/14/10	1730	Pt. alert and oriented to person, place,
		and time. Finished 80% of dinner tray.
		No difficulty swallowing. Feeds self
		with minimal effort. Full ROM upper
		extremities. Strong bilateral hand-
		grip. Weakness in left leg unchanged,
		muscle strength 3/5 left leg and 5/5
		right leg. Son visiting with patient.
		Mary Petty, RN

Shoulder, arm, wrist, and hand strength

Have the patient extend the arms, palms up, for 30 seconds to test the strength of the shoulder girdle. If the patient cannot lift both arms equally and keep the palms up, or if one arm drifts down, there is probably shoulder girdle weakness on that side.

Next, have the patient hold both arms in front with the elbows bent. To test bicep strength, pull down on the flexor surface of the forearm as the patient resists. To test triceps strength, have the patient try to straighten both arms as you push upward against the extensor surface of the forearm.

Assess the strength of the patient's flexed wrist by pushing against it. Test the strength of the extended wrist by pushing down on it. Test the strength of finger abduction, thumb opposition, and handgrip the same way.

Leg strength

Ask the patient to lie in a supine position on the examination table or bed and lift both legs at the same time. Note whether the patient lifts both legs at the same time and to the same distance. To test quadriceps strength, have the patient lower both legs and raise them again while you press down on the anterior thighs.

Finally, assess ankle strength by having the patient push down with each foot against your resistance and then pull each foot up as you try to hold it down.

Skill check

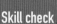

Testing muscle strength

To test specific muscle groups, ask the patient to move the muscles while you apply resistance; then compare the contralateral muscle groups. Use the techniques shown here to test the muscle strength of your patient's arm and ankle muscles.

Biceps strength

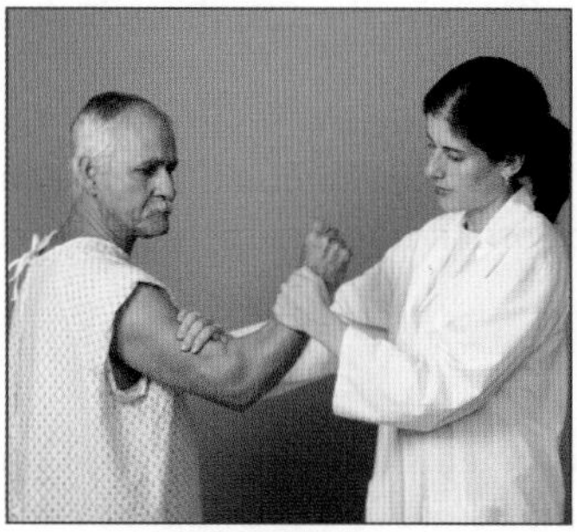

Triceps strength

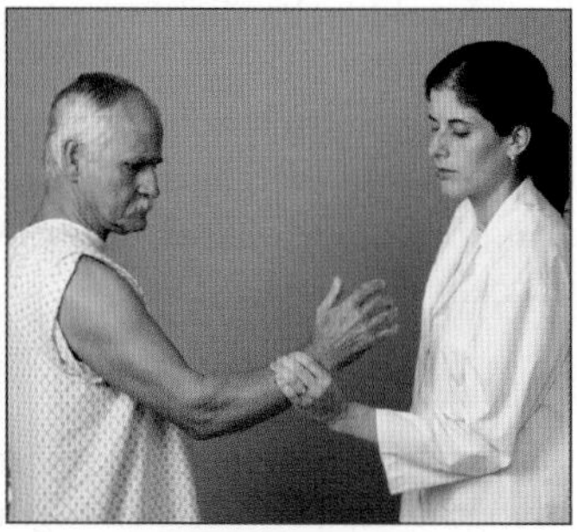

Ankle strength: Plantar flexion

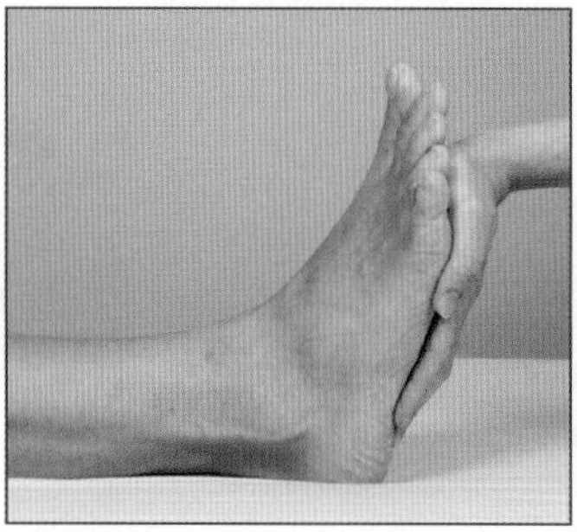

Ankle strength: Dorsiflexion

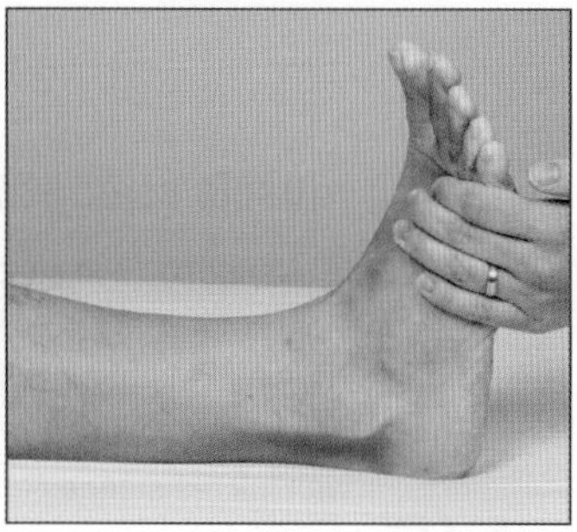

Testing handgrip strength

- Face the patient.
- Extend the first and second fingers of each hand, and ask the patient to grasp your fingers and squeeze.
- Don't extend fingers with rings on them; a strong handgrip on those fingers can be painful.

Abnormal findings

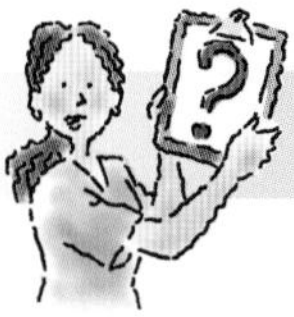

Outside the norm

Common musculoskeletal abnormalities

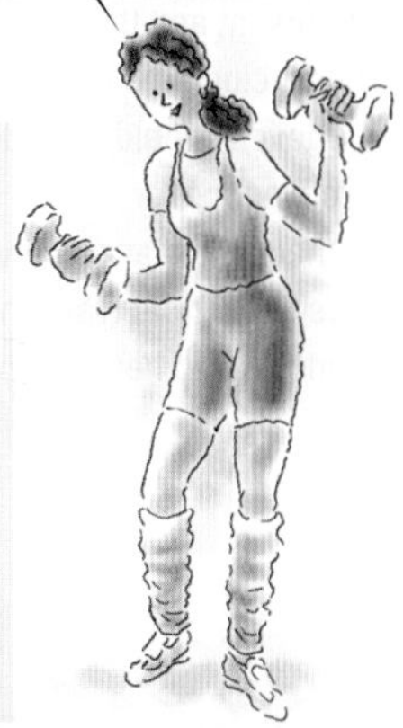
Pump up your assessment skills by familiarizing yourself with these abnormal musculoskeletal findings.

Footdrop

Footdrop—plantar flexion of the foot with the toes bent toward the instep—is a characteristic sign of certain peripheral nerve or motor neuron disorders. It results from weakness or paralysis of the dorsiflexor muscles of the foot and ankle. Footdrop may also stem from prolonged immobility.

Muscle spasms

Muscle spasms, or cramps, are strong, painful contractions. They can occur in virtually any muscle but are most common in the calf and foot. Muscle spasms typically result from simple muscle fatigue, exercise, electrolyte imbalances, neuromuscular disorders, and pregnancy.

Muscle atrophy

Muscle atrophy, or muscle wasting, results from denervation or prolonged muscle disuse. Some muscle atrophy also occurs with aging.

Crepitus

Crepitus is an abnormal crunching or grating you can hear and feel when a joint with roughened articular surfaces moves. It occurs in patients with rheumatoid arthritis or osteoarthritis or when broken pieces of bone rub together.

Muscle weakness

Muscle weakness can result from a malfunction in the cerebral hemispheres, brainstem, spinal cord, nerve roots, peripheral nerves, or myoneural junctions and within the muscle itself.

Traumatic injury

Traumatic injuries include fractures, dislocations, amputations, crush injuries, and serious lacerations. To swiftly assess a musculoskeletal injury, remember the 5 Ps: pain, paresthesia, paralysis, pallor, and pulse.

Pain

Arm pain (pain anywhere from the hand to the shoulder) and leg pain usually result from musculoskeletal disorders, but they can also stem from neurovascular, cardiovascular, or neurologic disorders.

memory board

The 5 Ps of musculoskeletal injury

Pain—Does the patient feel pain? If so, assess its location, severity, and quality.
Paresthesia—Assess for loss of sensation by touching the injured area with the tip of an open safety pin. Abnormal sensation or loss of sensation indicates neurovascular involvement.
Paralysis—Can the patient move the affected area? If not, the patient may have nerve or tendon damage.
Pallor—Paleness, discoloration, and coolness on the injured side may indicate neurovascular compromise.
Pulse—Check all pulses distal to the injury site. If a pulse is decreased or absent, blood supply to the area is reduced.

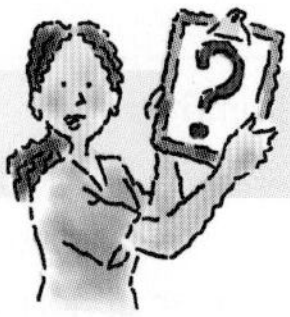

Outside the norm

Scoliosis

In a patient with scoliosis, lateral deviation of the spine is present and the patient leans to the side. Other findings include the following:

- uneven shoulder blade height and shoulder blade prominence
- unequal distance between the arms and the body
- asymmetrical waistline
- uneven hip height

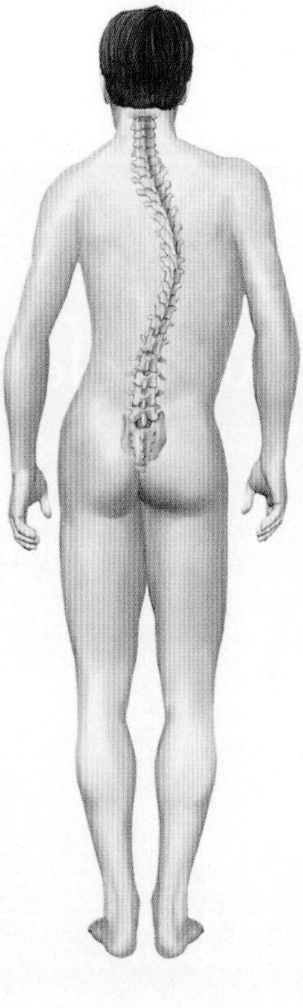

Kyphosis and lordosis

Kyphosis

If the patient has pronounced kyphosis, the thoracic curve is abnormally rounded, as shown below.

Lordosis

If the patient has pronounced lordosis, the lumbar spine is abnormally concave, as shown below. Lordosis (as well as a waddling gait) is normal in pregnant women and young children.

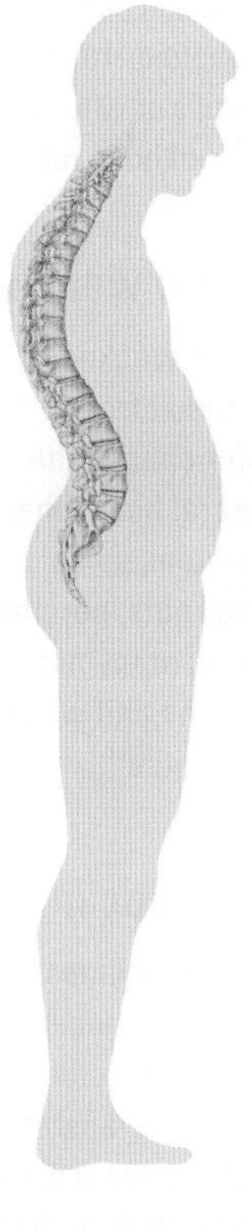

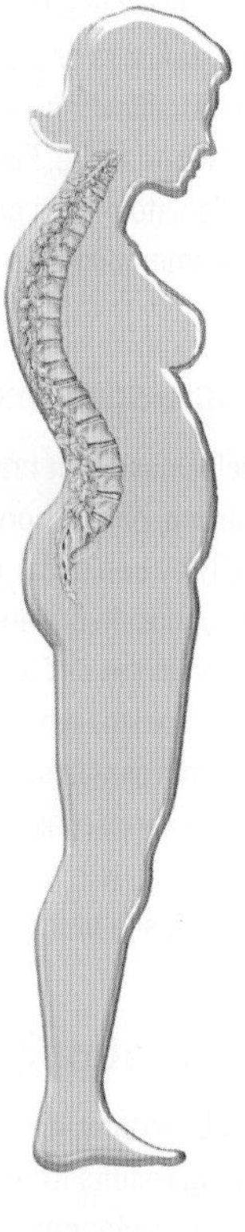

Heberden and Bouchard nodes

Heberden and Bouchard nodes are typically seen in patients with osteoarthritis, a chronic deterioration of the joint cartilage that commonly occurs in the hips, knees, and joints of the fingers. The nodes may be red, swollen, and painful initially. Eventually, they become painless but are associated with limited joint mobility.

Heberden nodes

Heberden nodes are hard, bony, and cartilaginous enlargements that appear on the distal interphalangeal joints.

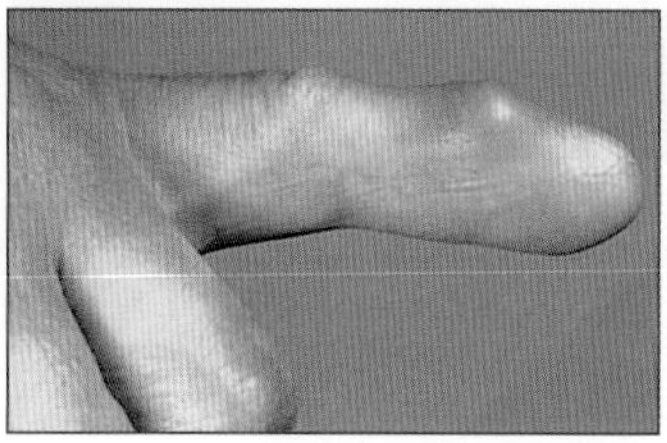

Bouchard nodes

Bouchard nodes are similar but less common and appear on the proximal interphalangeal joints.

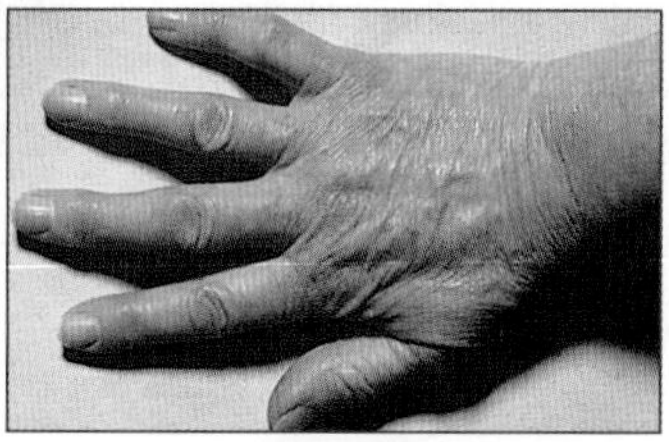

Ganglion

A ganglion is a round, enlarged, fluid-filled cyst commonly found on the dorsal side of the wrist. A ganglion may be nontender, but when it develops near a tender sheath, it may be painful and may limit joint mobility.

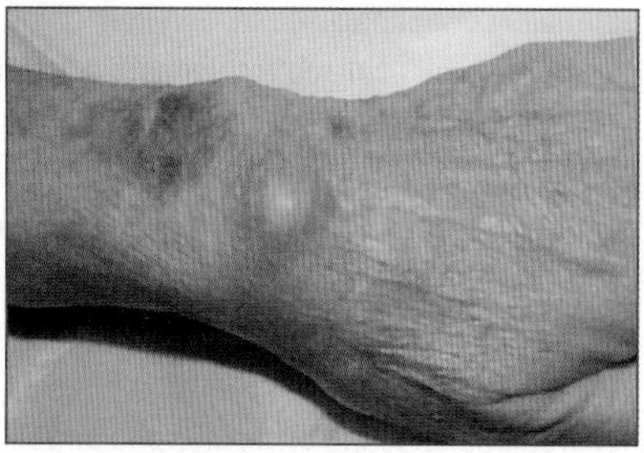

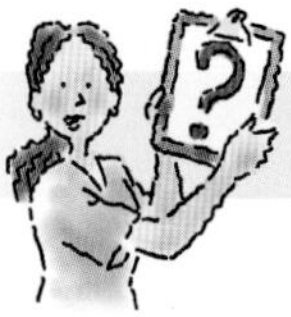

Outside the norm

Rheumatoid arthritis

A chronic, systemic inflammatory immune disorder, rheumatoid arthritis commonly affects bilateral joints of the fingers, wrists, elbows, knees, or ankles as well as surrounding muscles, tendons, ligaments, and blood vessels. Spontaneous remissions and unpredictable exacerbations mark the course of this potentially crippling disease. Swollen, painful, and stiff joints, especially of the hands, are typical in acute rheumatoid arthritis.

As the disease progresses, bone atrophy and misalignment cause visible deformities, restriction of movement, and muscle atrophy. In chronic rheumatoid arthritis, deformities of the interphalangeal joints develop. Swan-neck deformity—hyperextension of the proximal interphalangeal joints with flexion of the distal interphalangeal joints—may occur. A less common deformity is the boutonnière deformity—flexion of the proximal interphalangeal joint with hyperextension of the distal interphalangeal joint.

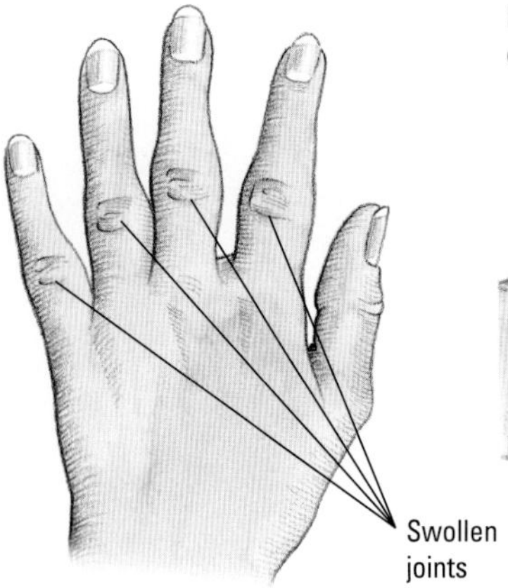
Swollen joints

Acute rheumatoid arthritis

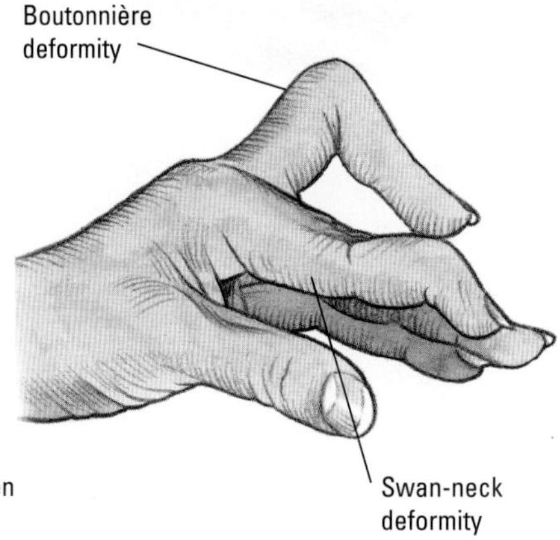
Boutonnière deformity
Swan-neck deformity

Chronic rheumatoid arthritis

Gout

Gout is a metabolic disorder in which uric acid deposits in the joints cause the joints to become painful, arthritic, red, and swollen. Skin temperature may be elevated due to the irritation and inflammation.

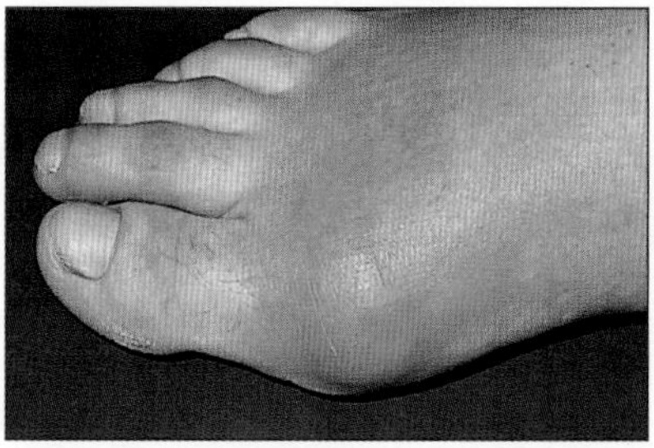

Muscular dystrophy

Muscular dystrophy is a group of congenital disorders characterized by progressive symmetrical wasting of skeletal muscles without neural or sensory defects. The most common form is Duchenne (pseudohypertrophic) muscular dystrophy. Duchenne occurs during early childhood; onset is insidious and occurs between ages 3 and 5. The disorder initially affects the legs, pelvis, and shoulders. Findings include the following:

- enlarged, firm calf muscles
- waddling gait, toe-walking, lumbar lordosis, and positive Gower sign
- difficulty climbing stairs
- history of frequent falls

Gower sign

A positive Gower sign—an inability to lift the trunk without using the hands and arms to brace and push—indicates pelvic muscle weakness, as occurs in muscular dystrophy and spinal muscle atrophy. To check for Gower sign, place the patient in the supine position and ask the patient to rise.

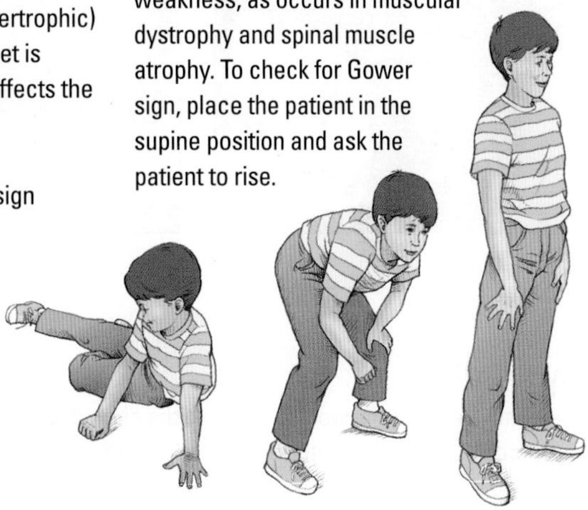

Muscles affected by Duchenne

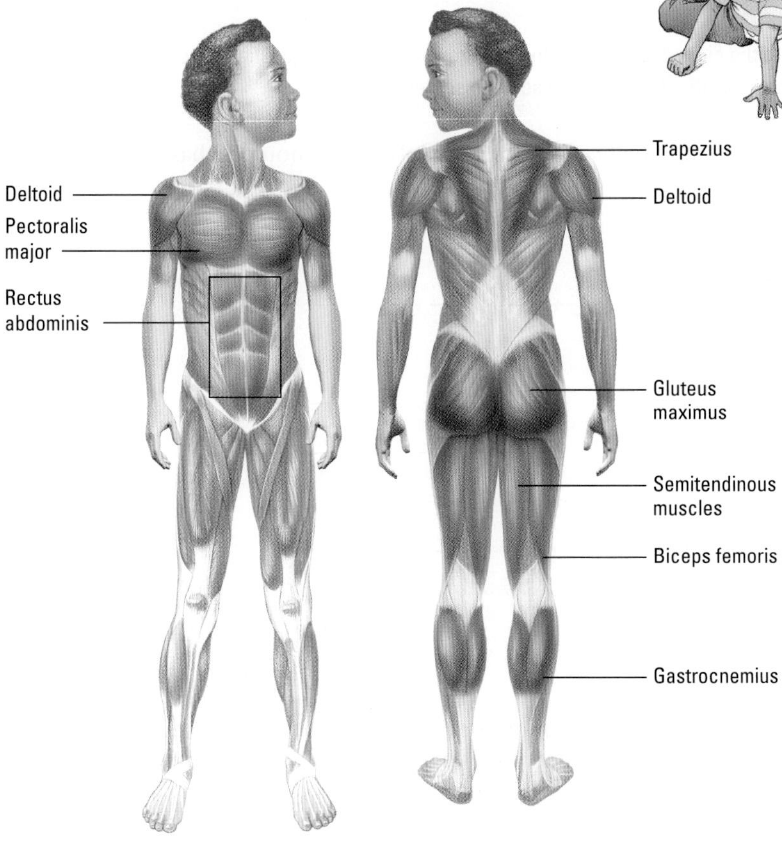
Deltoid
Pectoralis major
Rectus abdominis
Trapezius
Deltoid
Gluteus maximus
Semitendinous muscles
Biceps femoris
Gastrocnemius

Q&A

Show and tell

Name and describe the assessment techniques shown for testing muscle strength.

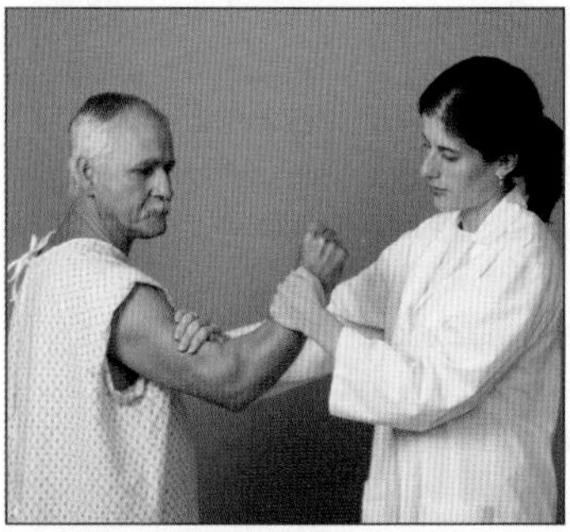

1. ____________________

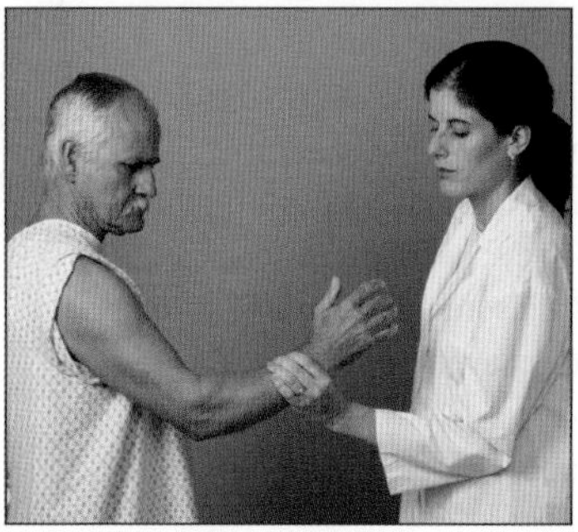

2. ____________________

My word!

Unscramble each of the words. Then use the circled letters from those words to answer the question posed here. Hint: The words listed are all related to the muscles affected by this muscular disorder.

Question: What muscular disorder that initially affects the legs, pelvis, and shoulders has an insidious onset that occurs between ages and 5?

1. diedlot _ _ _ _ _ _ (_)
2. alicesport jarom _ _ (_) _ _ _ _ _ _ _   _ _ _ _ _
3. azuretips _ _ _ _ (_) _ _ _ _
4. useglut summaxi _ _ _ _ _ _ (_)   _ _ _ _ _ _ _
5. custer biasdimno _ _ _ _ _ _   _ _ _ _ _ _ (_) _ _
6. piesbc semifor _ _ _ (_) _ _   _ _ _ _ _ _ _
7. anecgissumrot _ _ _ _ _ _ _ (_) _ _ _ (_) _
8. dothyspry _ _ _ _ _ _ _ (_) _

Answer: _ _ _ _ _ _ _ _ ' _

Answers: Show and tell 1. Biceps strength—The examiner pulls down on the flexor surface of the patient's forearm as the patient resists, 2. Triceps strength—The patient straightens the arm as the examiner pushes upward against the extensor surface of the forearm; My word! 1. Deltoid, 2. Pectoralis major, 3. Trapezius, 4. Gluteus maximus, 5. Rectus abdominis, 6. Biceps femoris, 7. Gastrocnemius, 8. Dystrophy; Question: Duchenne.

Selected References

Beighton, P., Grahame, R., & Bird, H. (2012). Assessment of hypermobility. In *Hypermobility of joints* (pp. 11–26). London: Springer.

Drakonaki, E. E., Allen, G. M., & Wilson, D. J. (2014). Ultrasound elastography for musculoskeletal applications. *Ultrasound, 85*(1019).

Kennedy, I., & Caldwell, K. (2014). A cross-sectional postal survey of musculoskeletal physiotherapists' current practice of cervical pain assessment in relation to vertebrobasilar artery insufficiency, attitudes toward guidelines, and manual therapy practice. *International Musculoskeletal Medicine, 36*(4), 137–149.

Naraghi, A., & White, L. M. (2012). Three-dimensional MRI of the musculoskeletal system. *American Journal of Roentgenology, 199*(3), W283–W293.

Nicolaou, S., Liang, T., Murphy, D. T., Korzan, J. R., Ouellette, H., & Munk, P. (2012). Dual-energy CT: A promising new technique for assessment of the musculoskeletal system. *American Journal of Roentgenology, 199*(5_supplement), S78–S86.

Rimondi, E., Rossi, G., Bartalena, T., Ciminari, R., Alberghini, M., Ruggieri, P., … Mercuri, M. (2011). Percutaneous CT-guided biopsy of the musculoskeletal system: Results of 2027 cases. *European Journal of Radiology, 77*(1), 34–42.

Roman-Liu, D. (2013). External load and the reaction of the musculoskeletal system—A conceptual model of the interaction. *International Journal of Industrial Ergonomics, 43*(4), 356–362.

Vincent, H. K., Raiser, S. N., & Vincent, K. R. (2012). The aging musculoskeletal system and obesity-related considerations with exercise. *Ageing Research Reviews, 11*(3), 361–373.

Vlaeyen, J. W., & Linton, S. J. (2012). Fear-avoidance model of chronic musculoskeletal pain: 12 years on. *Pain, 153*(6), 1144–1147.

Wolf, J. M., Cameron, K. L., & Owens, B. D. (2011). Impact of joint laxity and hypermobility on the musculoskeletal system. *Journal of the American Academy of Orthopaedic Surgeons, 19*(8), 463–471.

Chapter 10

Neurologic system

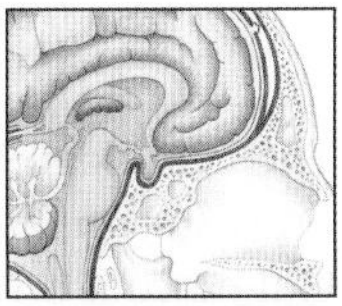
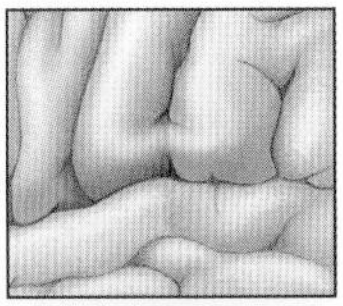
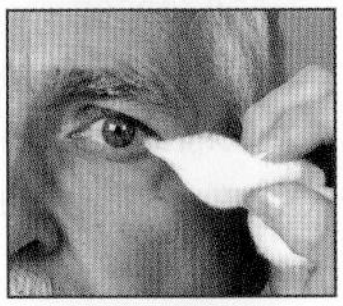
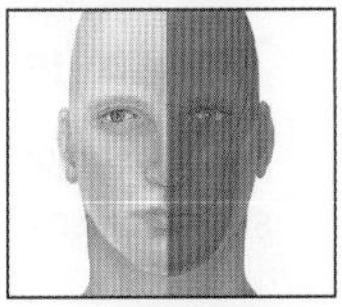
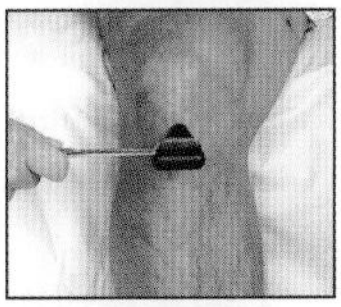
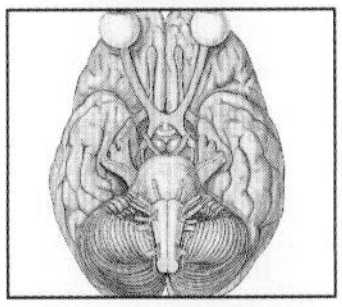
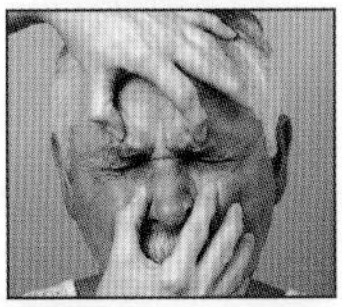
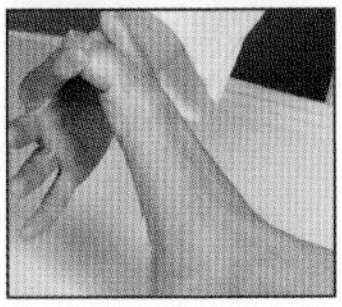
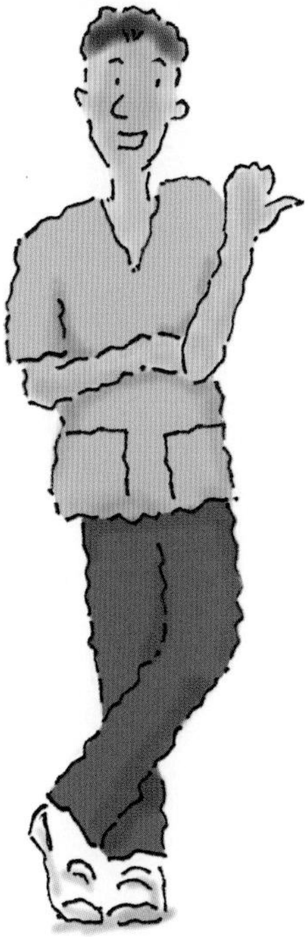

Anatomy

The neurologic system controls body function and is related to every other body system. It's divided into the central nervous system (CNS), the peripheral nervous system, and the autonomic nervous system.

Cerebrum

- Controls ability to think and reason
- Enclosed by three meninges (dura mater, arachnoid mater, and pia mater)

Thalamus

- Relay station for sensory impulses

Brain stem

- Controls heart rate and rate of breathing

Cerebellum

- Contains major motor and sensory pathways
- Helps maintain equilibrium
- Controls muscle coordination

Hypothalamus

- Controls regulatory functions, including temperature control, pituitary hormone production, and water balance

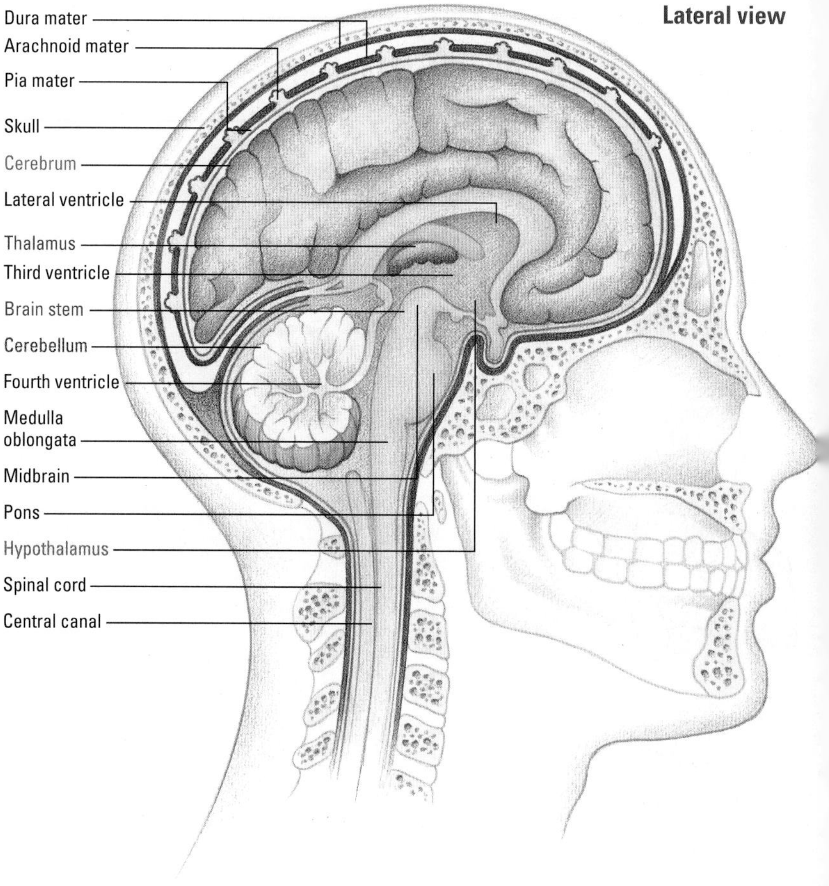
Lateral view
Dura mater
Arachnoid mater
Pia mater
Skull
Cerebrum
Lateral ventricle
Thalamus
Third ventricle
Brain stem
Cerebellum
Fourth ventricle
Medulla oblongata
Midbrain
Pons
Hypothalamus
Spinal cord
Central canal

Central nervous system

The CNS includes the brain and spinal cord. These two structures collect and interpret voluntary and involuntary motor and sensory stimuli.

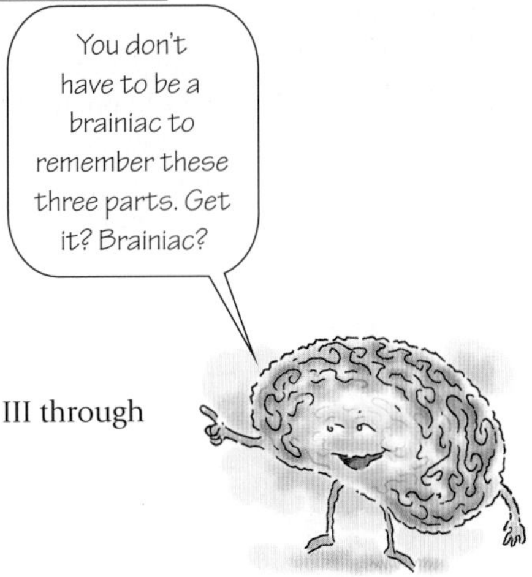
You don't have to be a brainiac to remember these three parts. Get it? Brainiac?

Brain

The brain consists of the cerebrum (or *cerebral cortex*), brain stem, and cerebellum. The diencephalon, a division of the cerebrum, contains the thalamus and hypothalamus. The brain stem, which lies below the diencephalon, contains cranial nerves III through XII and regulates automatic body functions, such as heart rate, breathing, and swallowing.

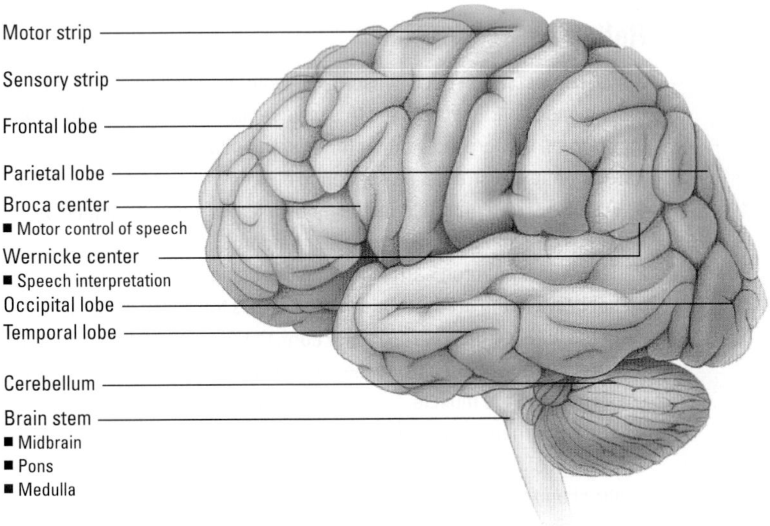
Motor strip
Sensory strip
Frontal lobe
Parietal lobe
Broca center
■ Motor control of speech
Wernicke center
■ Speech interpretation
Occipital lobe
Temporal lobe
Cerebellum
Brain stem
■ Midbrain
■ Pons
■ Medulla

Cerebral lobes and hemispheres

The cerebrum is divided into four lobes and two hemispheres. The right hemisphere controls the left side of the body, and the left hemisphere controls the right side of the body.

Frontal lobe
- Motor control of voluntary muscles
- Personality
- Concentration
- Organization
- Problem solving

Temporal lobe
- Hearing
- Memory of hearing and vision

Parietal lobe
- Sensory areas for touch, pain, and temperature
- Understanding of speech and language
- Thought expression

Occipital lobe
- Visual recognition
- Focus of the eye

Spinal cord

The spinal cord is the primary pathway for messages traveling between the peripheral areas of the body and the brain. It also mediates the sensory-to-motor transmission path known as the *reflex arc*. Because the reflex arc enters and exits the spinal cord at the same level, reflex pathways don't need to travel up and down the way other stimuli do. The spinal cord extends from the upper border of the first cervical vertebra to the lower border of the first lumbar vertebra. It's encased and protected by a continuation of the meninges and cerebrospinal fluid of the brain. It's also protected by the bony vertebrae of the spine.

Lateral view

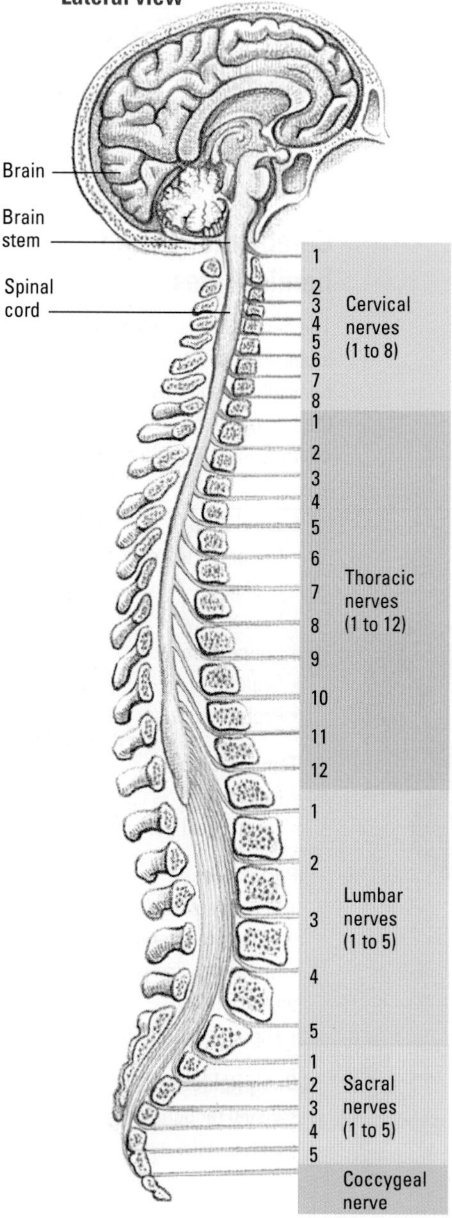
Brain
Brain stem
Spinal cord
1 2 3 4 5 6 7 8
Cervical nerves (1 to 8)
1 2 3 4 5 6 7 8 9 10 11 12
Thoracic nerves (1 to 12)
1 2 3 4 5
Lumbar nerves (1 to 5)
1 2 3 4 5
Sacral nerves (1 to 5)
Coccygeal nerve

Matter of impulse

The dorsal white matter within the spinal cord contains the ascending tracts that carry impulses up the spinal cord to higher sensory centers. The ventral white matter within the spinal cord contains the descending motor tracts that transmit motor impulses down from the higher motor centers to the spinal cord.

Reflex arc

Spinal nerves, which have sensory and motor portions, control deep tendon and superficial reflexes. A simple reflex arc requires a sensory (or *afferent*) neuron and a motor (or *efferent*) neuron. The knee-jerk, or *patellar,* reflex illustrates the sequence of events in a normal reflex arc:

1. A **sensory receptor** detects the mechanical stimulus produced by the reflex hammer striking the patellar tendon.
2. The sensory neuron carries the impulse along its axon by way of the **spinal nerve** to the **dorsal root**, where it enters the spinal column.
3. In the **anterior horn of the spinal cord,** the sensory neuron joins with a motor neuron, which carries the impulse along its axon by way of a spinal nerve to the muscle.
4. The motor neuron transmits the impulse to the muscle fibers through stimulation of the **motor end plate.** This impulse triggers the muscle to contract and the leg to extend.

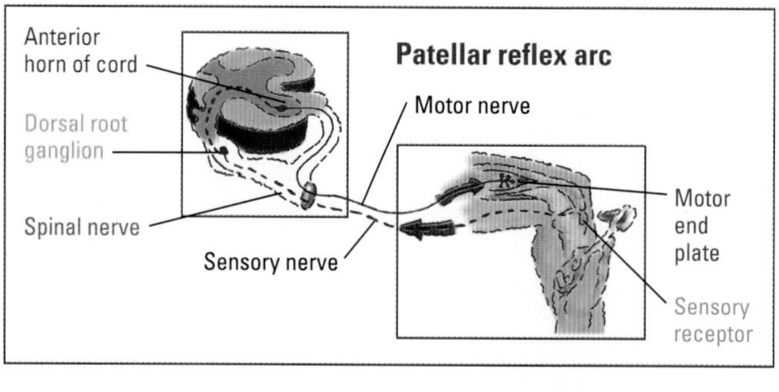
Patellar reflex arc
Anterior horn of cord
Dorsal root ganglion
Spinal nerve
Sensory nerve
Motor nerve
Motor end plate
Sensory receptor

Peripheral nervous system

The peripheral nervous system includes the peripheral and cranial nerves:

- Peripheral sensory nerves transmit stimuli to the posterior horn of the spinal cord from sensory receptors located in the skin, muscles, sensory organs, and viscera. The area of skin that's innervated by each sensory nerve is called a *dermatome*.
- The 12 pairs of cranial nerves are the primary motor and sensory pathways between the brain, head, and neck.

Cranial nerves

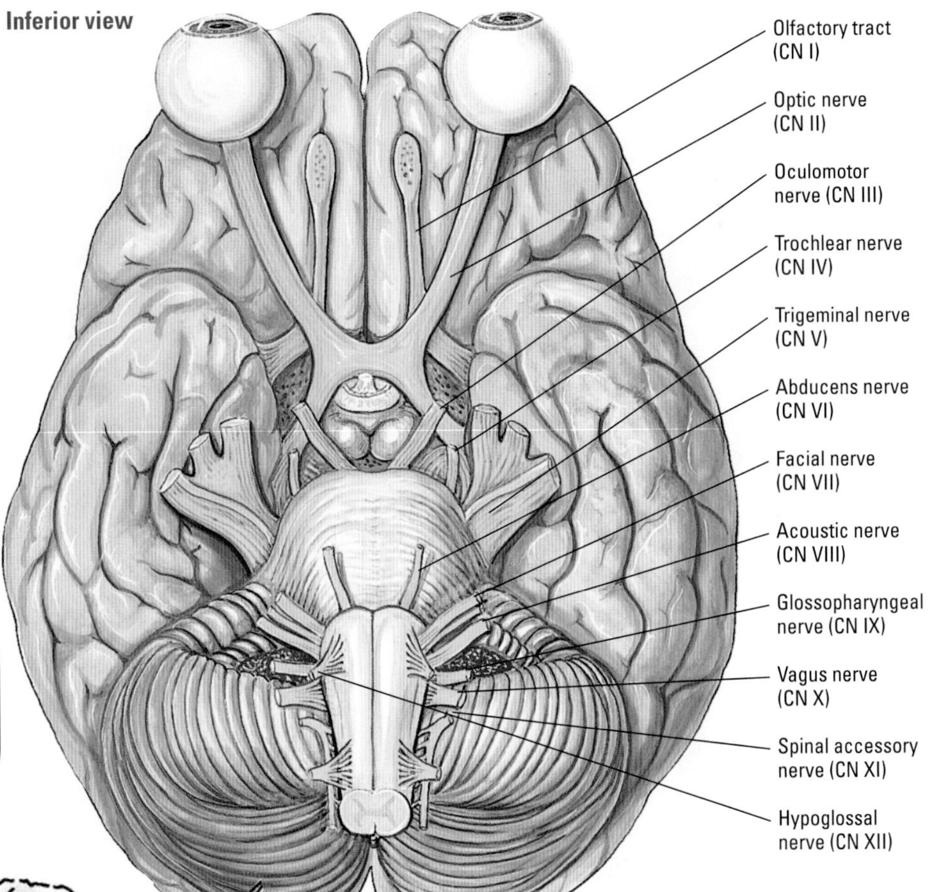
Inferior view
Olfactory tract (CN I)
Optic nerve (CN II)
Oculomotor nerve (CN III)
Trochlear nerve (CN IV)
Trigeminal nerve (CN V)
Abducens nerve (CN VI)
Facial nerve (CN VII)
Acoustic nerve (CN VIII)
Glossopharyngeal nerve (CN IX)
Vagus nerve (CN X)
Spinal accessory nerve (CN XI)
Hypoglossal nerve (CN XII)

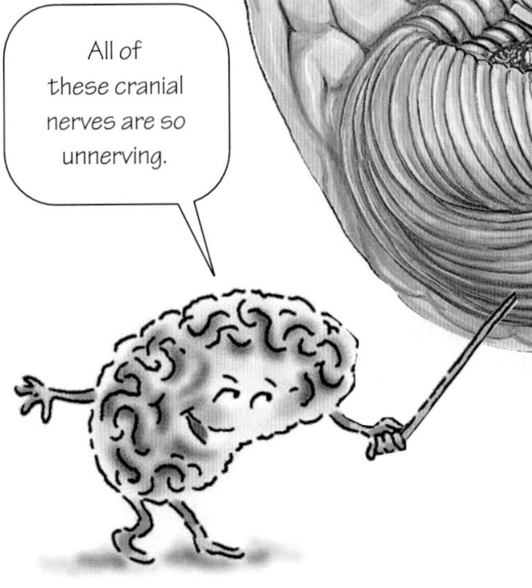
All of these cranial nerves are so unnerving.

Dermatomes

For the purpose of documenting sensory function, the body is divided into dermatomes. Each dermatome represents an area supplied with sensory nerve fibers from an individual spinal root—cervical (C), thoracic (T), lumbar (L), or sacral (S).

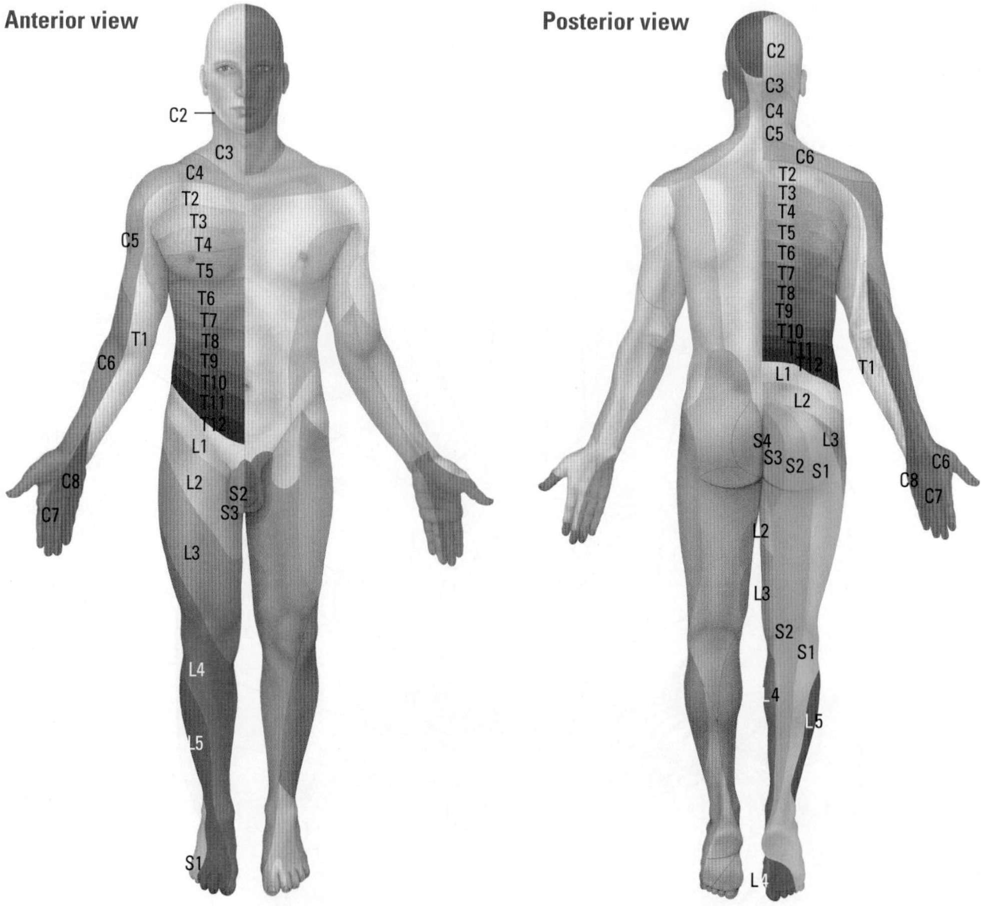
Anterior view
C2
C3
C4
T2
T3
C5
T4
T5
T6
T7
T1
T8
C6
T9
T10
T11
T12
L1
C8
L2
S2
C7
S3
L3
L4
L5
S1
Posterior view
C2
C3
C4
C5
C6
T2
T3
T4
T5
T6
T7
T8
T9
T10
T11
T12
T1
L1
L2
S4
L3
S3
S2
S1
C6
C8
C7
L2
L3
S2
S1
L4
L5
L4

Autonomic nervous system

The autonomic nervous system contains motor neurons that regulate the activities of the visceral organs and affect the smooth and cardiac muscles and glands. It consists of two parts:

- sympathetic division, which controls fight-or-flight reactions
- parasympathetic division, which maintains baseline body functions

Assessment

A complete neurologic examination is long and detailed, and you probably won't perform one in its entirety. However, if your initial screening examination suggests a neurologic problem, you may want to perform a detailed assessment.

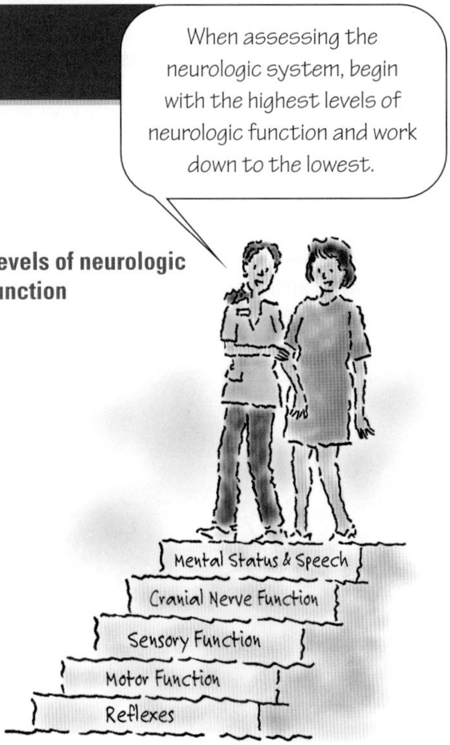
When assessing the neurologic system, begin with the highest levels of neurologic function and work down to the lowest.
Mental Status & Speech
Cranial Nerve Function
Sensory Function
Motor Function
Reflexes

Levels of neurologic function

Assessing mental status and speech

Mental status assessment begins during the health history. How the patient responds to your questions gives clues to the patient's orientation and memory. Be sure to ask questions that require more than "yes" or "no" answers. Otherwise, confusion or disorientation may not be immediately apparent. If you have doubts about a patient's mental status, perform a screening examination.

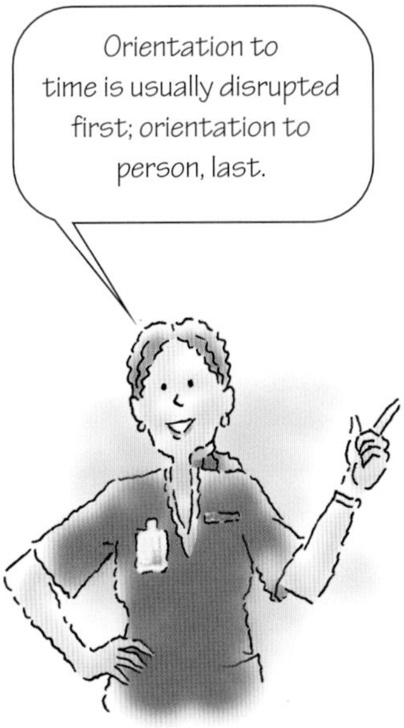
Orientation to time is usually disrupted first; orientation to person, last.

A quick check of mental status

To quickly screen a patient for disordered thought processes, ask the questions below. An incorrect answer to any question may indicate the need for a complete mental status examination.

Question	Function screened
What's your name?	Orientation to person
What's your mother's name?	Orientation to other people
What year is it?	Orientation to time
Where are you now?	Orientation to place
How old are you?	Memory
Where were you born?	Remote memory
What did you have for breakfast?	Recent memory
Who's currently the US president?	General knowledge
Can you count backward from 20 to 1?	Attention span and calculation skills

Level of consciousness

To assess level of consciousness (LOC), clearly describe the patient's response to various stimuli.

Alert

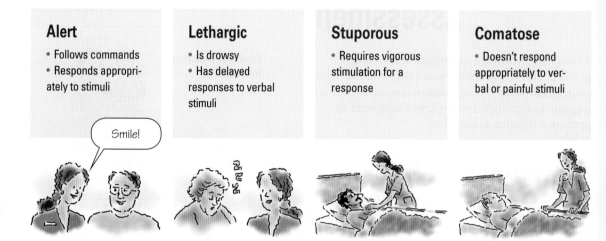

- Follows commands
- Responds appropriately to stimuli

Smile!

Lethargic

- Is drowsy
- Has delayed responses to verbal stimuli

Stuporous

- Requires vigorous stimulation for a response

Comatose

- Doesn't respond appropriately to verbal or painful stimuli

Appearance and behavior

Are the patient's appearance and behavior inappropriate? Is the patient's personal hygiene poor? If so, discuss your findings with the family to determine whether this is a change or if this is their baseline. Even subtle changes in behavior can signal new onset of a chronic disease or a more acute change that involves the frontal lobe.

Speech

Listen to how well the patients can express themselves. Is the patient's speech fluent or fragmented? Note the pace, volume, clarity, and spontaneity of the speech. To assess for dysarthria (difficulty forming words), ask the patient to repeat the phrase "No ifs, ands, or buts."

Cognitive function

Test orientation, memory, and attention span using the mental status questions on page 195. Note the patient's ability to pay attention.

Content clarity

Assess thought content by evaluating the clarity and cohesiveness of the patients' ideas. Do they use logical transitions between ideas? Does the patient have hallucinations (sensory perceptions that lack appropriate stimuli) or delusions (beliefs not supported by reality)?

Proverbial test

Test the patient's ability to think abstractly by asking the patient to interpret a common proverb such as "A stitch in time saves nine." A patient with dementia may interpret this proverb literally. If the patient's primary language isn't English, have a family member ask the patient to explain a saying in the patient's native language, if possible.

Let's say…

Test judgment by asking the patient how he or she would respond to a hypothetical situation. For example, what would the patient do if while in a public building and the fire alarm sounded? Evaluate the appropriateness of the answer.

In the mood

Throughout the interview, note the patient's mood, emotional lability or stability, and the appropriateness of emotional responses.

Constructional ability

Observe the patient's ability to perform simple tasks and use various objects. Constructional disorders affect this ability.

Not a numbers person?

When testing attention span and calculation skills, keep in mind that lack of mathematical ability and anxiety can affect the patient's performance. If the patient has difficulty with numerical computation, ask the patient to spell the word "world" backward.

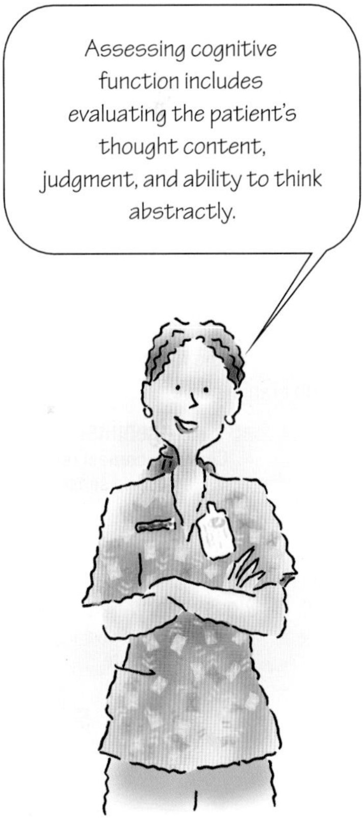
Assessing cognitive function includes evaluating the patient's thought content, judgment, and ability to think abstractly.

Assessing cranial nerve function

Cranial nerve assessment reveals valuable information about the condition of the CNS, especially the brain stem. Because of their location, some cranial nerves are more vulnerable to the effects of increasing intracranial pressure (ICP). Therefore, cranial nerve assessment focuses on four key nerves. Evaluate other nerves if the patient's history or symptoms indicate a potential CNS disorder or when performing a complete nervous system assessment.

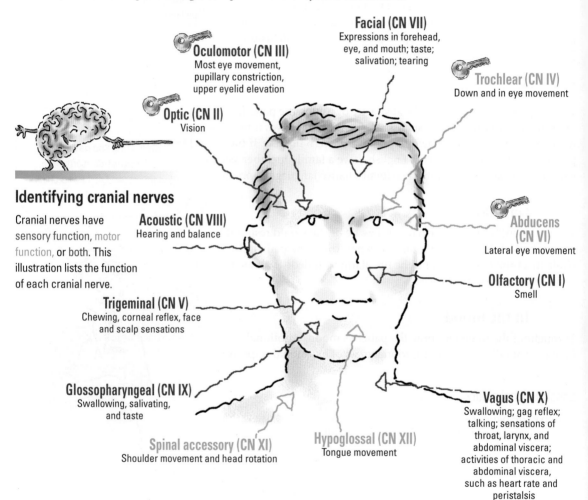

Identifying cranial nerves

Cranial nerves have sensory function, motor function, or both. This illustration lists the function of each cranial nerve.

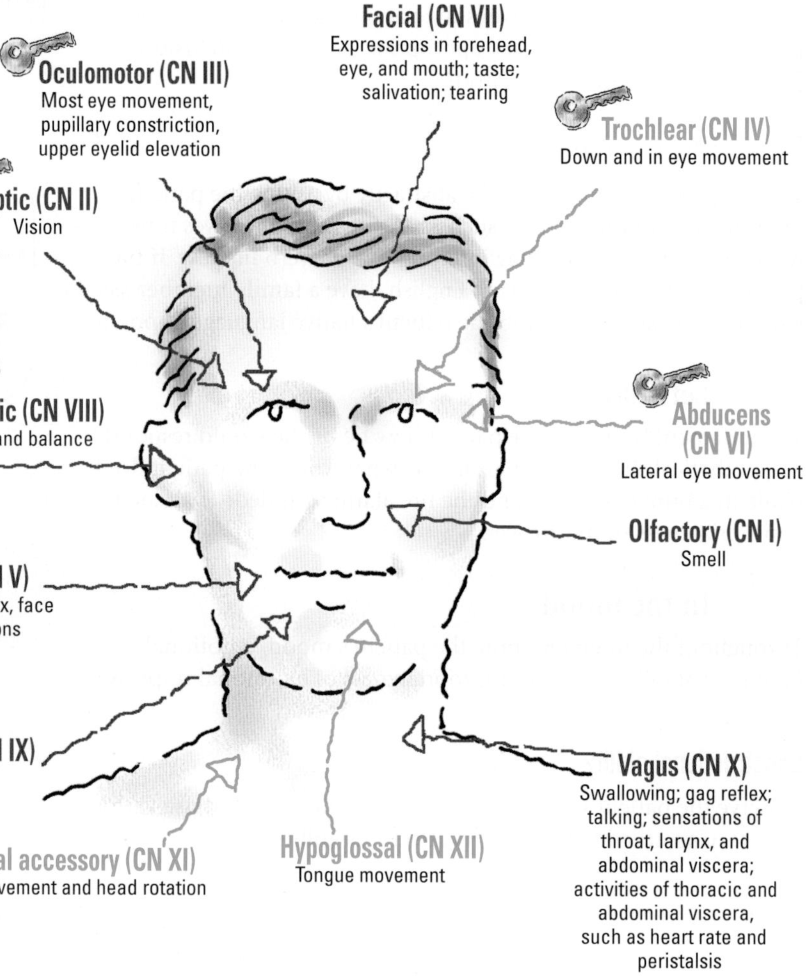
Facial (CN VII)
Expressions in forehead, eye, and mouth; taste; salivation; tearing
Oculomotor (CN III)
Most eye movement, pupillary constriction, upper eyelid elevation
Trochlear (CN IV)
Down and in eye movement
Optic (CN II)
Vision
Acoustic (CN VIII)
Hearing and balance
Abducens (CN VI)
Lateral eye movement
Olfactory (CN I)
Smell
Trigeminal (CN V)
Chewing, corneal reflex, face and scalp sensations
Glossopharyngeal (CN IX)
Swallowing, salivating, and taste
Vagus (CN X)
Swallowing; gag reflex; talking; sensations of throat, larynx, and abdominal viscera; activities of thoracic and abdominal viscera, such as heart rate and peristalsis
Spinal accessory (CN XI)
Shoulder movement and head rotation
Hypoglossal (CN XII)
Tongue movement

Olfactory nerve

Ask the patient to identify at least two common substances, such as coffee and cinnamon. Make sure the patient's nostrils are patent before performing this test.

Optic nerve

Test visual acuity with a Snellen chart and the Rosenbaum near-vision card. Use confrontation to assess visual fields. Then perform an examination of the optic fundi.

Oculomotor nerve, trochlear nerve, and abducens nerve

Assess these nerves together using the corneal light reflex test, six cardinal positions of gaze, and cover-uncover test (see page 39). Also, inspect the size, shape, and symmetry of the pupils and pupillary reactions to light.

Trigeminal nerve

To assess the sensory component of the trigeminal nerve, ask the patient to close the eyes and then touch the patient with a wisp of cotton on the forehead, cheek, and jaw on each side. Next, test pain perception by touching the tip of a safety pin to the same three areas. Ask the patient to describe and compare both sensations.

To test the motor component, ask the patient to clench the teeth while you palpate the temporal and masseter muscles. Note the strength of the muscle contraction; it should be equal bilaterally. Then test the corneal reflex.

Skill check

Trigeminal nerve assessment sites

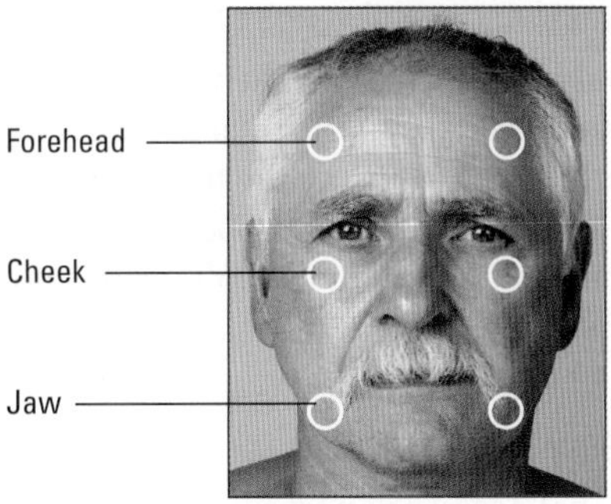
Forehead
Cheek
Jaw

Skill check

Assessing corneal reflex

To test the corneal reflex, touch a wisp of cotton from a cotton ball to the cornea, as shown. The patient should blink. If the patient doesn't, he or she may have suffered damage to the sensory fibers of cranial nerve V or to the motor fibers controlled by cranial nerve VII.

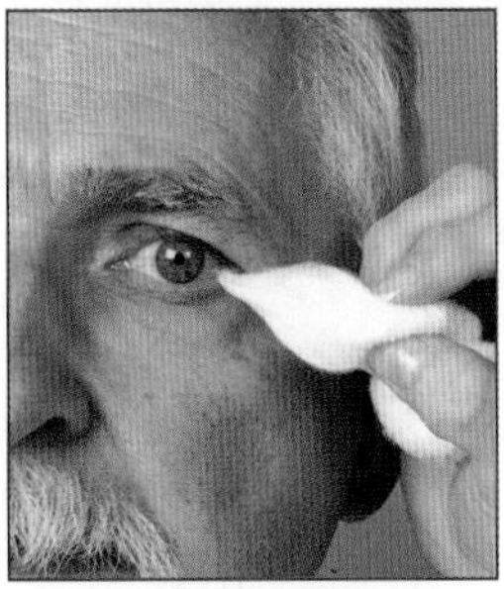

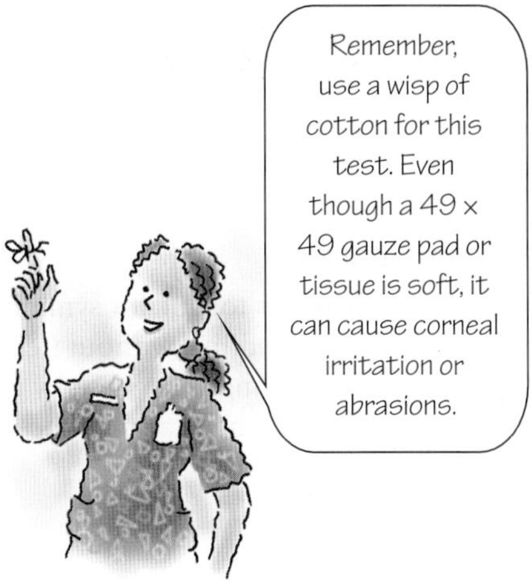
Remember, use a wisp of cotton for this test. Even though a 49 x 49 gauze pad or tissue is soft, it can cause corneal irritation or abrasions.

Facial nerve

To assess the sensory component, test taste by placing items with various tastes on the anterior portion of the patient's tongue—for example, sugar (sweet), salt, lemon juice (sour), and quinine (bitter). Assess motor function as described at right.

Acoustic nerve

To assess this nerve, use the Weber test and the Rinne test (see pages 44 and 45).

Skill check

Testing motor function of the facial nerve

To test motor function, observe the patient's face for symmetry at rest and while he or she smiles, frowns, and raises the eyebrows. Then have the patient close both eyes tightly. Test muscle strength by attempting to open the eyes, as shown.

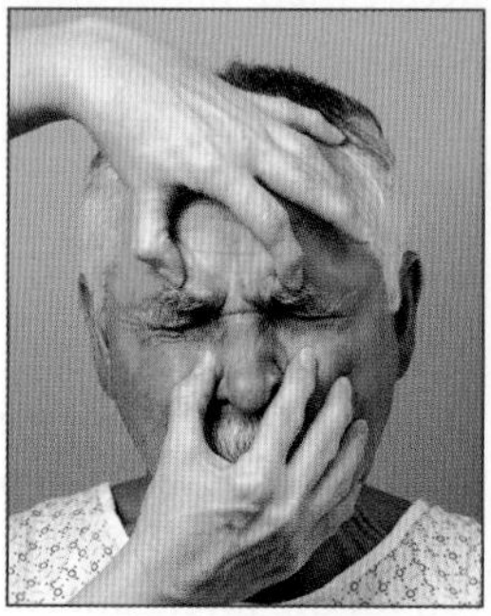

Glossopharyngeal nerve and vagus nerve

The glossopharyngeal nerve and the vagus nerve are tested together because their innervation overlaps in the pharynx. Listen to the patient's voice. Then check the gag reflex by touching the tip of a tongue blade against the posterior pharynx and asking the patient to open wide and say "ah." Watch for the symmetrical upward movement of the soft palate and uvula and for the midline position of the uvula.

Spinal accessory nerve

Assess the spinal accessory nerve by testing the strength of the sternocleidomastoid muscles and the upper portion of the trapezius muscle.

Skill check

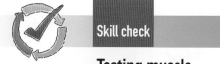

Testing muscle strength

- Place your palm against the patient's cheek.
- Ask the patient to turn the head against your resistance, as shown.
- Place your hands on the patient's shoulder and ask to shrug the shoulders against your resistance.
- Repeat each test on the other side, comparing muscle strength.

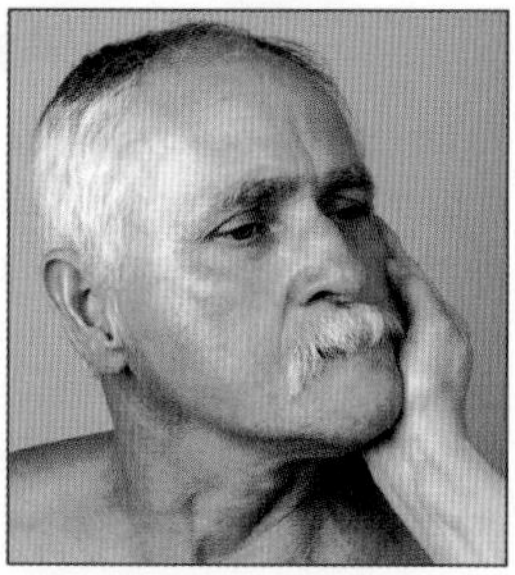

Hypoglossal nerve

Observe the patient's tongue for symmetry. The tongue should be midline, without tremors or fasciculations. Test tongue strength by asking the patient to push the tongue against the cheek as you apply resistance.

Assessing sensory function

Pain

Have the patient close the eyes; then touch all the major dermatomes, first with the sharp end of a safety pin and then with the dull end. Proceed in this order: 1 fingers, 2 shoulders, 3 toes, 4 thighs, and 5 trunk. Ask the patient to identify when he or she feels the sharp stimulus.

If the patient has major deficits, start in the area with the least sensation and move toward the area with the most sensation to help you determine the level of deficit.

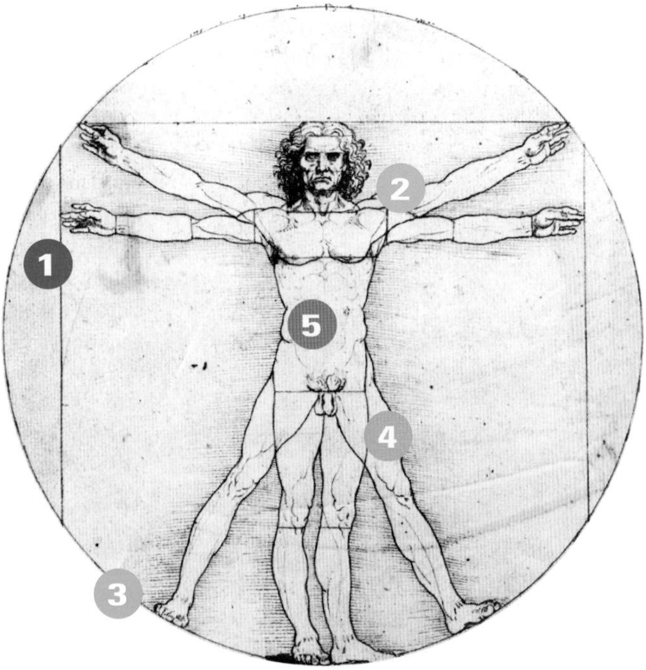
1
2
3
4
5

Light touch

To test for the sense of light touch, follow the same routine as above but use a wisp of cotton. A patient with a peripheral neuropathy might retain sensation for light touch after he or she has lost pain sensation.

Vibration

Apply a vibrating tuning fork over bony prominences while the patient keeps the eyes closed. Start at the distal interphalangeal joint of the index finger and move proximally. Then repeat the test over the interphalangeal joint of the big toe. Test only until the patient feels the vibration because everything above that level will be intact. If vibratory sense is intact, you won't have to check position sense because the same pathway carries both senses.

Skill check

Evaluating vibratory sense

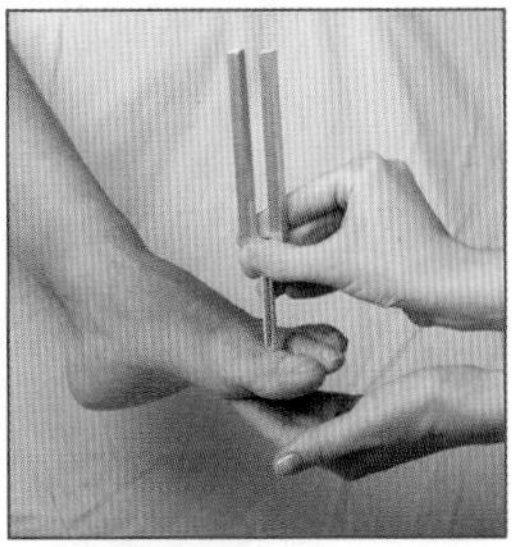

To evaluate vibratory sense, apply the base of a vibrating tuning fork to the interphalangeal joint of the patient's great toe, as shown.

Ask the patient what he or she feels. If the patient feels the sensation, he or she will typically report a feeling of buzzing or vibration. If the patient doesn't feel the sensation at the toe, try the medial malleolus. Then continue moving proximally until the patient feels the sensation. Note where the patient feels it, and then repeat the process on the other leg.

Position

To be tested for position sense, the patient needs intact vestibular and cerebellar function.

Skill check

Assessing position sense

Ask the patient to close the eyes. Then grasp the sides of the big toe, move the toe up and down, and ask the patient what position it's in. To test the patient's upper extremities, grasp the sides of the index finger and move it back and forth.

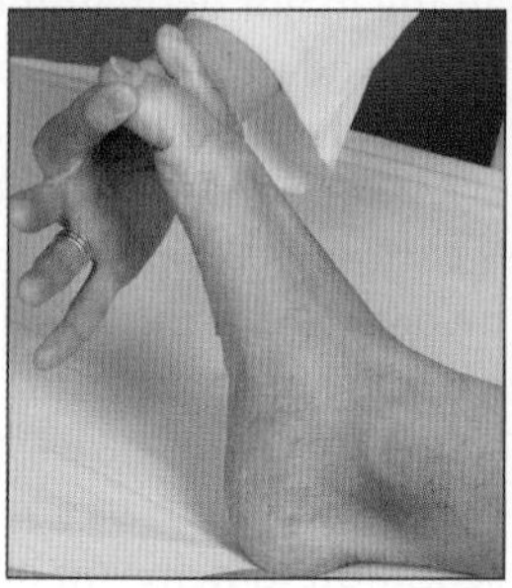

Discrimination

Discrimination testing assesses the ability of the cerebral cortex to interpret and integrate information. *Stereognosis* is the ability to discriminate the shape, size, weight, texture, and form of an object by touching and manipulating it.

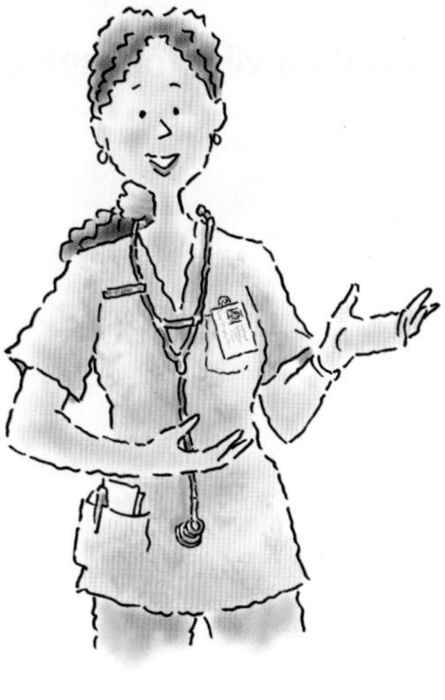

Skill check

Assessing discrimination

Ask the patient to close the eyes and open the hand. Place a common object, such as a key, in the hand and ask for the patient to identify it. If the patient can't identify the object, test graphesthesia—the ability to recognize figures or numbers written on the skin. Have the patient keep the eyes closed and hold out the hand while you trace a large number on the palm, as shown. Ask the patient to identify the number.

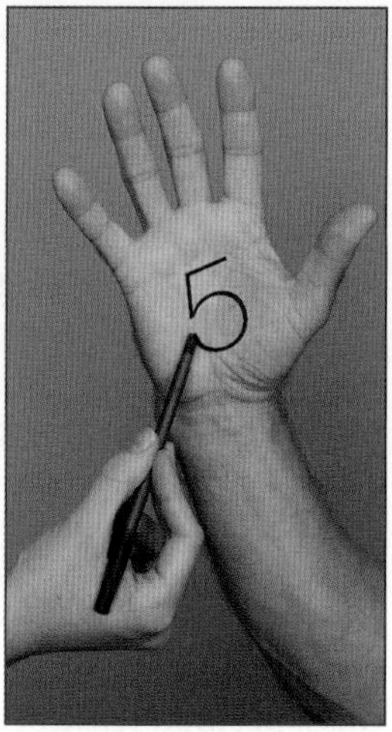
5

Assessing motor function

To assess motor function, inspect the muscles and test muscle tone and strength. Also conduct cerebellar testing because the cerebellum plays a role in smooth-muscle movements, such as tics, tremors, and fasciculations.

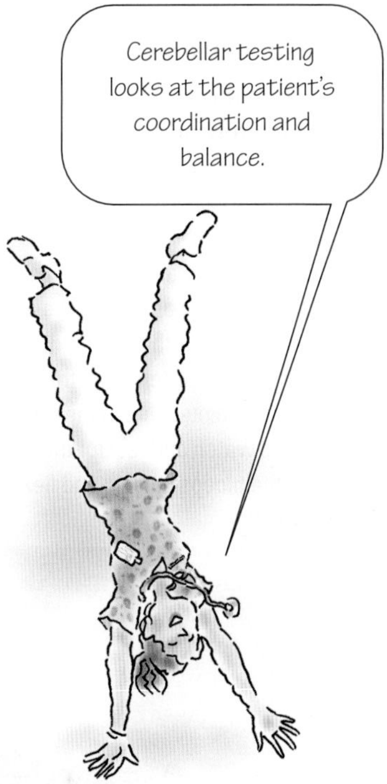
Cerebellar testing looks at the patient's coordination and balance.

Muscle tone

To test arm muscle tone, move the patient's shoulder through passive range-of-motion (ROM) exercises. You should feel a slight resistance. Then let the arm drop to the patient's side. It should fall easily.

To test leg muscle tone, guide the hip through passive ROM exercises; then let the leg fall to the bed. The leg shouldn't fall into an externally rotated position.

Muscle strength

Observe the patient's gait and motor activities. Then ask the patient to move major muscles and muscle groups against resistance.

Cerebellum

If the patients can sit and stand without support, observe them as they walk across the room, turn, and walk back. Note imbalances or abnormalities. A wide-based, unsteady gait indicates cerebellar dysfunction. Deviation to one side may indicate a cerebellar lesion on that side.

Ask the patients to walk heel to toe, and observe their balance. Then perform the Romberg test, as described at right.

1, 2, 3...

To assess rapid alternating movements, ask the patient to touch the thumb of the right hand to the right index finger and then to each of the remaining fingers. Next, ask the patient to sit with both palms resting on both thighs. Tell the patient to turn the palms up and down, gradually increasing the speed. These movements should be accurate and smooth.

Romberg test

- Observe the patient's balance as he or she stands with the eyes open, feet together, and arms at their sides.
- Ask the patient to close the eyes.
- Hold your arms out on either side of the patient to protect the patient if he or she sways.
- If the patient falls to one side, the result of the Romberg test is positive.

Assessing reflexes

Evaluating reflexes involves testing deep tendon and superficial reflexes and observing for primitive reflexes, such as grasp and sucking reflexes.

Deep tendon reflexes

Test deep tendon reflexes by moving from head to toe and comparing side to side.

Skill check

Biceps reflex

Position the patient's arm so the elbow is flexed at a 45-degree angle and the arm is relaxed. Place your thumb or index finger over the biceps tendon. Strike your finger with the pointed end of the reflex hammer, and watch and feel for the contraction of the biceps muscle and flexion of the forearm.

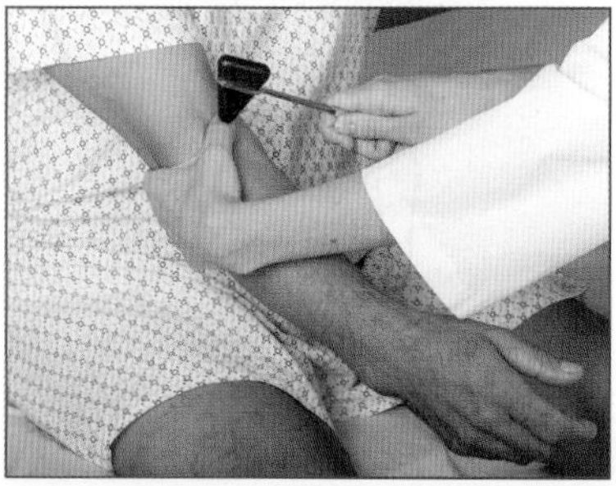

Triceps reflex

Ask the patient to adduct the arm and place the forearm across the chest. Strike the triceps tendon about 2″ (5 cm) above the olecranon process on the extensor surface of the upper arm. Watch for contraction of the triceps muscle and extension of the forearm.

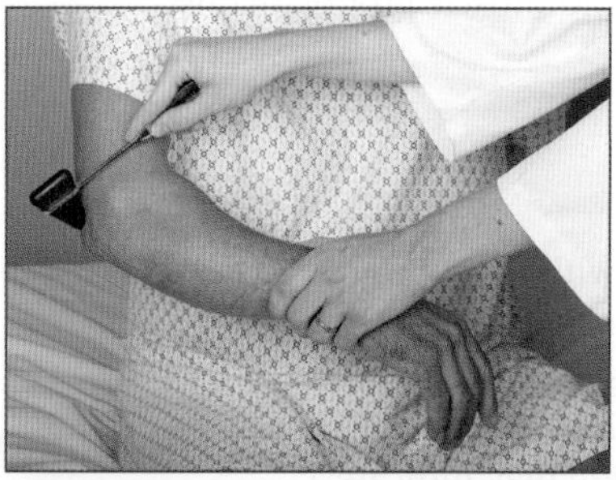

Brachioradialis reflex

Ask the patient to rest the ulnar surface of the hand on their abdomen or lap with the elbow partially flexed. Strike the radius, and watch for supination of the hand and flexion of the forearm at the elbow.

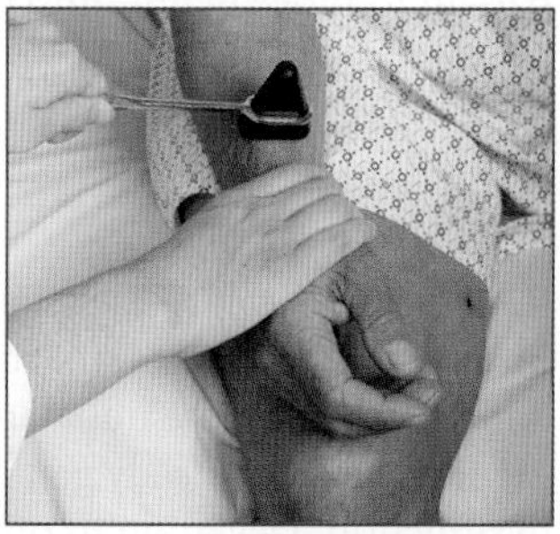

Patellar reflex

Ask the patient to sit with legs dangling freely. If the patient can't sit up, flex the knee at a 45-degree angle and place your nondominant hand behind it for support. Strike the patellar tendon just below the patella, and look for contraction of the quadriceps muscle in the thigh with extension of the leg.

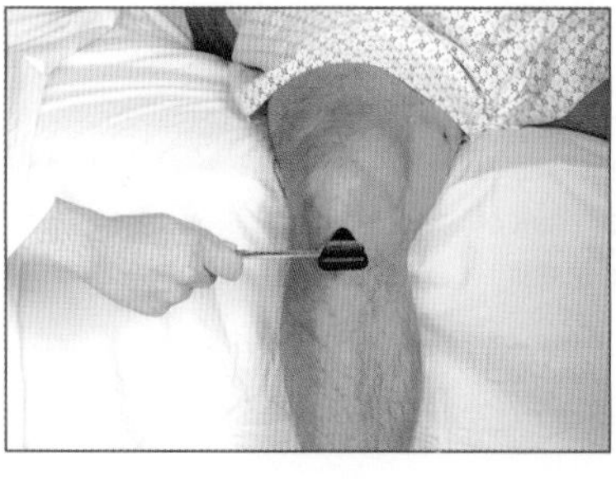

Achilles reflex

Ask the patient to flex the foot. Strike the Achilles tendon, and watch for plantar flexion of the foot at the ankle.

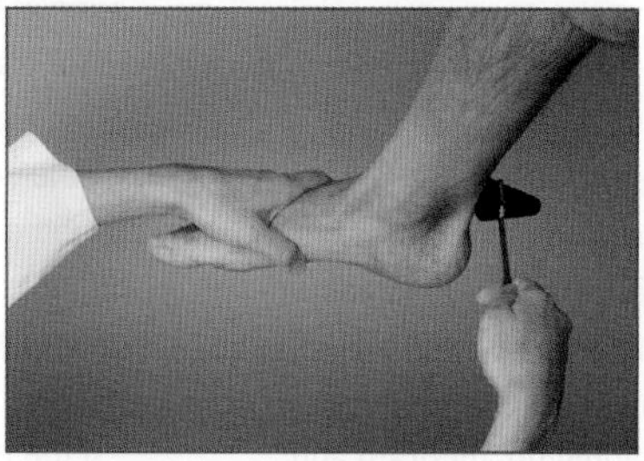

Making the grade

Grade deep tendon reflexes using this scale.

0 = Absent impulses
+1 = Diminished impulses
+2 = Normal impulses
+3 = Increased impulses
+4 = Hyperactive impulses

Superficial reflexes

Stimulating the skin or mucous membranes is a method of testing superficial reflexes. Because superficial reflexes are cutaneous reflexes, the more you try to elicit them in succession, the less of a response you'll get. Carefully observe for a response the first time you stimulate. Assess for plantar response and abdominal reflexes.

Test the abdominal reflexes with the patient in the supine position with arms at sides and the patient's knees slightly flexed. Briskly stroke both sides of the abdomen above and below the umbilicus, moving from the periphery toward the midline. Movement of the umbilicus toward the stimulus is normal.

In men, also assess for the cremasteric reflex. Use an applicator stick to stimulate the inner thigh. Normal reaction is contraction of the cremaster muscle and elevation of the testicle on the side of the stimulus.

Skill check

Testing for plantar response

To test for plantar response, use an applicator stick or tongue blade and slowly stroke the lateral side of the patient's sole from the heel to the great toe. The normal response in an adult is plantar flexion of the toes.

Dorsiflexion or upward movement of the great toe and fanning of the little toes is called the *Babinski reflex,* an abnormal response that may occur with upper motor neuron lesions.

Plantar response

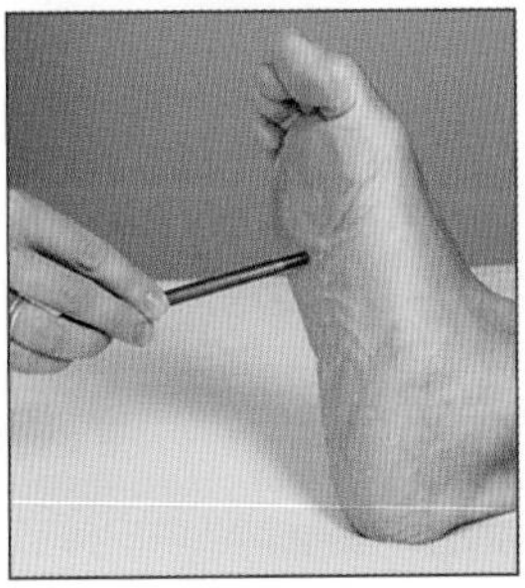

Babinski reflex

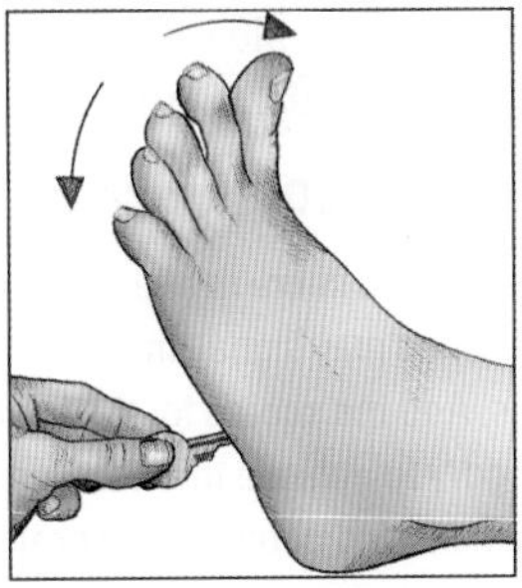

Primitive reflexes

Primitive reflexes are abnormal in an adult but normal in an infant, whose CNS is immature.

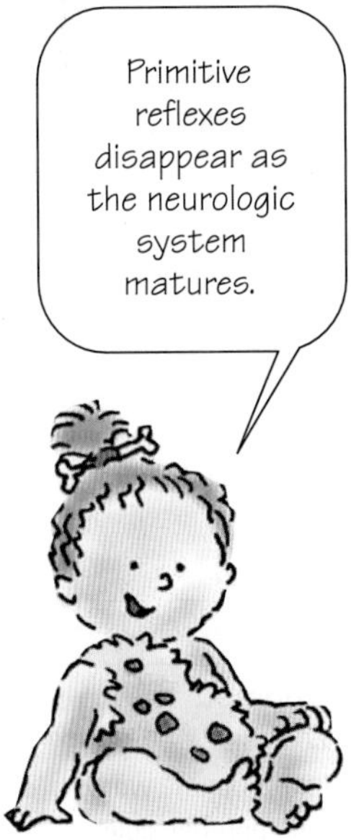
Primitive reflexes disappear as the neurologic system matures.

Grasp reflex

Apply gentle pressure to the patient's palm with your fingers. If the patient grasps your fingers between his or her index finger and thumb, suspect cortical or premotor cortex damage.

Snout reflex

Lightly tap on the patient's upper lip. Pursing of the lip is a positive snout reflex that indicates frontal lobe damage.

Sucking reflex

Observe the patients while you're feeding them, or, if the patient has an oral airway or endotracheal tube in place, observe the oral area. If you see a sucking motion, this indicates cortical damage. This reflex is commonly seen in patients with advanced dementia.

Glabella response

The glabella response is elicited by repeatedly tapping the bridge of the patient's nose. Persistent blinking indicates diffuse cortical dysfunction.

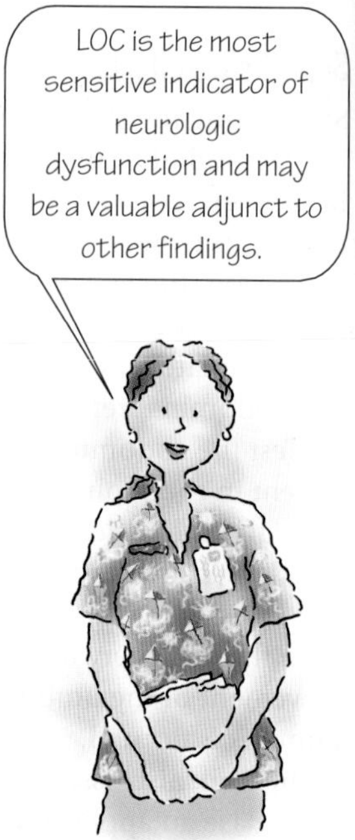
LOC is the most sensitive indicator of neurologic dysfunction and may be a valuable adjunct to other findings.

Abnormal findings

Abnormal neurologic findings include altered LOC, cranial nerve impairment, abnormal gaits, and meningeal irritation.

Altered level of consciousness

Consciousness may be impaired by any disorder that affects the cerebral hemisphere of the brain stem. When assessing LOC, make sure that you provide a stimulus that's strong enough to get a true picture of the patient's baseline. The Glasgow Coma Scale offers an objective way to assess the patient's LOC. Decerebrate and decorticate postures are indicators of severe neurologic damage.

Glasgow Coma Scale

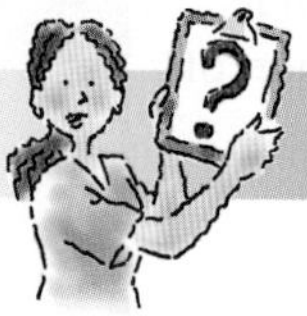

A decreased score in one or more of the following categories may signal an impending neurologic crisis. Add the scores for the best response in each category to achieve the total score. A total score of less than 9 indicates severe brain injury.

Test	Score	Patient's response
Eye opening		
Spontaneously	4	Opens eyes spontaneously
To speech	3	Opens eyes to verbal command
To pain	2	Opens eyes to painful stimulus
None	1	Doesn't open eyes in response to stimulus
Motor response		
Obeys	6	Reacts to verbal command
Localizes	5	Identifies localized pain
Withdraws	4	Assumes a decorticate position
Abnormal flexion	3	Assumes a decorticate position
Abnormal extension	2	Assumes a decerebrate position
None	1	No response; lies flaccid
Verbal response		
Oriented	5	Is oriented and converses
Confused	4	Is disoriented and confused
Inappropriate words	3	Replies randomly with incorrect words
Incomprehensible	2	Moans or screams
None	1	No response

Outside the norm

Decerebrate posture

In a decerebrate posture, the arms are adducted and extended, with the wrists pronated and the fingers flexed. The legs are stiffly extended, with plantar flexion of the feet. This posture results from damage to upper brain stem.

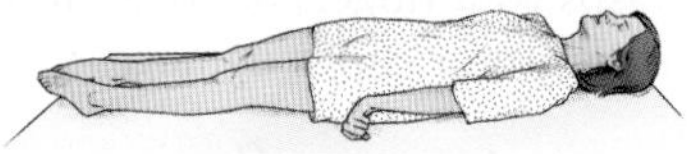

Decorticate posture

In a decorticate posture, the arms are adducted and flexed, with the wrists and fingers flexed on the chest. The legs are stiffly extended and internally rotated, with plantar flexion of the feet. This posture results from damage to one or both corticospinal tracts.

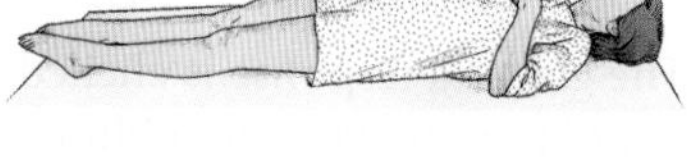

Cranial nerve impairment

Olfactory impairment

If the patient can't detect odors with both nostrils, he or she may have a dysfunction in CN I. This dysfunction can result from any condition that affects the olfactory tract, such as a tumor, hemorrhage, or, more commonly, a facial bone fracture that crosses the cribriform plate.

Vision impairment

Visual field defects may result from tumors or infarcts of the optic nerve head, optic chiasm, or optic tracts. If the patient's pupillary response to light is affected, the patient may have damage to the oculomotor nerve. Pupils are also sensitive indicators of neurologic dysfunction.

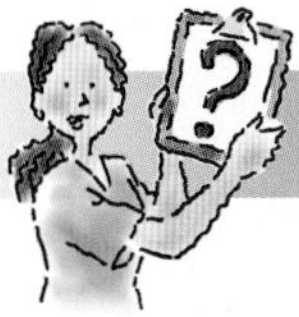

Outside the norm

Visual field defects

Here are some examples of visual field defects. The black areas represent vision loss.

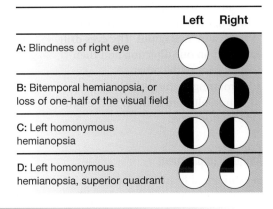

	Left	Right
A: Blindness of right eye		
B: Bitemporal hemianopsia, or loss of one-half of the visual field		
C: Left homonymous hemianopsia		
D: Left homonymous hemianopsia, superior quadrant		

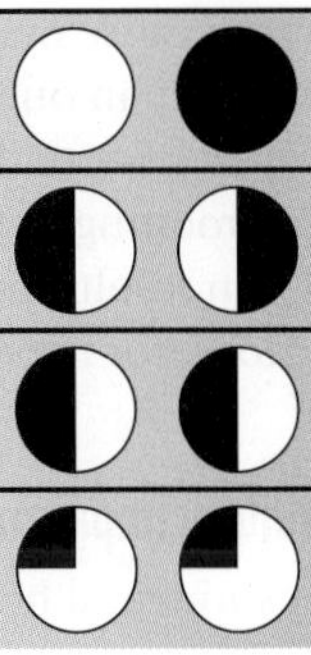

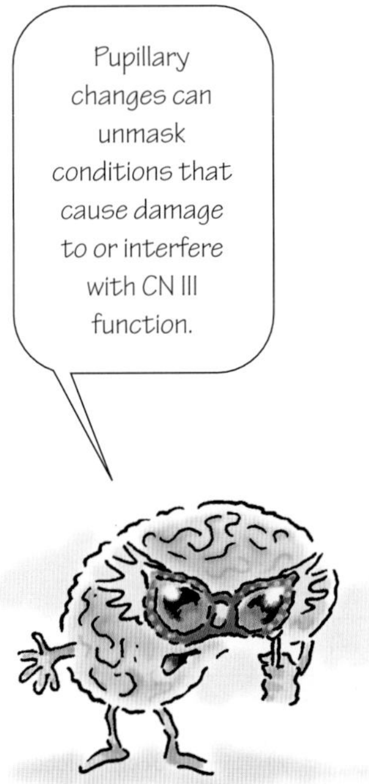
Pupillary changes can unmask conditions that cause damage to or interfere with CN III function.

Keeping an eye on pupils

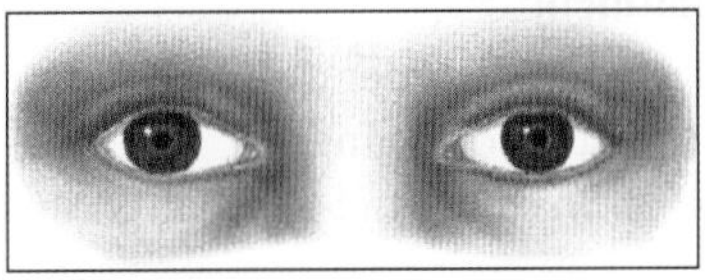

Small pupils
Small pupils indicate disruption of sympathetic nerve supply to the head caused by spinal cord lesion above T1.

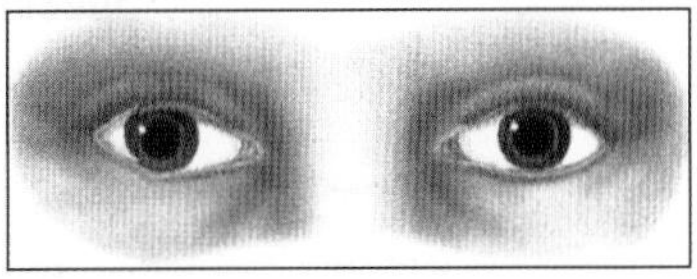

Large pupils
Bilaterally fixed and dilated pupils indicate severe midbrain damage, hypoxia caused by cardiopulmonary arrest, or anticholinergic poisoning.

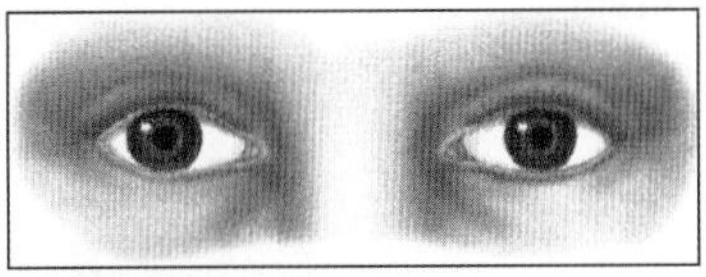

Midposition fixed pupils
Midposition, or slightly dilated, fixed pupils are characteristic of midbrain involvement caused by edema, hemorrhage, infarctions, or contusions.

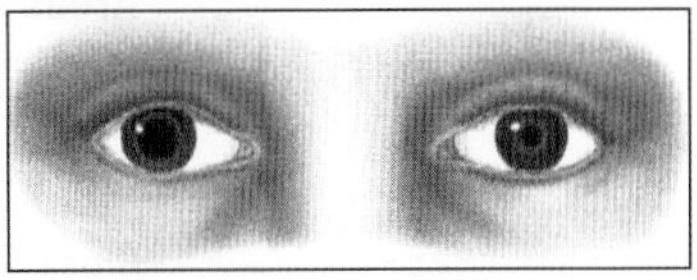

One large pupil
Fixation and dilation of only one pupil is a warning sign for herniation of the temporal lobe, which can cause CN III compression. It may also indicate brain stem compression from an aneurysm, increased ICP, or head trauma with subsequent subdural or epidural hematoma.

Other cranial nerve impairments

- Weakness or paralysis of the eye muscles can result from cranial nerve damage.
- Damage to the peripheral labyrinth, brain stem, or cerebellum can cause nystagmus. The eyes drift slowly in one direction and then jerk back to the other.
- Drooping of the eyelid, or *ptosis,* can result from a defect in the oculomotor nerve.

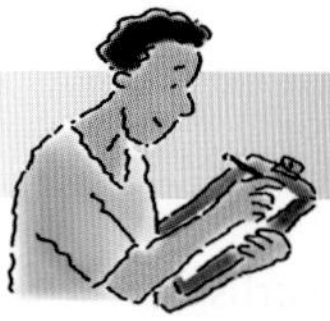

Take note

Documenting pupillary changes

4/06/10 0400 Received pt. from ED with #7 ETT in place, on ventilator with TV 750 cc; FIO_2 80%; GCS 3; pupils fixed, dilated, and nonreactive to light; BP 100/60 mm Hg; HR 116; RR 22 breaths/min, with no assist. Family at bedside.

Brittany James, RN

Auditory impairment

Sensorineural hearing loss can result from acoustic nerve lesions. A patient with this type of hearing loss may have trouble hearing high-pitched sounds or may have total loss of hearing in the affected ear.

Speech impairment

Aphasia is a speech disorder caused by injury to the cerebral cortex. Types of aphasia include the following:

- *expressive* or *Broca aphasia*—impaired fluency and difficulty finding words
- *receptive* or *Wernicke aphasia*—inability to understand written words or speech and the use of made-up words
- *global aphasia*—lack of expressive and receptive language

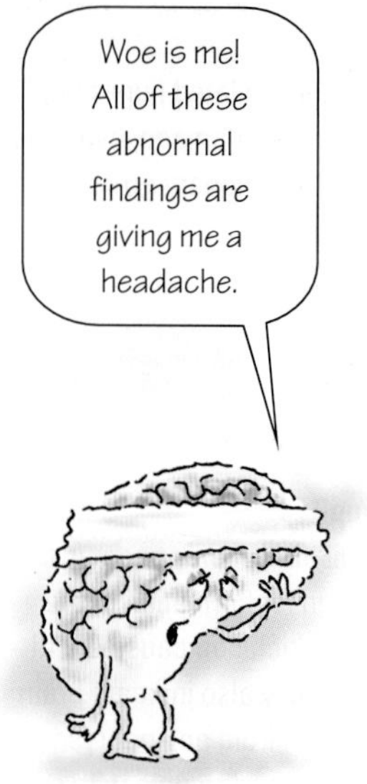
Woe is me! All of these abnormal findings are giving me a headache.

Areas of the brain affected by aphasia

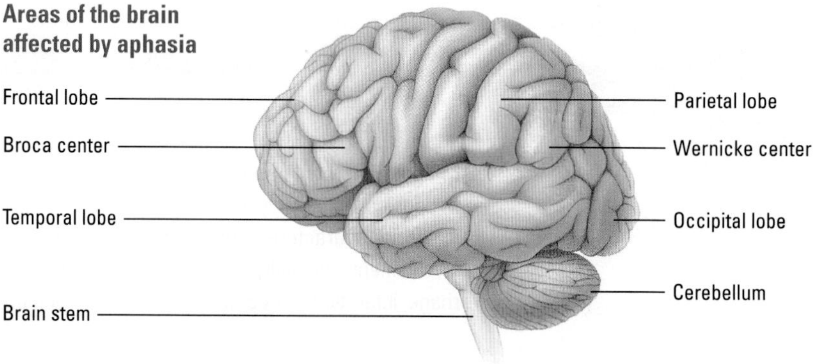
Frontal lobe
Broca center
Temporal lobe
Brain stem
Parietal lobe
Wernicke center
Occipital lobe
Cerebellum

Abnormal gaits

Gait abnormalities may result from disorders of the cerebellum, posterior columns, corticospinal tract, basal ganglia, and lower motor neurons.

Spastic gait

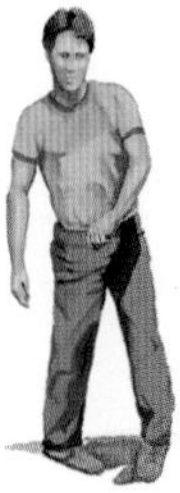

- Stiff, foot-dragging walk caused by unilateral leg muscle hypertonicity

Scissors gait

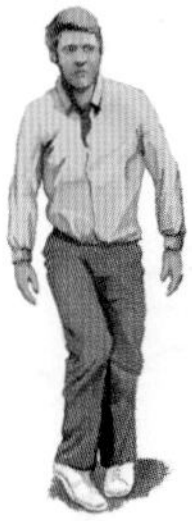

- Adduction of thighs with each step, causing knees to hit or cross in a scissor-like movement
- Results from bilateral spastic paresis

Propulsive gait

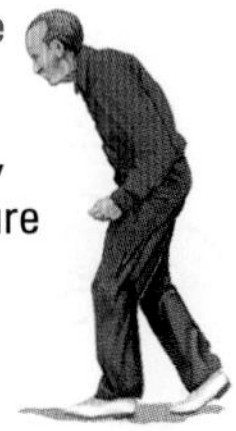

- Stooped, rigid posture
- Cardinal sign of advanced Parkinson disease

Steppage gait

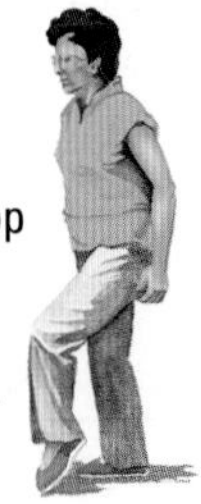

- Results from footdrop (usually caused by lower motor neuron disease), which causes outward rotation of hip and exaggerated flexion of knee
- Toes hit ground first, producing an audible slap

Waddling gait

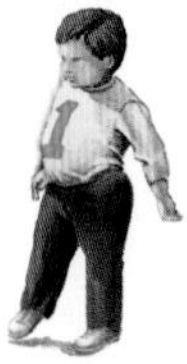

- Distinctive duck-like walk
- Results from deterioration of the pelvic girdle muscles

Meningeal irritation

Positive Brudzinski and Kernig signs indicate meningeal irritation, which may occur with meningitis.

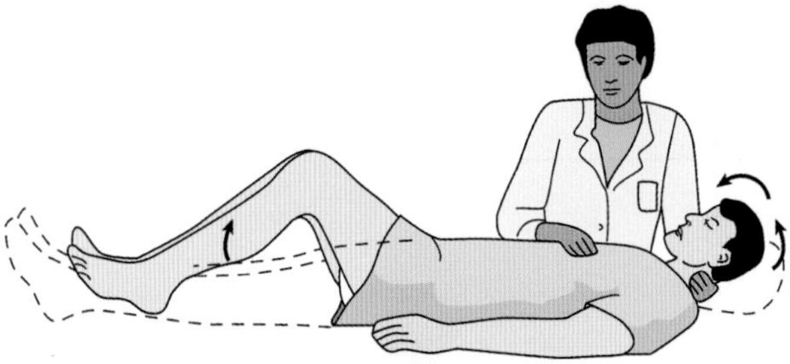

Brudzinski sign

Ask the patient to lie in the supine position. Then place your hand under the patient's neck, and flex it forward, chin to chest. The test is positive if the patient flexes the ankles, knees, and hips bilaterally. The patient typically complains of pain when the neck is flexed.

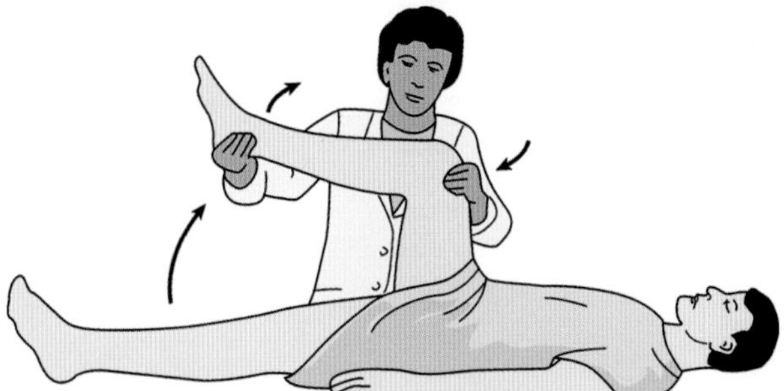

Kernig sign

Ask the patient to lie in the supine position. Flex the patient's hip and knee to form a 90-degree angle. Then attempt to extend this leg. If the patient exhibits pain or resistance to extension and spasm of the hamstring, the test is positive.

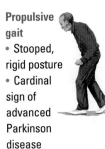

Q&A

Able to label?

Identify the cranial nerves indicated on this illustration.

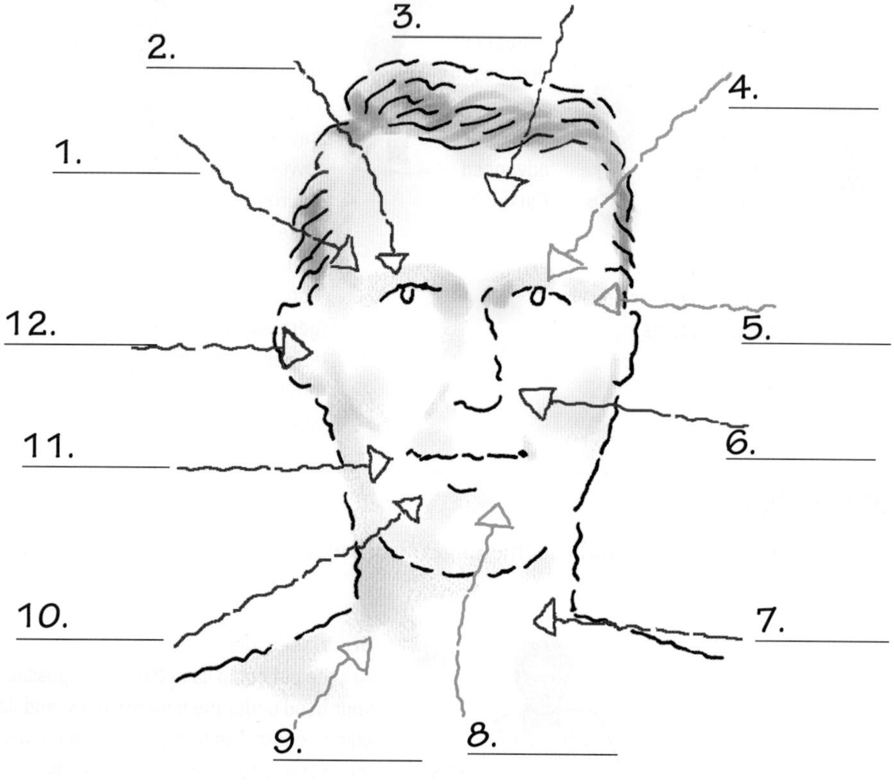
1. ____
2. ____
3. ____
4. ____
5. ____
6. ____
7. ____
8. ____
9. ____
10. ____
11. ____
12. ____

Show and tell

Identify and explain the procedure shown below.

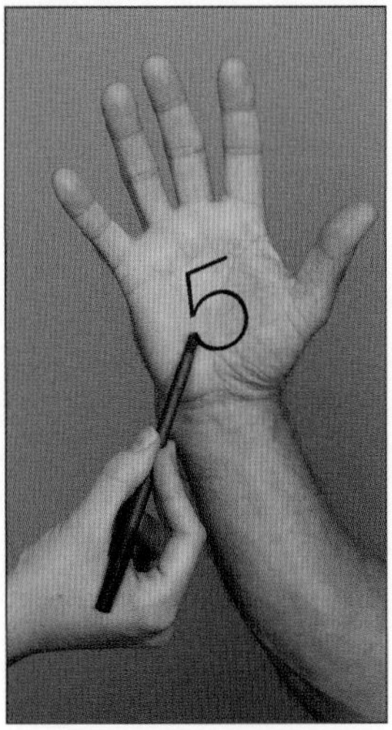
5

Answers: Able to label? 1. Optic, 2. Oculomotor, 3. Facial, 4. Trochlear, 5. Abducens, 6. Olfactory, 7. Vagus, 8. Hypoglossal, 9. Spinal accessory, 10. Glossopharyngeal, 11. Trigeminal, 12. Acoustic; Show and tell The procedure shown assesses graphesthesia. With the patient's eyes closed, hold out the patient's hand while you trace a large number on his or her palm. Ask the patient to identify the number.

Selected References

Buttaro, T. M., Trybulski, J., Bailey, P., & Sandburg-Cook, J. (2013). *Primary care: A collaborative practice* (4th ed.). St. Louis, MO: Elsevier Mosby.

Goroll, A. H., & Mulley, A. G. (2014). *Primary care medicine: Office evaluation and management of the adult patient* (7th ed.). China: Wolters Kluwer.

Chapter 11

Genitourinary system

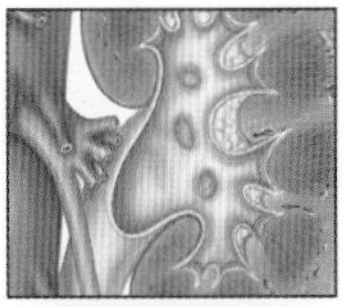

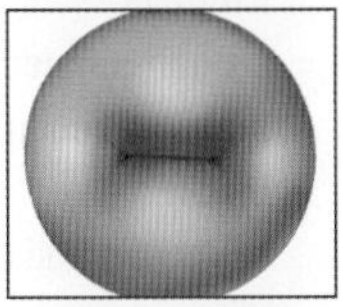

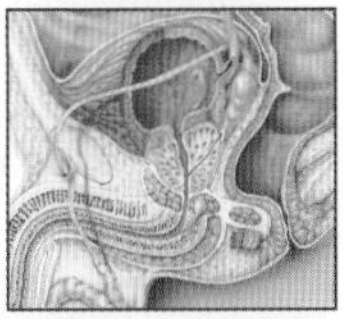

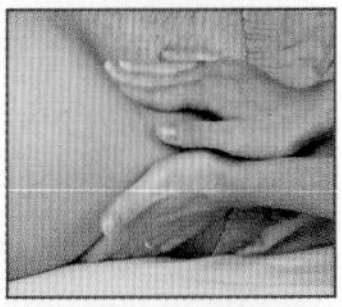

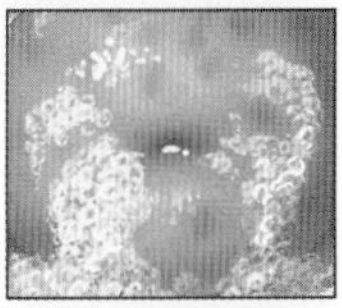

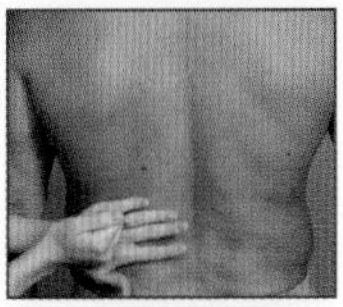

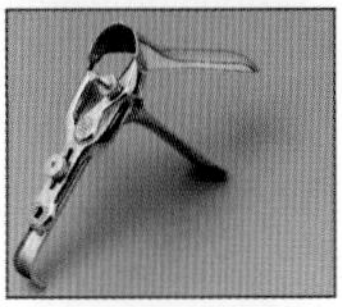

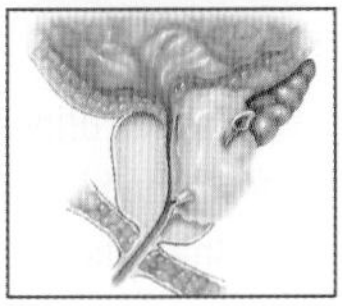

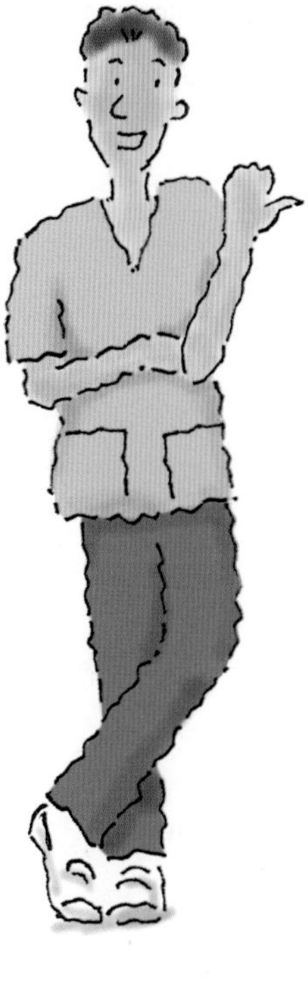

Anatomy

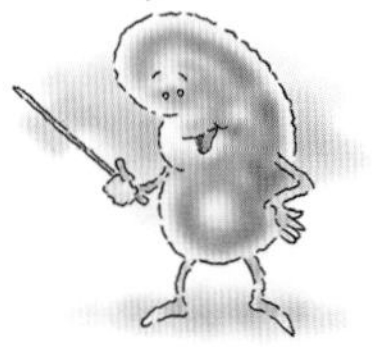
The right kidney extends slightly lower than does the left because it's crowded by the liver. As a result, the right ureter is slightly shorter than the left one.

Kidneys
- Bean-shaped highly vascular organ
- Filters blood and eliminates waste

Renal pelvis
- Receives urine

Ureters
- Carry urine from the kidneys to the bladder by peristaltic contractions that occur one to five times per minute

Bladder
- Hollow and muscular
- Container for urine collection

External meatus
- Passageway for urine (and sperm in men)

Aorta
- Supplies blood to the renal arteries

Urethra
- Carries urine from the bladder to the outside of the body

Urinary system

The urinary system consists of the kidneys, ureters, bladder, and urethra. The kidneys form urine to remove waste from the body; maintain acid-base, fluid, and electrolyte balance; and assist in blood pressure control.

Each kidney contains roughly one million nephrons. Urine gathers in the collecting tubules and ducts of the nephrons and eventually drains into the ureters, down into the bladder and, when urination occurs, out through the urethra.

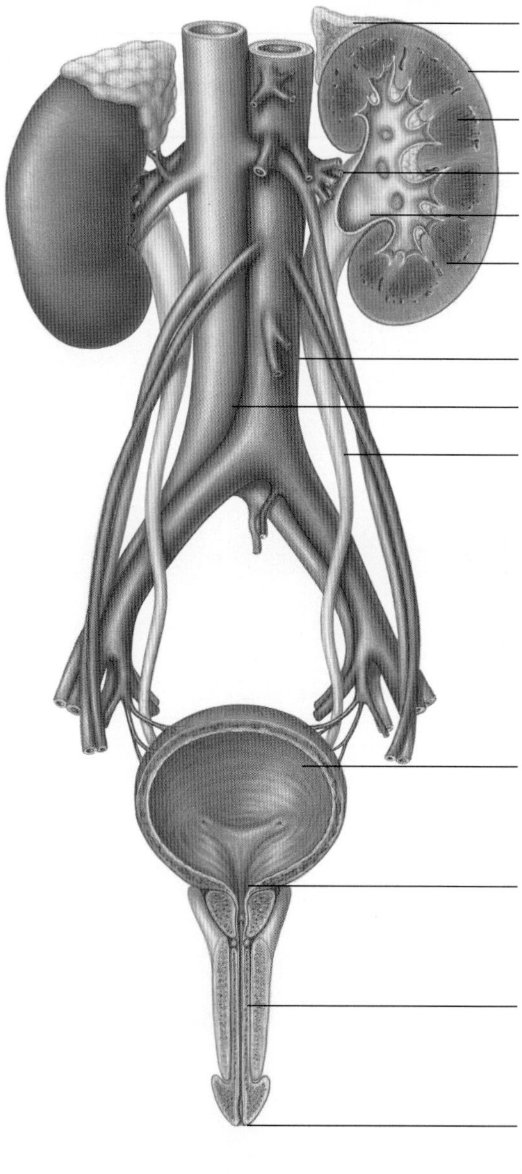
Adrenal gland
Kidney
Renal papilla
Renal artery
Renal pelvis
Renal parenchyma
Aorta
Inferior vena cava
Ureter
Bladder
Bladder neck
Urethra
External meatus

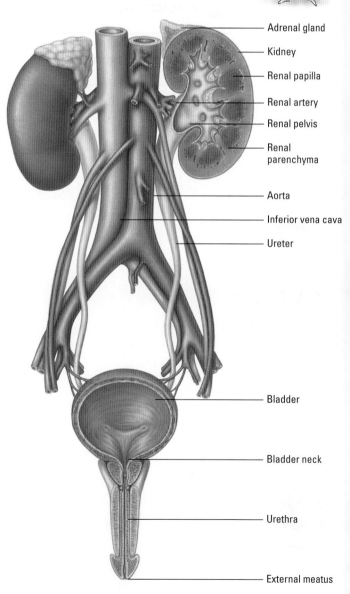

Female reproductive system

External genitalia

The external genitalia, collectively called the *vulva,* include the mons pubis, labia majora, labia minora, clitoris, vaginal orifice, urethra, and Skene and Bartholin glands.

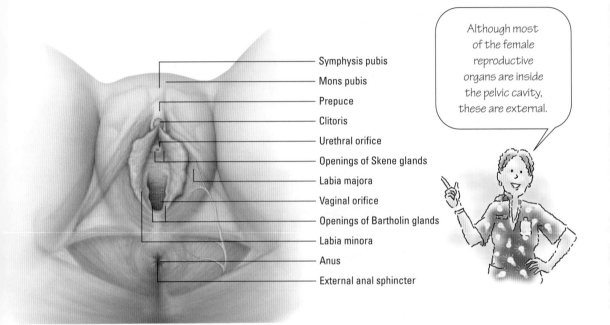

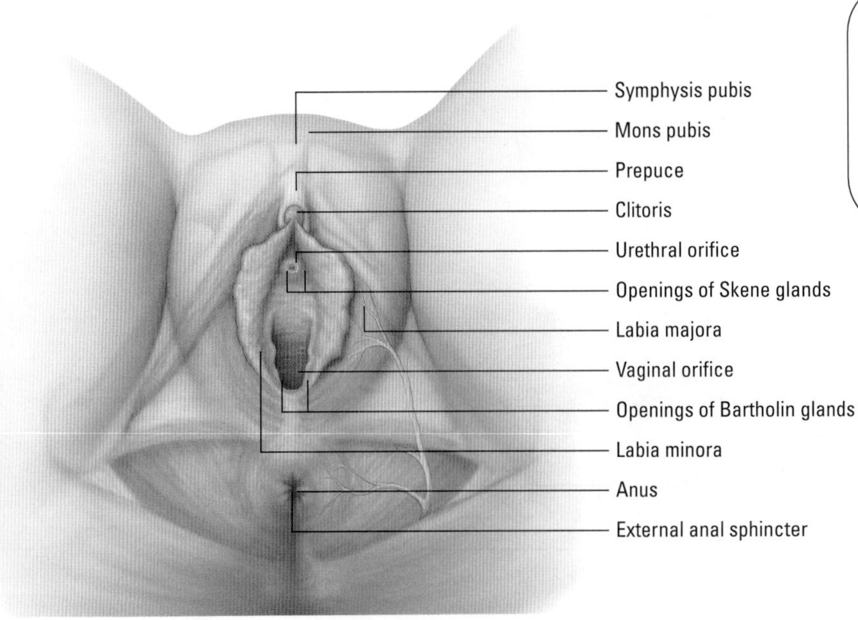
Symphysis pubis
Mons pubis
Prepuce
Clitoris
Urethral orifice
Openings of Skene glands
Labia majora
Vaginal orifice
Openings of Bartholin glands
Labia minora
Anus
External anal sphincter

Although most of the female reproductive organs are inside the pelvic cavity, these are external.

Prepuce
- Caps the clitoris

Vestibule
- Contains urethral and vaginal orifices

Mons pubis
- Mound of adipose tissue

Clitoris
- Composed of erectile tissue

Vaginal orifice
- Thin, vertical slit in women who have intact hymens (the thin fold of mucous membrane that partially covers the vaginal opening)
- Large with irregular edges in women whose hymens have been perforated

Labia majora
- Two rounded folds of adipose tissue
- Extend from the mons pubis to the perineum

Labia minora
- Inner vulval lips
- Form the prepuce

Openings of Skene glands and Bartholin glands
- Contain ducts that open into the vulva
- Produce lubricating fluids important for the reproductive process

Internal genitalia

The internal genitalia include the vagina, uterus, ovaries, and fallopian tubes.

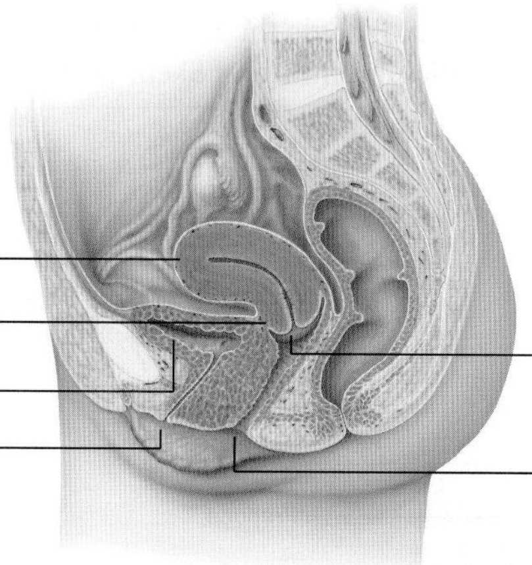
Uterus
Cervix
Urinary bladder
Urethra
External cervical os
Vagina

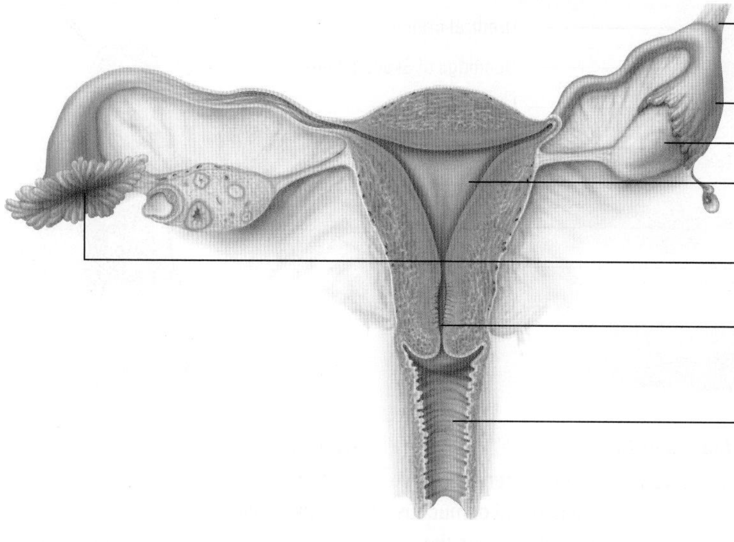
Suspensory ligament of ovary
Fallopian tube
Ovary
Cavity of uterus
Abdominal opening of fallopian tube
Cervical canal
Vagina

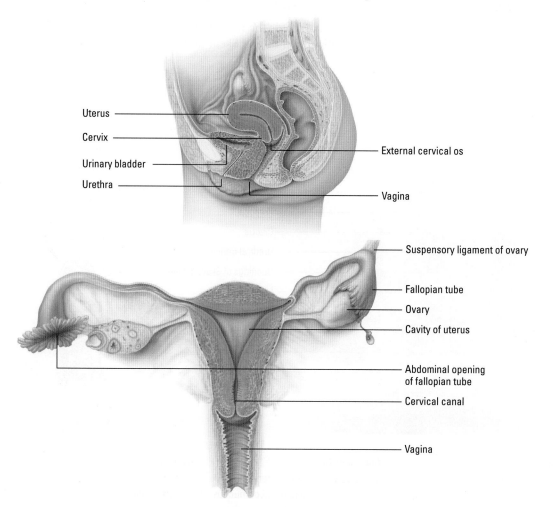

Uterus
- Hollow, pear shaped, and muscular
- Divided into the fundus (upper portion) and cervix
- Accommodates the growing fetus during pregnancy

Fallopian tube
- During ovulation, helps guide the ova to the uterus after expulsion from the ovaries

Cervix
- Contains mucus-secreting glands that aid reproduction and protect the uterus from pathogens

Vagina
- Pink, hollow, collapsed tube
- Route of passage for childbirth and menstruation
- Accommodates penis during coitus

Ovary
- Located in the lower abdominal cavity (one on each side of the uterus)
- Produces ova
- Releases estrogen and progesterone
- Fully develops after puberty and shrinks after menopause

Male reproductive system

The male reproductive system includes the penis, scrotum, testes, epididymides, urethra, vas deferens, seminal vesicles, and prostate gland.

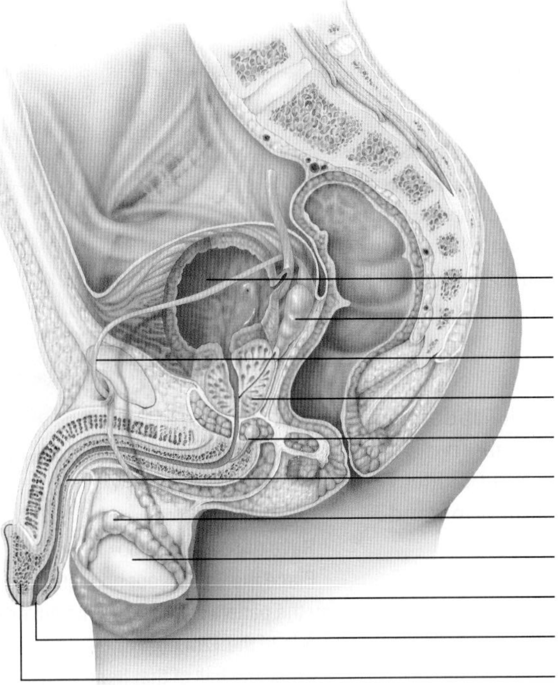
Urinary bladder
Seminal vesicles
Vas deferens
Prostate gland
Bulbourethral gland
Urethra
Epididymis
Testis
Scrotum
Urethral meatus
Glans penis

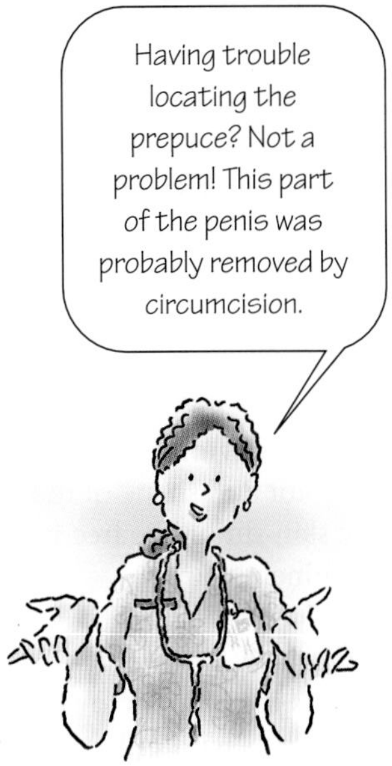
Having trouble locating the prepuce? Not a problem! This part of the penis was probably removed by circumcision.

Prepuce
- Foreskin that surrounds and protects the penis

Penis
- Consists of the shaft, glans, urethral meatus, corona, and prepuce (foreskin)
- Can discharge sperm and semen when erect

Scrotum
- Loose, wrinkled, deeply pigmented sac
- Has two compartments, each containing a testicle, an epididymis, and portions of the spermatic cord

Testes
- Oval and rubbery
- Produce testosterone and sperm

Epididymides
- Reservoirs for maturing sperm

Urethra
- Passage for ejection of sperm and semen during sexual activity

Vas deferens
- Storage site and pathway for sperm

- **Seminal vesicles**
- Saclike glands
- Produce secretions that help form seminal fluid

Prostate gland
- Produces a thin, milky, alkaline fluid that mixes with seminal fluid during ejaculation to enhance sperm activity

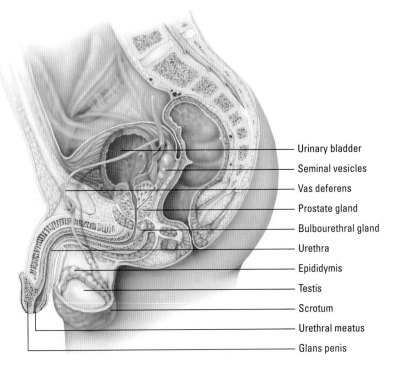

Assessment

Examining the urinary system

First evaluate your patient's vital signs, weight, and mental status. These observations can provide clues about renal dysfunction. For example, an elevated blood pressure can be the result of renal dysfunction or cause renal dysfunction. Elevated weight may be directly related to the inability of the renal system to eliminate fluid. Changes in mental status may be seen as a result of the renal system's failure to eliminate waste and toxins from the body.

Inspection

Inspect the abdomen with the patient lying supine. The abdomen should be symmetrical and smooth, flat, or concave. Observe the color and shape of the area around the kidneys and bladder. The skin should be free from lesions, bruises, discolorations, and prominent veins.

Percussion

Percuss the kidneys to check for costovertebral angle tenderness that occurs with inflammation.

To percuss the bladder, first ask the patient to empty it. Then have the patient lie in the supine position. Start at the symphysis pubis and percuss upward toward the bladder and over it. You should hear tympany. A dull sound signals retained urine.

Palpation

Because the kidneys lie behind other organs and are protected by muscle, they normally aren't palpable unless they're enlarged. If the kidneys feel enlarged, the patient may have hydronephrosis, cysts, or tumors.

In very thin patients, you may be able to feel the lower end of the right kidney as a smooth round mass that drops on inspiration. In elderly patients, you may be able to palpate both kidneys because of decreased muscle tone and elasticity.

You won't be able to palpate the bladder unless it's distended. With the patient in a supine position, use the fingers of one hand to palpate the lower abdomen in a light dipping motion. A distended bladder will feel firm and relatively smooth, extending above the symphysis pubis.

Skill check

Percussing the kidneys

- Have the patient sit up.
- Place the ball of your nondominant hand on the patient's back at the costovertebral angle of the 12th rib.
- Strike the ball of that hand with the ulnar surface of your other hand. Use just enough force to cause a painless but perceptible thud.

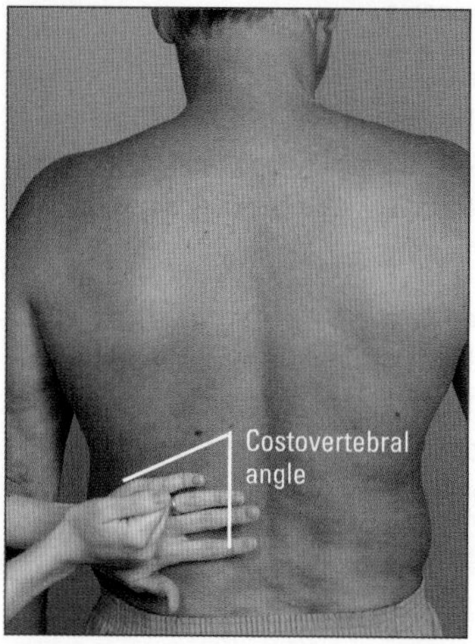
Costovertebral angle

Skill check

Palpating the kidneys

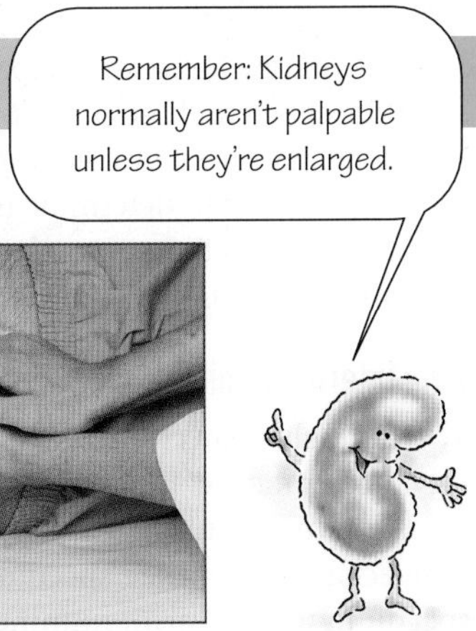
Remember: Kidneys normally aren't palpable unless they're enlarged.

Have the patient lie in a supine position. To palpate the right kidney, stand on the patient's right side. Place your left hand between the posterior rib cage and the iliac crest and place your right hand on the patient's abdomen. Instruct the patient to inhale deeply, so the kidney moves downward. As the patient inhales, press up with your left hand and down with your right, as shown.

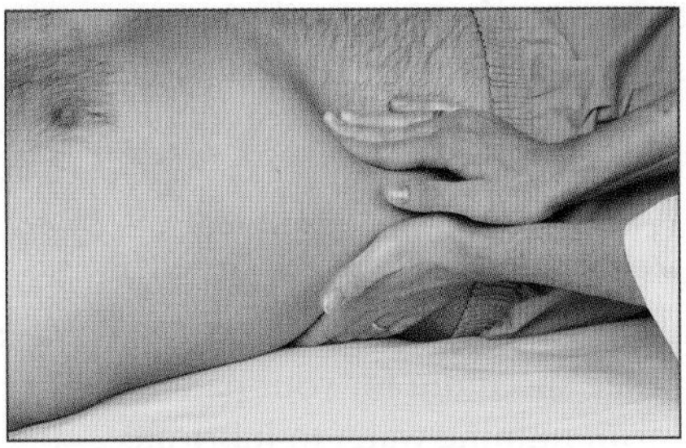

To palpate the left kidney, reach across the patient's abdomen, placing your left hand behind the patient's left flank. Place your right hand over the area of the left kidney. Ask the patient to inhale deeply again. As the patient does so, pull up with your left hand and press down with your right.

Examining the female reproductive system

First ask the patient to void. Provide privacy and then have her disrobe and put on an examination gown. Help her into the dorsal lithotomy position, and drape all areas not being examined. Explain the procedure to her before the examination.

Inspecting the external genitalia

Put on gloves. Using your index finger and thumb, gently spread the labia majora and minora. Locate the urethral meatus. It should be a pink, irregular, slitlike opening at the midline, just above the vagina. Note the presence of discharge or ulcerations. Inspect for pubic hair and assess sexual maturity.

The labia should be moist and free from lesions. Normal discharge varies from clear before ovulation to white and opaque after ovulation. It should be odorless and nonirritating to the mucosa.

Examine the vestibule. Check for swelling, redness, lesions, discharge, and unusual odor. Inspect the vaginal opening, noting whether the hymen is intact or perforated.

Skill check

Inspecting the genitalia

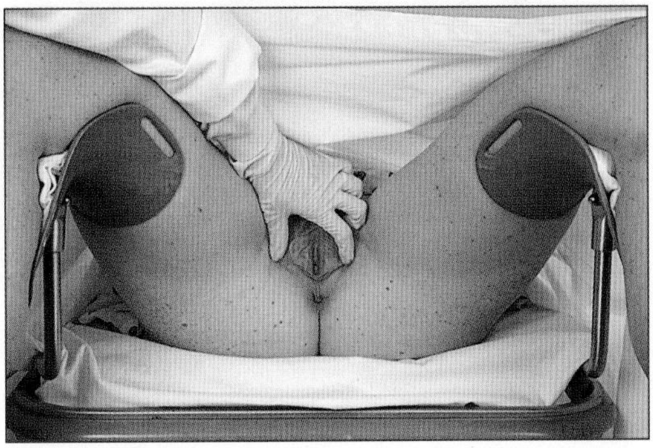

Palpating the external genitalia

Spread the labia with one hand and palpate with the other. The labia should feel soft and the patient shouldn't feel any pain. Note swelling, hardness, or tenderness. If you detect a mass or lesion, palpate it to determine its size, shape, and consistency. If you find swelling or tenderness, see if you can palpate the Bartholin glands, which normally aren't palpable.

Inspecting the internal genitalia

Nurses don't routinely inspect internal genitalia unless they're in advanced practice. However, you may be asked to assist with this examination.

To start, select an appropriate speculum for your patient. Hold the speculum under warm, running water to lubricate and warm the blades. Don't use other lubricants because many of them can alter Papanicolaou (Pap) test results.

A look at specula

Specula come in various shapes and sizes. Choose an appropriate one for your patient. The illustrations below show a typical speculum and three types of specula available.

Skill check

Palpating Bartholin glands

- Insert your gloved index finger carefully into the patient's posterior introitus, as shown.
- Place your thumb along the lateral edge of the swollen or tender labium.
- Gently squeeze the labium. If discharge from the duct results, culture it.

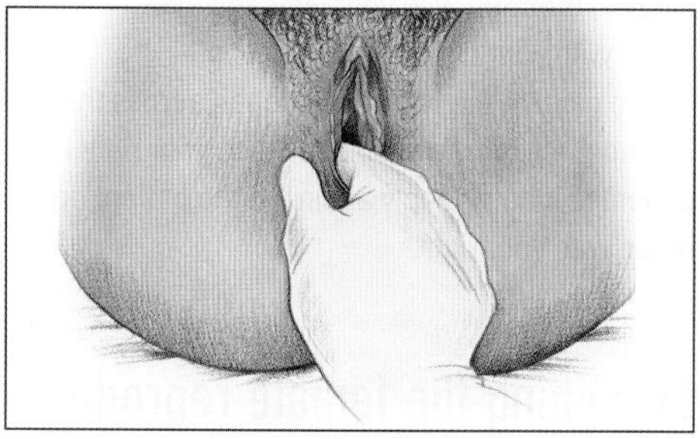

Parts of a speculum

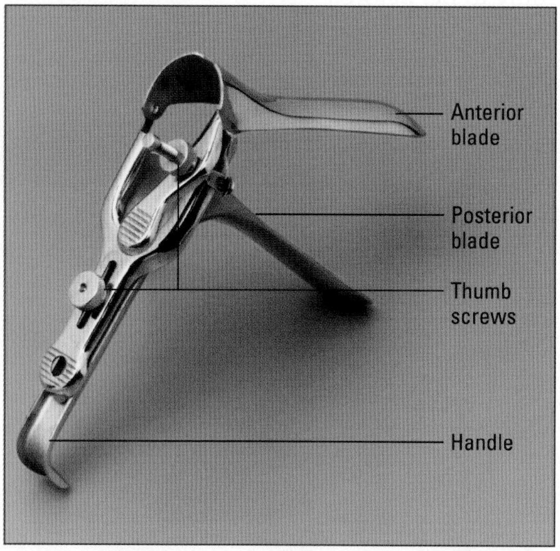
Anterior blade
Posterior blade
Thumb screws
Handle

Types of specula

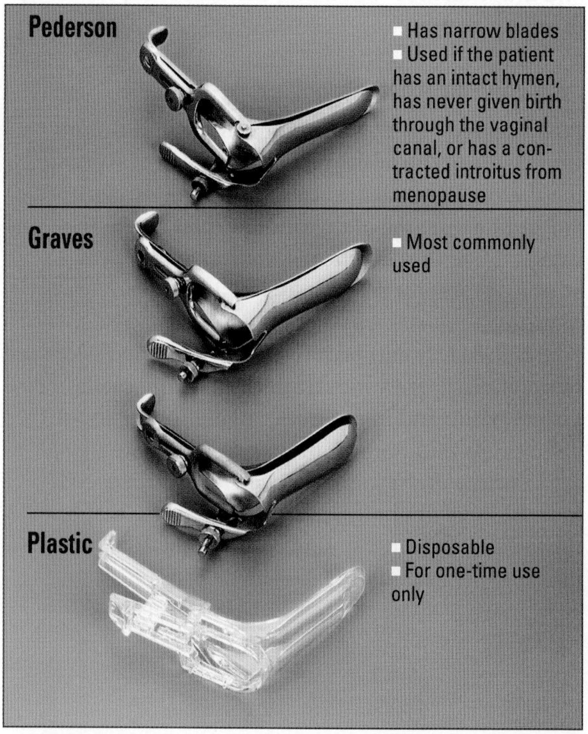
Pederson
Has narrow blades
Used if the patient has an intact hymen, has never given birth through the vaginal canal, or has a contracted introitus from menopause
Graves
Most commonly used
Plastic
Disposable
For one-time use only

Tell the patient she'll feel internal pressure and possibly some slight, transient discomfort during insertion of the speculum. Encourage the patient to take slow, deep breaths during insertion to relax her abdominal muscles.

Skill check

Inserting a speculum

1 Initial insertion

Put on gloves. Place the index and middle fingers of your nondominant hand about 1" (2.5 cm) into the vagina. Spread the fingers to exert pressure on the posterior vagina. Hold the speculum in your dominant hand, and insert the blades between your fingers, as shown below.

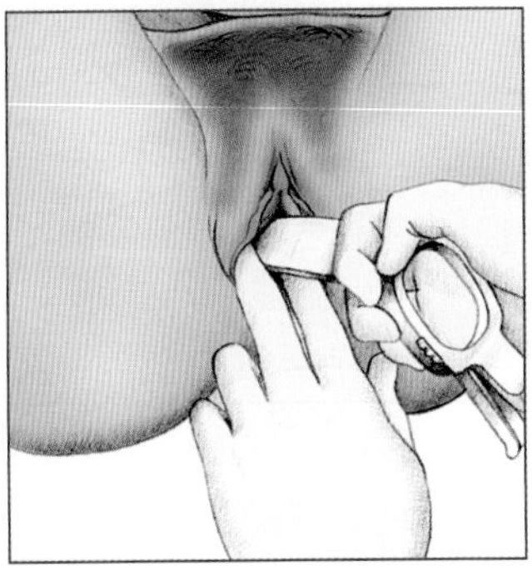

2 Deeper insertion

Ask the patient to bear down to open the introitus and relax the perineal muscles. Point the speculum slightly downward, and insert the blades until the base of the speculum touches your fingers, inside the vagina.

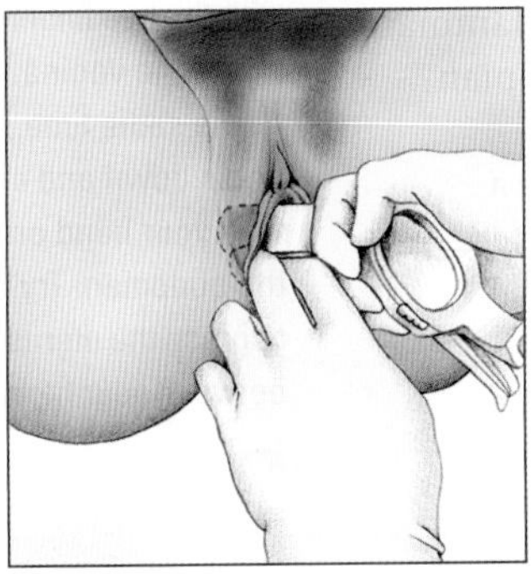

3 Rotate and open

Rotate the speculum in the same plane as the vagina, and withdraw your fingers. Using the thumb of the hand holding the speculum, press the lower lever to open the blades. Open the blades as far as possible and lock them by tightening the thumbscrew above the lever. You should now be able to view the cervix clearly.

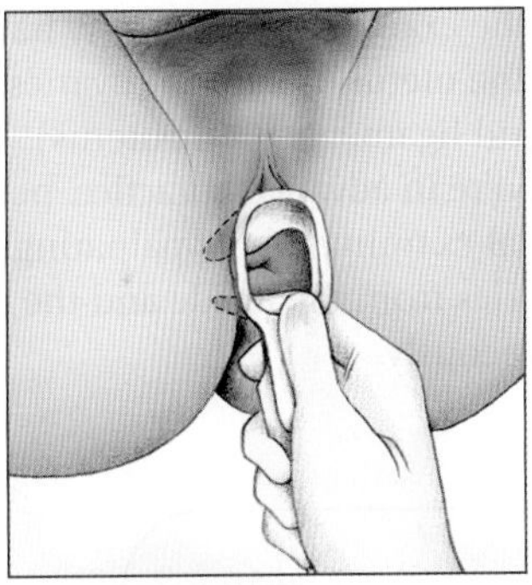

After inserting the speculum, observe the color, texture, and integrity of the vaginal lining. A thin, white, odorless discharge on the vaginal walls is normal. Examine the cervix for color, position, size, shape, mucosal integrity, and discharge. It should be smooth and round. Then inspect the central cervical opening, or cervical os. Expect to see a clear, watery cervical discharge during ovulation and a slightly bloody discharge just before menstruation.

Obtain a specimen for a Pap test. Finally, unlock and close the blades and withdraw the speculum.

Skill check

The normal os

The os is circular in a woman who hasn't given birth vaginally (nulliparous) and a horizontal slit in a woman who has (parous).

Nulliparous

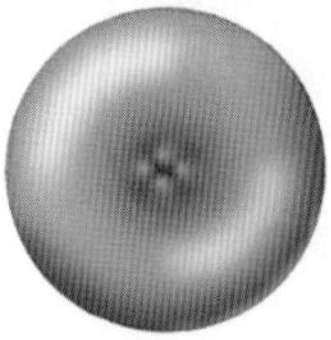

Parous

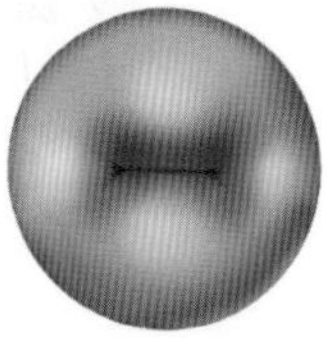

Palpating the internal genitalia

To palpate the internal genitalia, lubricate the index and middle fingers of your gloved dominant hand. Use the thumb and index finger of your other hand to spread the labia majora. Insert your two lubricated fingers into the vagina, exerting pressure posteriorly to avoid irritating the anterior wall and urethra.

When your fingers are fully inserted, note tenderness or nodularity in the vaginal wall. Ask the patient to bear down so you can assess the support of the vaginal outlet. Bulging of the vaginal wall may indicate a cystocele or a rectocele.

To palpate the cervix, sweep your fingers from side to side across the cervix and around the os. The cervix should be smooth and firm. If you palpate nodules or irregularities, the patient may have cysts, tumors, or other lesions.

Next, place your fingers into the recessed area around the cervix. The cervix should move in all directions. If the patient reports pain during this part of the examination, she may have inflammation of the uterus or adnexa (ovaries, fallopian tubes, and ligaments of the uterus).

If you're in advanced practice, perform a bimanual examination by palpating the uterus and ovaries from the inside and the outside simultaneously.

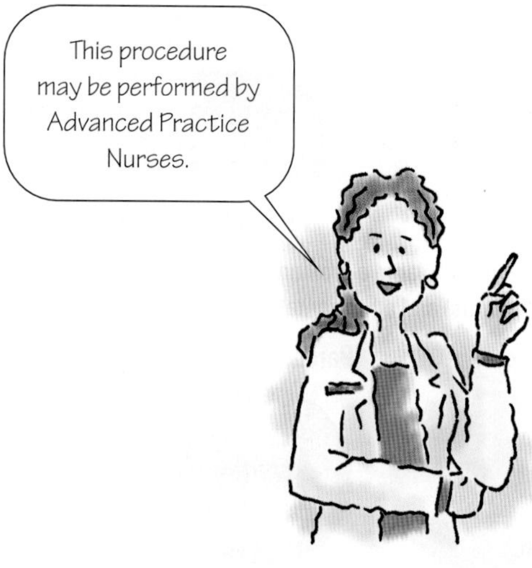
This procedure may be performed by Advanced Practice Nurses.

Skill check

Performing a bimanual examination

During a bimanual examination, palpate the uterus and ovaries from the inside and the outside simultaneously.

1

Proper position

Put on gloves. Place the index and third fingers of your dominant hand in the patient's vagina and move them up to the cervix. Place the fingers of your other hand on the patient's abdomen between the umbilicus and the symphysis pubis, as shown here.

Elevate the cervix and uterus by pressing upward with the two fingers inside the vagina. At the same time, press down and in with your hand on the abdomen. Try to grasp the uterus between your hands.

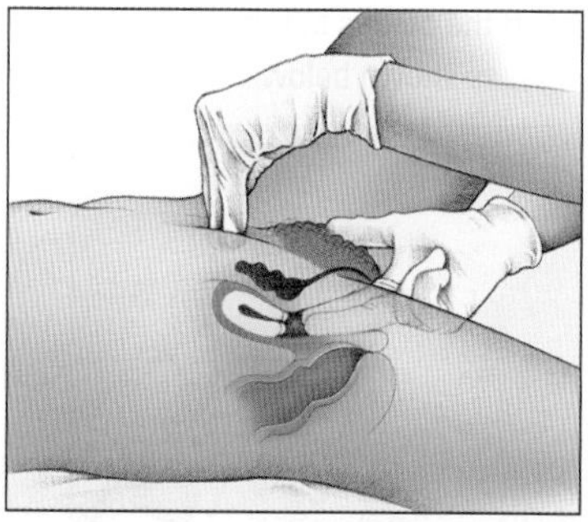

2

Note the position

Move your fingers into the posterior fornix, pressing upward and forward to bring the anterior uterine wall up to your nondominant hand. Use your dominant hand to palpate the lower portion of the uterine wall. Note the position of the uterus.

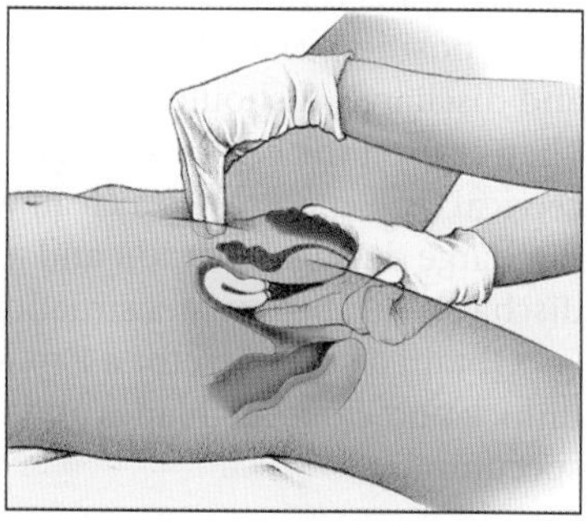

3

Palpate the walls

Slide your fingers farther into the anterior section of the fornix, the space between the uterus and cervix. You should feel part of the posterior uterine wall with this hand. You should feel part of the anterior uterine wall with the fingertips of your nondominant hand. Note the size, shape, surface characteristics, consistency, and mobility of the uterus as well as tenderness.

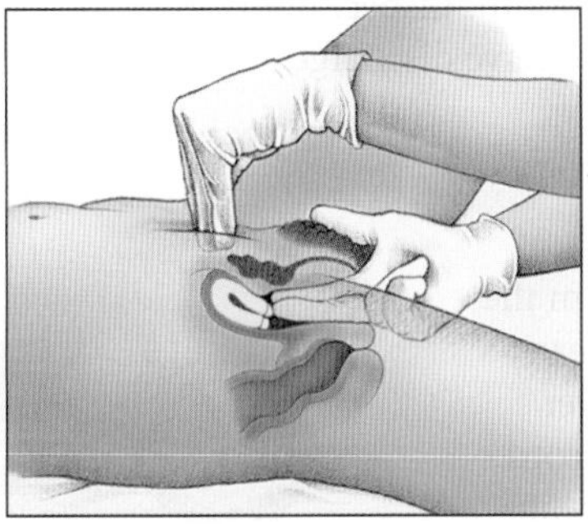

4

Palpate the ovaries

After palpating the anterior and posterior walls of the uterus, move your nondominant hand toward the right lower quadrant of the abdomen. Slip the fingers of your dominant hand into the right fornix and palpate the right ovary. Then palpate the left ovary. Note the size, shape, and contour of each ovary. The ovaries may not be palpable in women who aren't relaxed or who are obese. They shouldn't be palpable in postmenopausal women. Remove your hand from the patient's abdomen and your fingers from her vagina, and discard your gloves.

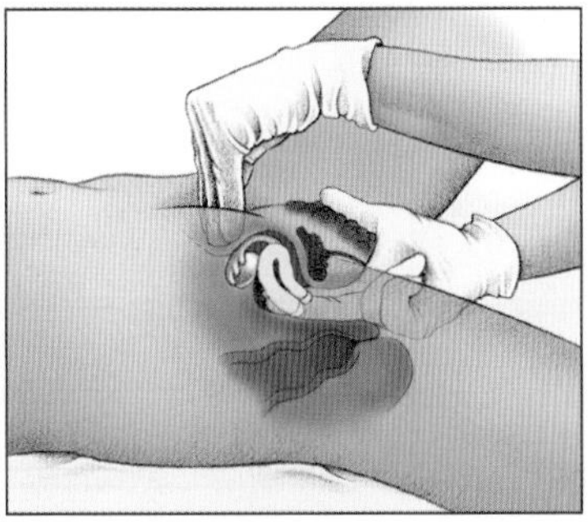

Rectovaginal palpation, the last step in a genital assessment, is used to examine the posterior part of the uterus and the pelvic cavity. Explain to the patient that this procedure may be uncomfortable. After performing rectovaginal palpation, help the patient to a sitting position and provide privacy for dressing and personal hygiene.

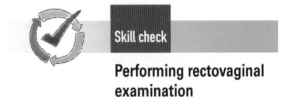

Skill check

Performing rectovaginal examination

1. Put on a pair of gloves and apply water-soluble lubricant to the index and middle fingers of your dominant hand.
2. Instruct the patient to bear down with her vaginal and rectal muscles; then insert your index finger a short way into her vagina and your middle finger into her rectum.
3. Use your middle finger to assess rectal muscle and sphincter tone.
4. Insert your middle finger deeper into the rectum, and palpate the rectal wall.
5. Sweep the rectum with your finger, assessing for masses or nodules.
6. Palpate the posterior wall of the uterus through the anterior wall of the rectum, evaluating the uterus for size, shape, tenderness, and masses. The rectovaginal septum (wall between the rectum and vagina) should feel smooth and springy.

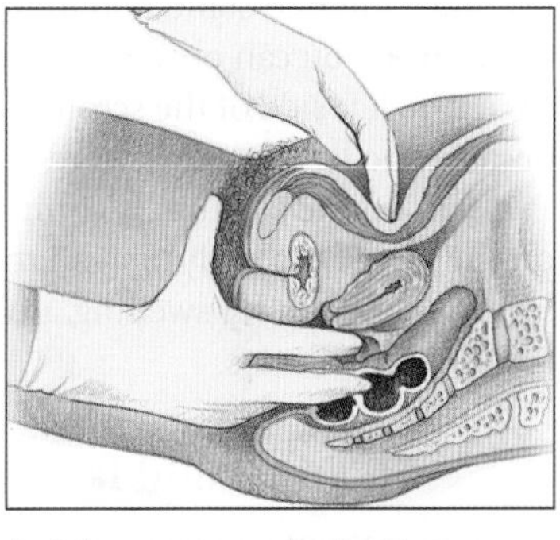

7. Place your nondominant hand on the patient's abdomen at the symphysis pubis. With your index finger in the vagina, palpate deeply to feel the posterior edge of the cervix and the lower posterior wall of the uterus, as shown.
8. If stool testing for occult blood is ordered, put on a new glove and apply water-soluble lubricant to your gloved index finger. Slide your index finger into the patient's anus to obtain a small stool sample. Withdraw your finger and test the stool for occult blood using a guaiac test.
9. When you're finished, discard the gloves and wash your hands.

Male reproductive system

Before examining the male reproductive system, put on gloves. Make the patient as comfortable as possible, and explain all procedures.

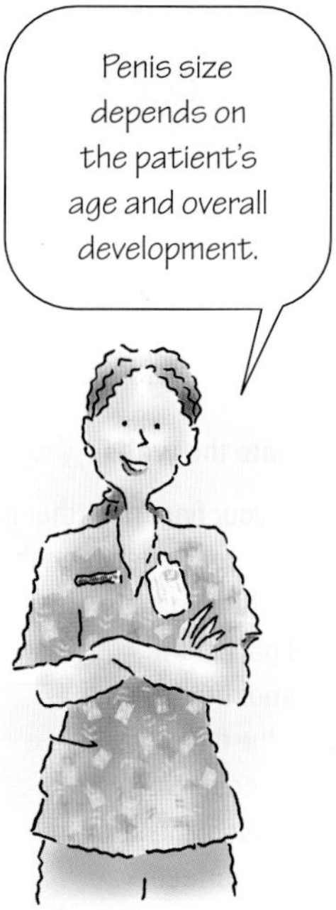
Penis size depends on the patient's age and overall development.

Inspection

Penis

The penile skin should be slightly wrinkled and pink to light brown in white patients and light brown to dark brown in black patients.

Check the penile shaft and glans for lesions, nodules, inflammations, and swelling. Inspect the glans of an uncircumcised penis by gently retracting the prepuce. Also check the glans for smegma, a cheesy secretion commonly found beneath the prepuce.

Gently compress the tip of the glans to open the urethral meatus. It should be located in the center of the glans and be pink and smooth. Inspect it for swelling, discharge, lesions, and inflammation. If you observe discharge, obtain a culture specimen.

Scrotum and testes

Ask the patient to stand and to hold the penis away from the scrotum so you can observe the scrotum's size and appearance. The left side of the scrotum normally appears lower because the left spermatic cord is longer than the right cord. The skin on the scrotum is commonly darker than the skin on the rest of the body. Spread the surface skin of the scrotum, and inspect for swelling, nodules, redness, ulcerations, and distended veins.

Inguinal and femoral areas

With the patient still standing, ask him to hold his breath and bear down while you inspect the inguinal and femoral areas for bulges or hernias.

Skill check

Examining the urethral meatus

To inspect the urethral meatus, compress the tip of the glans, as shown below.

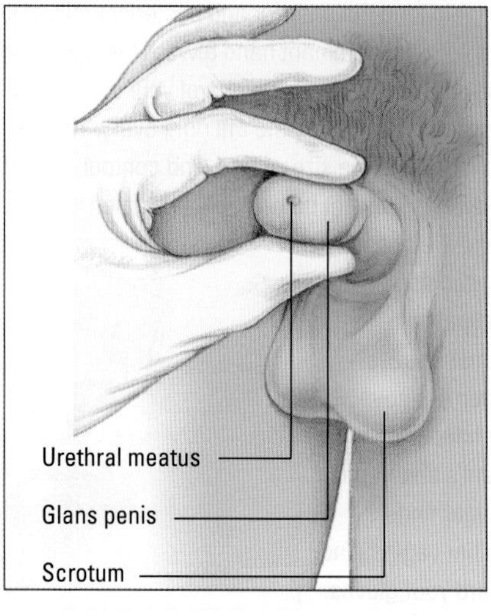
Urethral meatus
Glans penis
Scrotum

Palpation

Penis

Use your thumb and forefinger to palpate the penile shaft. It should be somewhat firm, and the skin should be smooth and movable. Note swelling, nodules, indurations, or discharge.

Testes

Starting at the base of the scrotal sac, rotate the testes between the thumb and first two fingers. The testes should be equal in size, move freely in the scrotal sac, and feel firm, smooth, and rubbery on palpation.

If you note hard, irregular areas or lumps, transilluminate them by darkening the room and pressing the head of a flashlight against the scrotum, behind the lump. The testis and any lumps, masses, warts, or blood-filled areas will appear as opaque shadows. Transilluminate the other testis to compare your findings.

Epididymides

Palpate the epididymides, which are usually located in the posterolateral area of the testes. They should be smooth, discrete, nontender, and free from swelling and induration.

Spermatic cords

Palpate both spermatic cords, one of which is located above each testis. Palpate from the base of the epididymis to the inguinal canal.

If you feel swelling, irregularity, or nodules, transilluminate the problem area. If serous fluid is present, you won't see a glow.

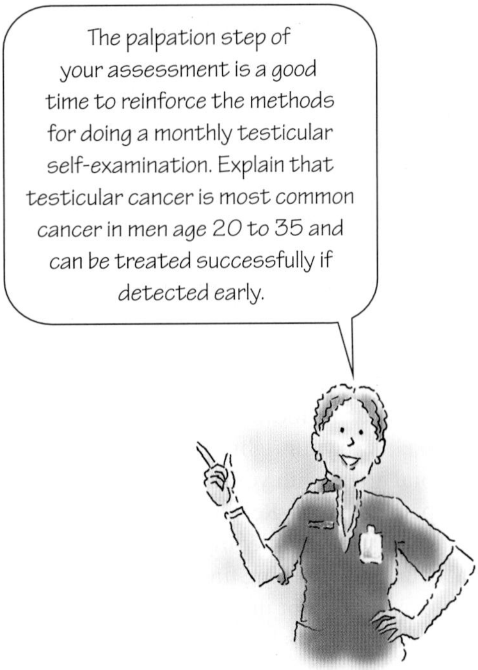
The palpation step of your assessment is a good time to reinforce the methods for doing a monthly testicular self-examination. Explain that testicular cancer is most common cancer in men age 20 to 35 and can be treated successfully if detected early.

Skill check

Palpating the testes

Gently palpate both testes between your thumb and first two fingers of your gloved hand. Assess their size, shape, and response to pressure. A normal response is a deep visceral pain.

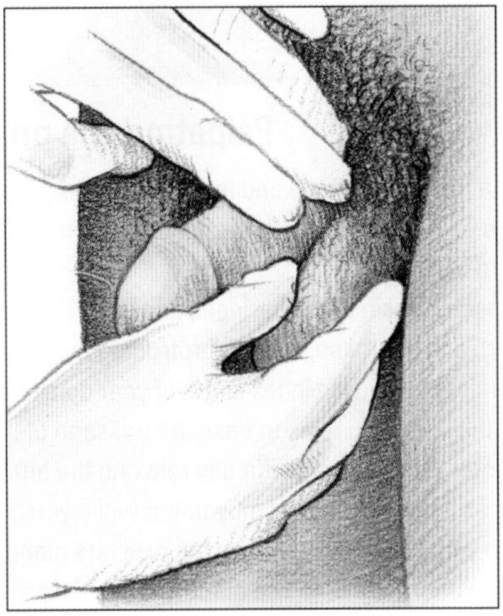

Inguinal area

To assess the patient for a direct inguinal hernia, place two fingers over each external inguinal ring and ask the patient to bear down. If he has a hernia, you'll feel a bulge.

To assess the patient for an indirect inguinal hernia, examine him while he's standing and then while he's in a supine position with his knee flexed on the side you're examining.

Femoral area

Although you can't palpate the femoral canal, you can estimate its location to help detect a femoral hernia. Place your right index finger on the right femoral artery with your finger pointing toward the patient's head. Keep your other fingers close together. Your middle finger will rest on the femoral vein, and your ring finger on the femoral canal. Note tenderness or masses. Use your left hand to check the patient's left side.

Prostate gland

Tell the patient that you need to place your finger in his rectum to examine his prostate gland. This exam is to assess for enlargement and nodules, which could indicate prostate cancer. According to the American Cancer Society, prostate screening should occur at age 50 for men at average risk and 40 to 45 for those considered higher than average risk.

Skill check

Palpating for an indirect inguinal hernia

Place your gloved finger on the neck of the scrotum and gently insert it into the inguinal canal, as shown below. When you've inserted your finger as far as possible, ask the patient to bear down or cough. A hernia feels like a mass of tissue that withdraws when it meets the finger.

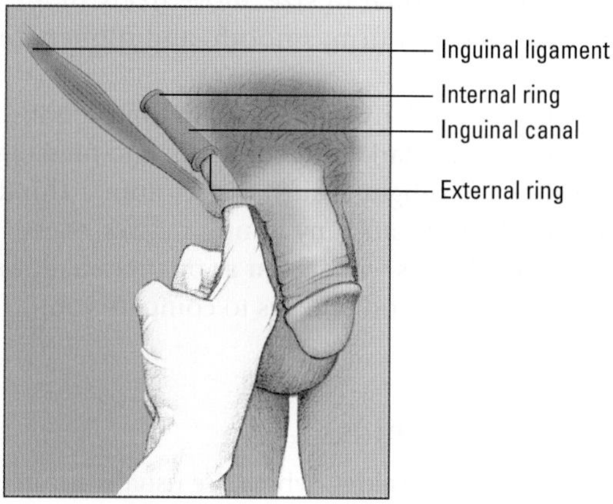
Inguinal ligament
Internal ring
Inguinal canal
External ring

Skill check

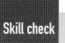

Palpating the prostate gland

- Have the patient stand and lean over the examination table. If he can't do this, have him lie on his left side, with his right knee and hip flexed or with both knees drawn toward his chest.
- Inspect the skin of the perineal, anal, and posterior scrotal areas. It should be smooth and unbroken, with no protruding masses.
- Lubricate the gloved index finger of your dominant hand and insert it into the rectum.
- Tell the patient to relax to ease the passage of the finger through the anal sphincter. If he's having difficulty relaxing the anal sphincter, ask him to bear down as if having a bowel movement while you gently insert your finger.
- With your finger pad, palpate the prostate gland on the anterior rectal wall just past the anorectal ring. The gland should feel smooth, rubbery, and about the size of a walnut.

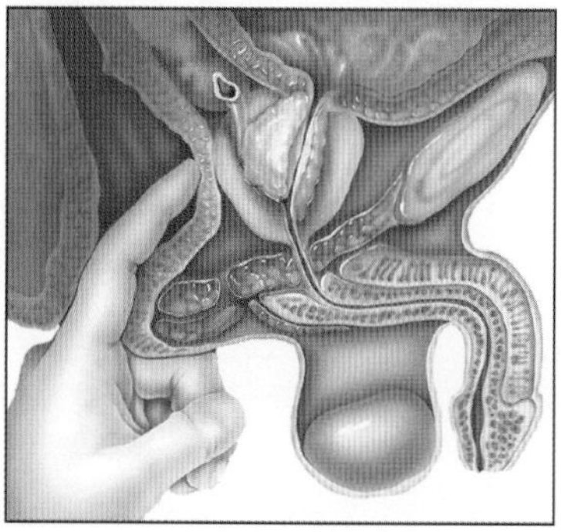

Abnormal findings

Urinary system abnormalities

Kidney enlargement

Kidney enlargement may indicate cysts, hydronephrosis, or tumors.

Urinary frequency

Urinary frequency is an increased incidence of the urge to urinate. It may be caused by bladder calculi, urinary tract infections (UTIs), and urethral stricture. In men, it may be caused by benign prostatic hyperplasia or prostate cancer, which can put pressure on the bladder.

Hematuria

Presence of blood in the urine, or *hematuria,* may indicate UTI, renal calculi, bladder cancer, or trauma to the urinary mucosa. It may also be a temporary condition after urinary tract surgery or urinary catheterization.

Nocturia

Excessive urination at night, or *nocturia,* is a common sign of renal or lower urinary tract disorders. It can result from endocrine or metabolic disorders or prostate cancer. It can also be an adverse effect of diuretics.

Urinary incontinence

Urinary incontinence may be transient or permanent. The amount of urine released may be small or large. Possible causes include stress incontinence, tumor, bladder cancer and calculi, and neurologic conditions, such as Guillain-Barré syndrome, multiple sclerosis, and spinal cord injury.

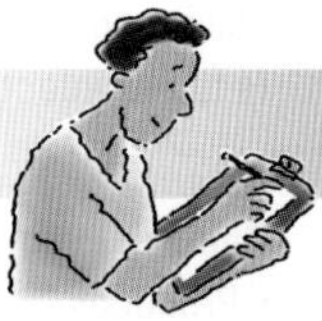

Take note

Documenting kidney palpation

3/25/10	0500	Pt. alert and oriented with c/o right flank pain, nausea, and vomiting. Pt. rates the pain 8/10 on a 0 to 10 pain scale. She reports hematuria, pain on urination, dribbling, and urinary hesitancy. Right kidney is palpable. Vital signs: BP 146/92, HR 110, RR 22, and temp. 100.4° F. Findings reported at 0445 to Dr. Renale, MD.
		Jane Stephens, RN

Female genital abnormalities

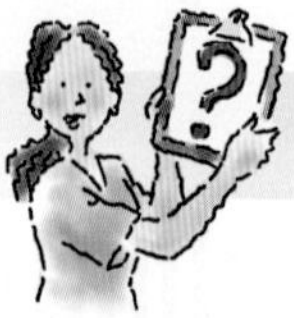

Outside the norm

Syphilitic chancre

In the early stages, syphilitic chancre causes a red, painless, eroding lesion with a raised, indurated border. The lesion usually appears inside the vagina but may also appear on the external genitalia.

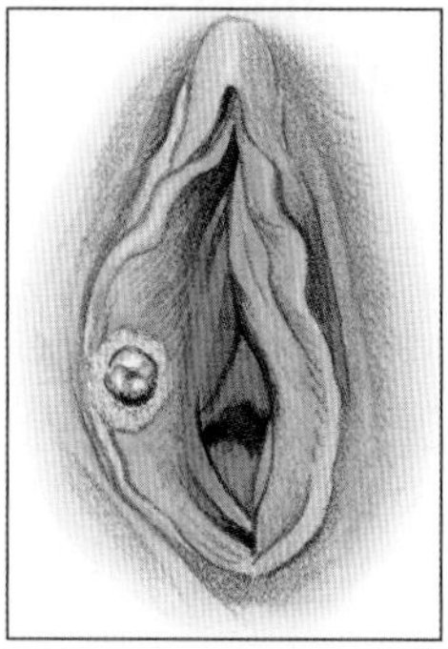

Vaginitis and abnormal discharge

Vaginitis usually results from an overgrowth of infectious organisms. It causes redness, itching, dyspareunia (painful intercourse), dysuria, and a malodorous discharge. Vaginitis occurs with bacterial vaginosis, *Candida albicans* infection (a fungal infection), trichomoniasis, and mucopurulent cervicitis.

Bacterial vaginosis

- Produces thin, grayish white discharge with fishy odor

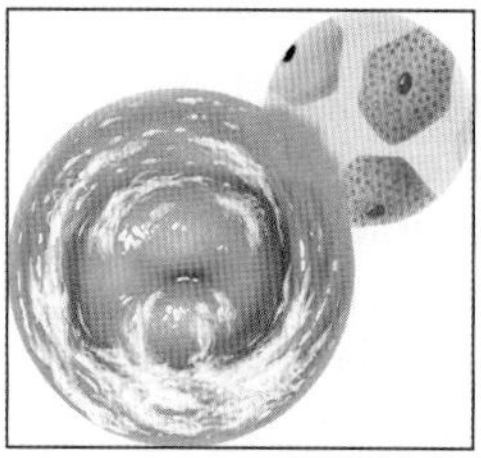

***Candida albicans* infection**

- Produces thick, white, curdlike discharge with a yeastlike odor
- Appears in patches on the cervix and vaginal walls

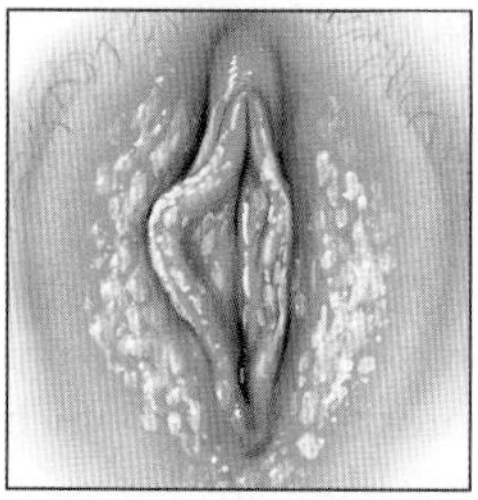

Mucopurulent cervicitis

- Produces purulent yellow discharge from the cervical os
- Occurs with chlamydia and gonorrhea

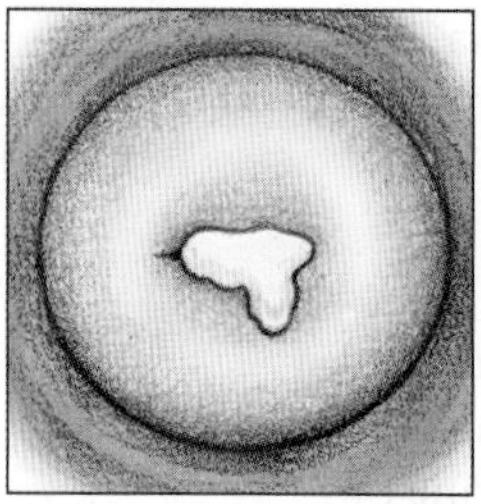

Trichomoniasis

- May produce a malodorous yellow or green, frothy or watery, foul-smelling discharge
- May also involve red papules on the cervix and vaginal walls, giving the tissue a "strawberry" appearance

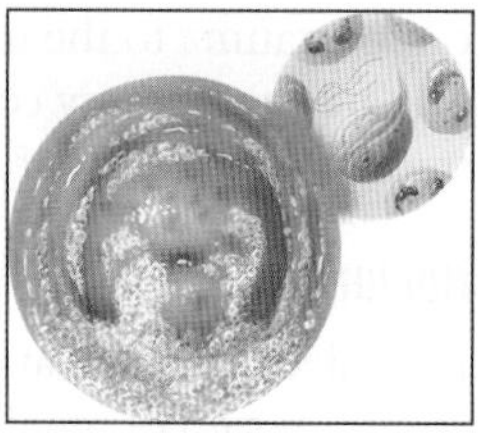

Causes of mucopurulent cervicitis

Chlamydia

Chlamydia is a common sexually transmitted disease caused by the organism *Chlamydia trachomatis*. Although 75% of women with chlamydia are asymptomatic, the disease may cause mucopurulent cervical discharge and cystitis.

Gonorrhea

Although gonorrhea commonly produces no symptoms, it may cause a purulent yellow discharge and cystitis.

Genital warts

Genital warts, a sexually transmitted disease caused by human papillomavirus, produce painless warts on the vulva, vagina, cervix, or anus. Warts start as tiny red or pink swellings that grow and develop stemlike structures. Multiple swellings with a cauliflower appearance are common.

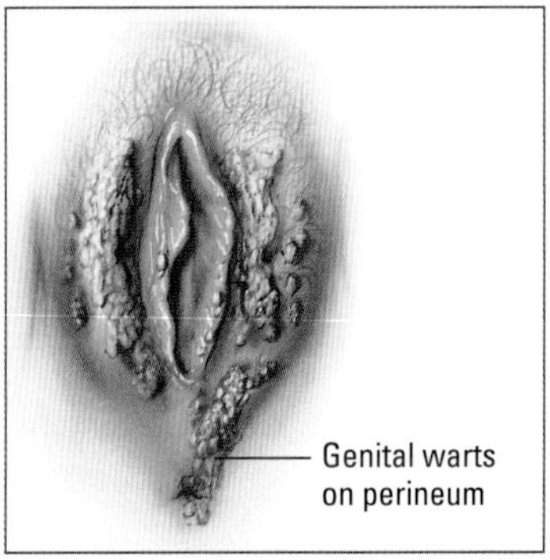
Genital warts on perineum

Genital herpes

Genital herpes produces multiple, shallow vesicles, lesions, or crusts inside the vagina, on the external genitalia, on the buttocks and, sometimes, on the thighs. Dysuria, regional lymph node inflammation, pain, edema, and fever may be present.

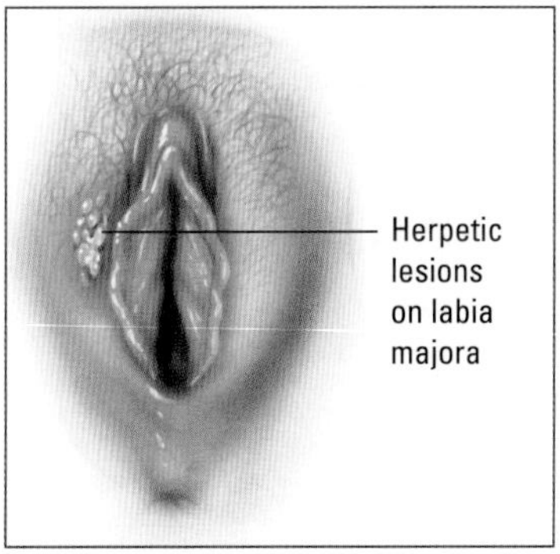
Herpetic lesions on labia majora

Vaginal and uterine prolapse

Also called *cystocele*, vaginal prolapse occurs when the anterior vaginal wall and bladder prolapse into the vagina. During speculum examination, you'll see a pouch or bulging on the anterior wall as the patient bears down. The uterus may prolapse into the vagina and even be visible outside the body.

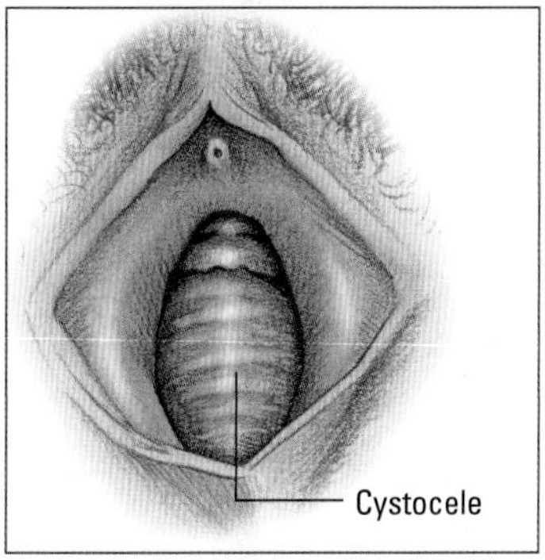
Cystocele

Cervical polyps

Cervical polyps are bright red, soft, and fragile. They're typically benign, but they may bleed. They usually arise from the endocervical canal.

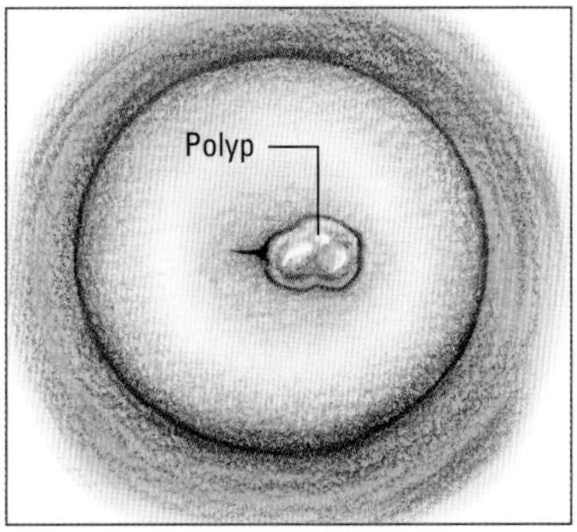
Polyp

Cervical cancer

During a speculum examination, you may detect hard, granular, friable lesions—signs of late-stage cervical cancer. In the early stages of cervical cancer, the cervix looks normal.

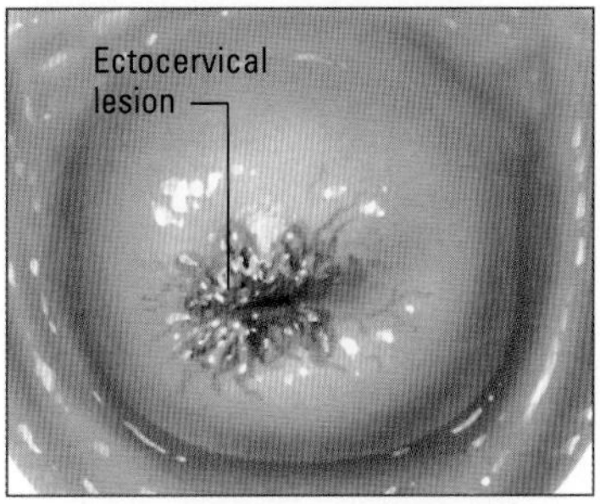
Ectocervical lesion

Rectocele

Rectocele is herniation of the rectum through the posterior vaginal wall. On examination, you'll see a pouch or bulging on the posterior wall as the patient bears down.

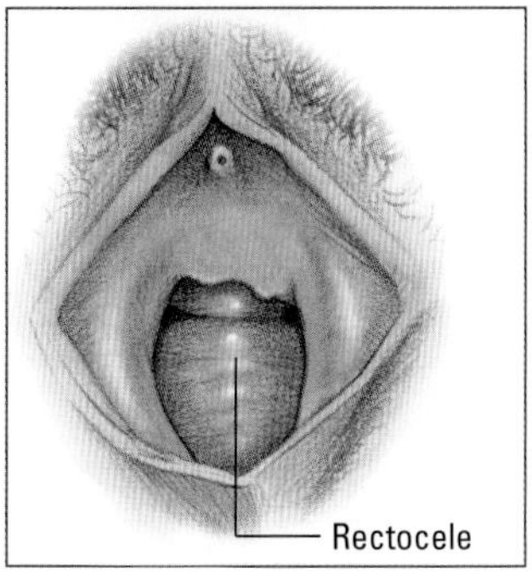
Rectocele

Male genital abnormalities

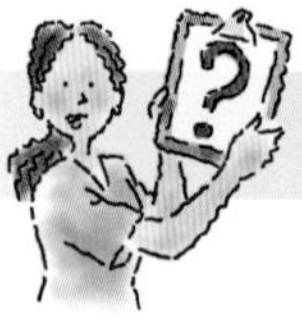

Outside the norm

Testicular tumor

A painless scrotal nodule that can't be transilluminated may be a testicular tumor, which could be benign or cancerous. The tumor can grow, enlarging the testis.

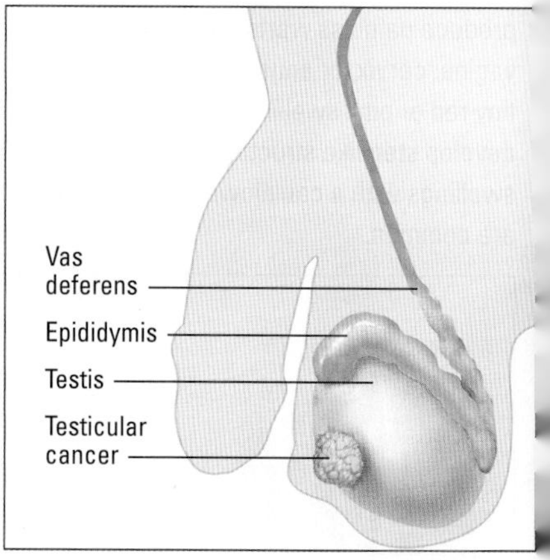
Vas deferens
Epididymis
Testis
Testicular cancer

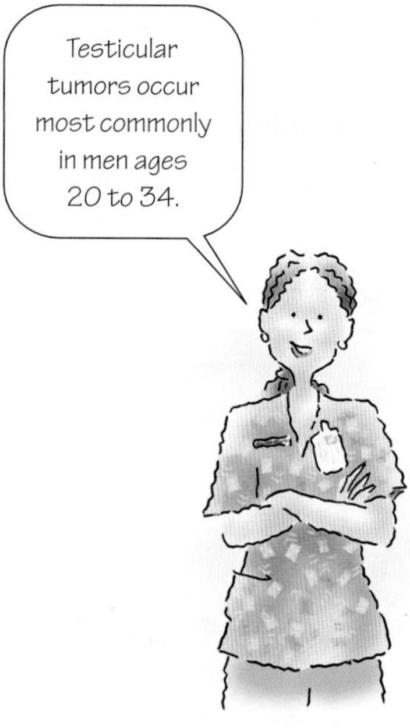
Testicular tumors occur most commonly in men ages 20 to 34.

Common male genital lesions

Penile cancer

Penile cancer causes a painless, ulcerative lesion on the glans or prepuce (foreskin), possibly accompanied by discharge.

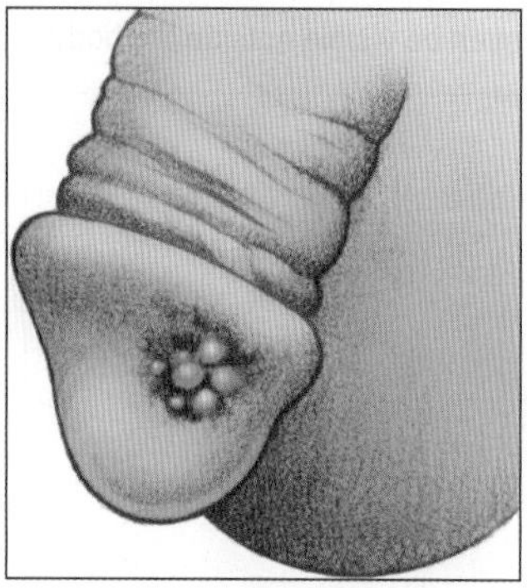

Genital warts

Genital warts are flesh-colored, soft, moist papillary growths that occur singly or in cauliflower-like clusters. They may be barely visible or several inches in diameter.

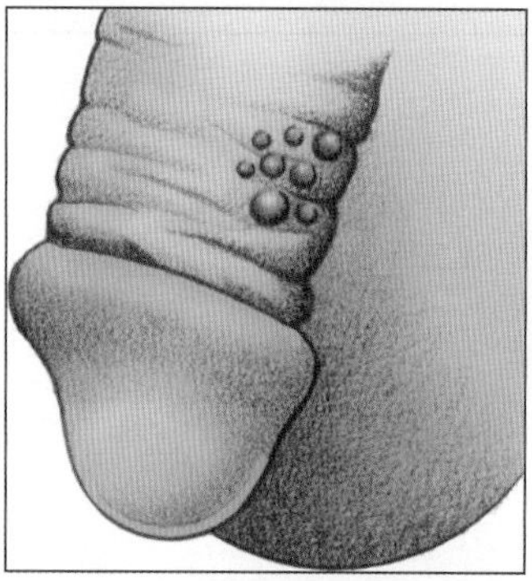

Genital herpes

Genital herpes causes a painful, reddened group of small vesicles or blisters on the prepuce, shaft, or glans. Lesions eventually disappear but tend to recur.

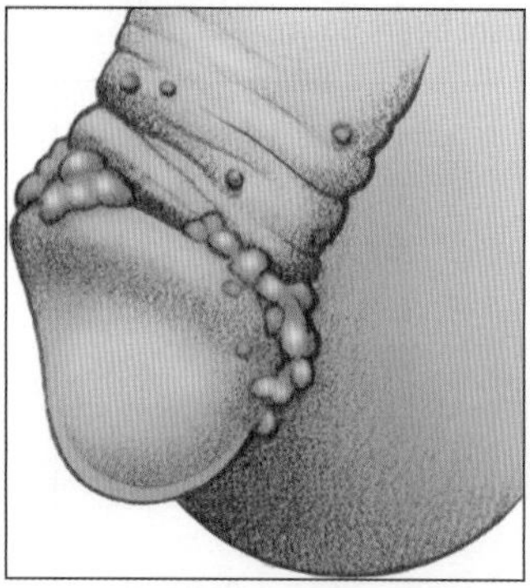

Syphilis

Syphilis causes a hard, round papule on the penis. When palpated, this syphilitic chancre may feel like a button. Eventually, the papule erodes into an ulcer. You may also note swollen lymph nodes in the inguinal area.

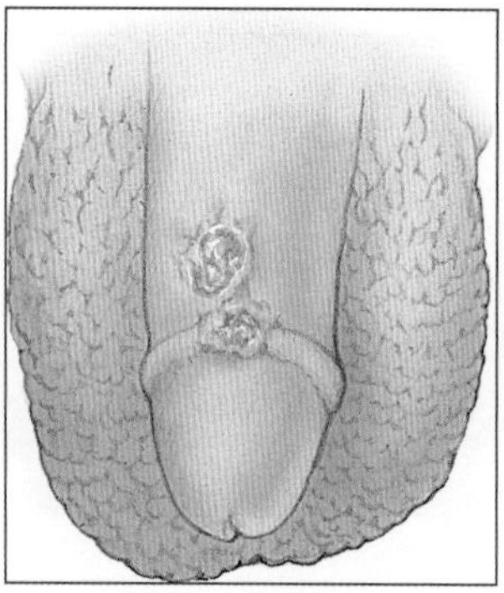

Prostate gland enlargement

A smooth, firm, symmetrical enlargement of the prostate gland indicates benign prostatic hyperplasia, which typically starts after age 50. This finding may be associated with nocturia, urinary hesitancy and frequency, and recurring urinary tract infections.

In acute prostatitis, the prostate gland is firm, warm, and extremely tender and swollen. Because bacterial infection causes the condition, the patient usually has a fever.

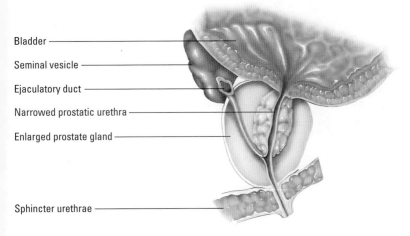

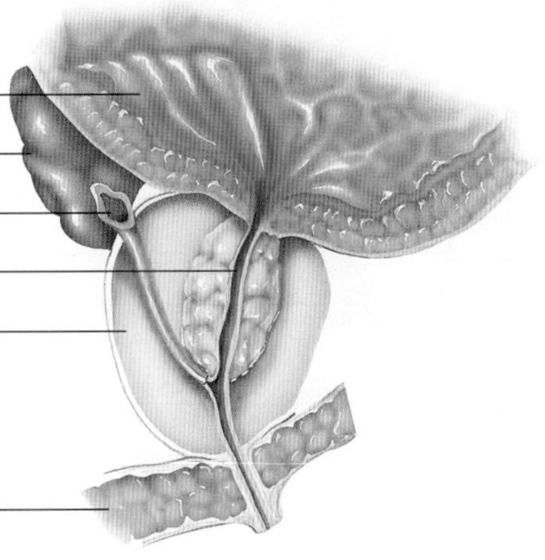
Bladder
Seminal vesicle
Ejaculatory duct
Narrowed prostatic urethra
Enlarged prostate gland
Sphincter urethrae

Prostate gland lesions

Hard, irregular, fixed lesions that make the prostate feel asymmetrical suggest prostate cancer. Palpation may be painful. This condition also causes urinary dysfunction. Back and leg pain may occur with bone metastases in advanced stages.

Prostate cancer

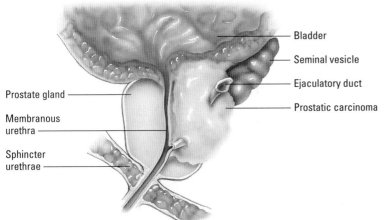

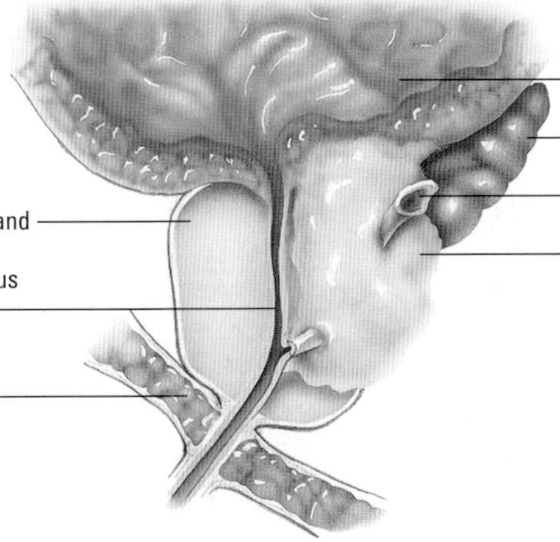
Bladder
Seminal vesicle
Ejaculatory duct
Prostatic carcinoma
Prostate gland
Membranous urethra
Sphincter urethrae

Hernia

A hernia is the protrusion of an organ through an abnormal opening in the muscle wall. It may be direct or indirect and inguinal or femoral.

A direct inguinal hernia emerges from behind the external inguinal ring and protrudes through it. This type of hernia seldom descends into the scrotum and usually affects men older than age 40.

An indirect inguinal hernia is the most common type of hernia; it occurs in men of all ages. It can be palpated in the internal inguinal canal with its tip in or beyond the canal or the hernia may descend into the scrotum.

Uncommon in men, a femoral hernia feels like a soft tumor below the inguinal ligament in the femoral area. It may be difficult to distinguish from a lymph node.

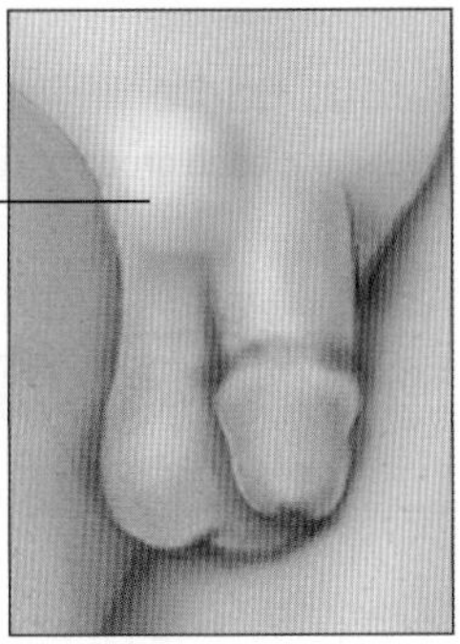
Inguinal hernia

Q&A

Able to label?

Identify the structures of the male reproductive system indicated on this illustration.

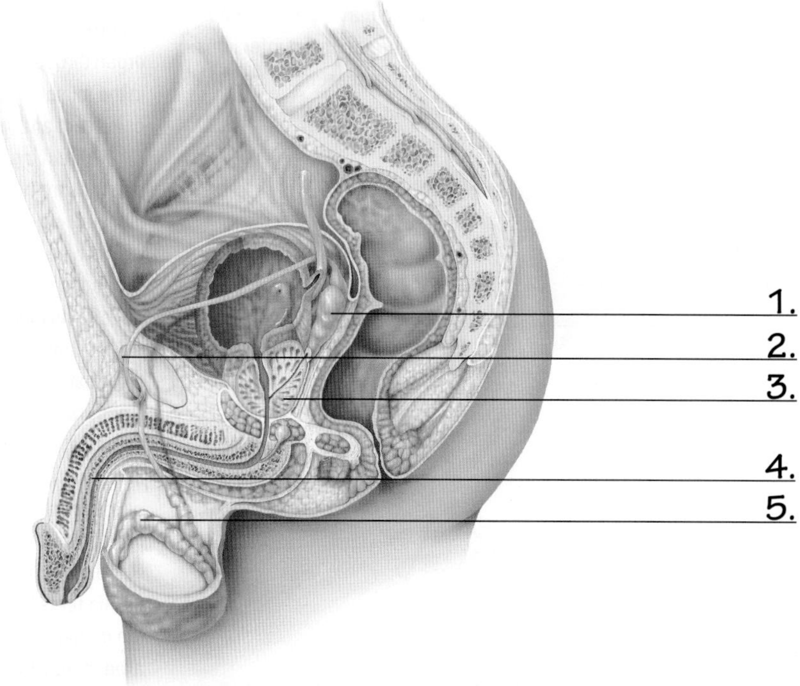
1.
2.
3.
4.
5.

Rebus riddle

Sound out each group of pictures and symbols to reveal information about the urinary system.

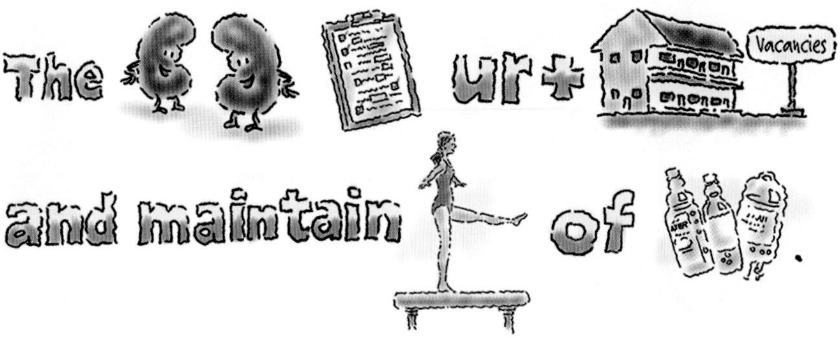
The
ur+
Vacancies
and maintain
of
.

Answers: Able to label? 1. Seminal vesicles, 2. Vas deferens, 3. Prostate gland, 4. Urethra, 5. Epididymis; Rebus riddle, The kidneys form urine and maintain balance of fluids.

Selected References

Bickley, L. S., & Szilagyi, P. G. (2013). *Bates' guide to physical examination and history taking* (11th ed.). Philadelphia, PA: Wolters Kluwer.

Lippincott. (2011). *Professional guide to pathophysiology* (3rd ed.). Philadelphia, PA: Wolters Kluwer.

Nettina, S. M. (2014). *Lippincott manual of nursing practice* (10th ed.). Philadelphia, PA: Wolters Kluwer.

Chapter 12

Pregnancy

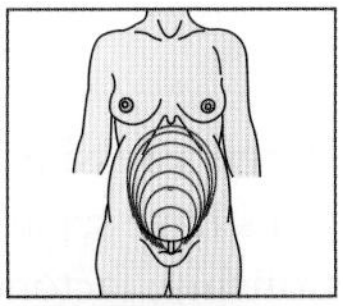

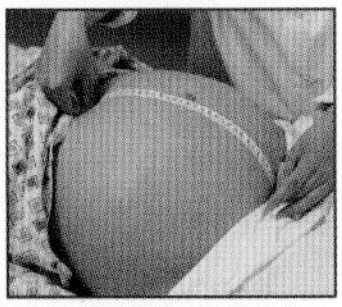

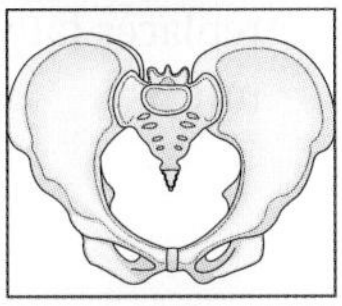

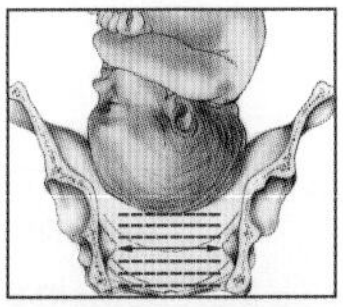

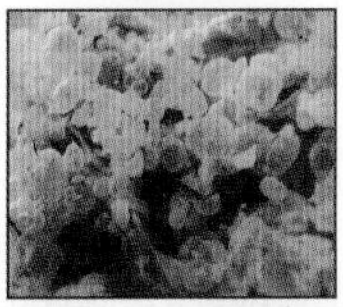

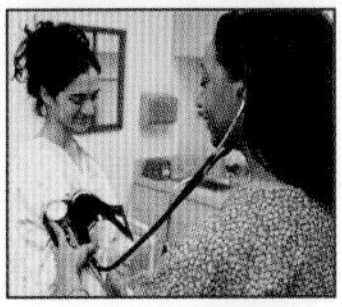

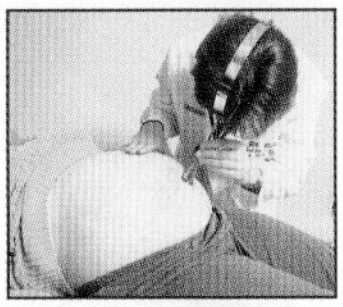

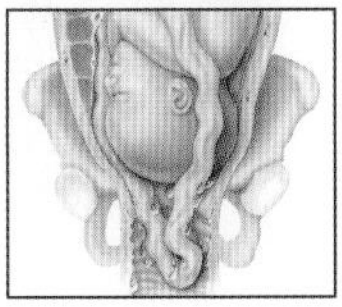

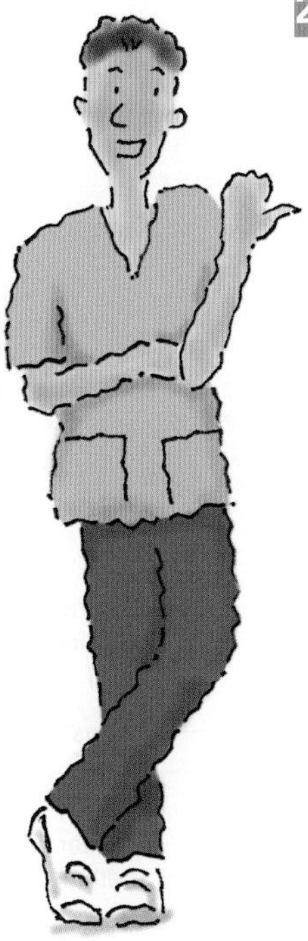

Anatomy

When assessing a pregnant patient, remember that although the mother and fetus have separate and distinct needs, they have an interdependent relationship; factors that influence the mother's health can also affect the fetus. Changes that occur in fetal well-being can also have an influence on the mother's physical and emotional health.

- The body undergoes many changes during pregnancy. For example, as a result of hormonal activity (estrogen and progesterone changes), the breasts may double in size and become more nodular. Glandular tissue replaces fatty tissue, and the mammary glands become capable of secreting milk.

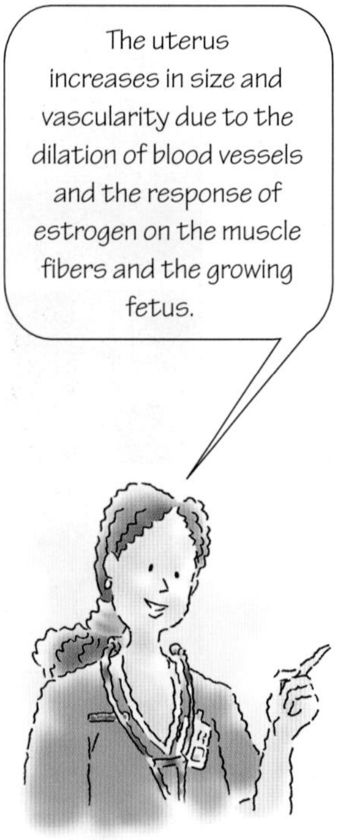
The uterus increases in size and vascularity due to the dilation of blood vessels and the response of estrogen on the muscle fibers and the growing fetus.

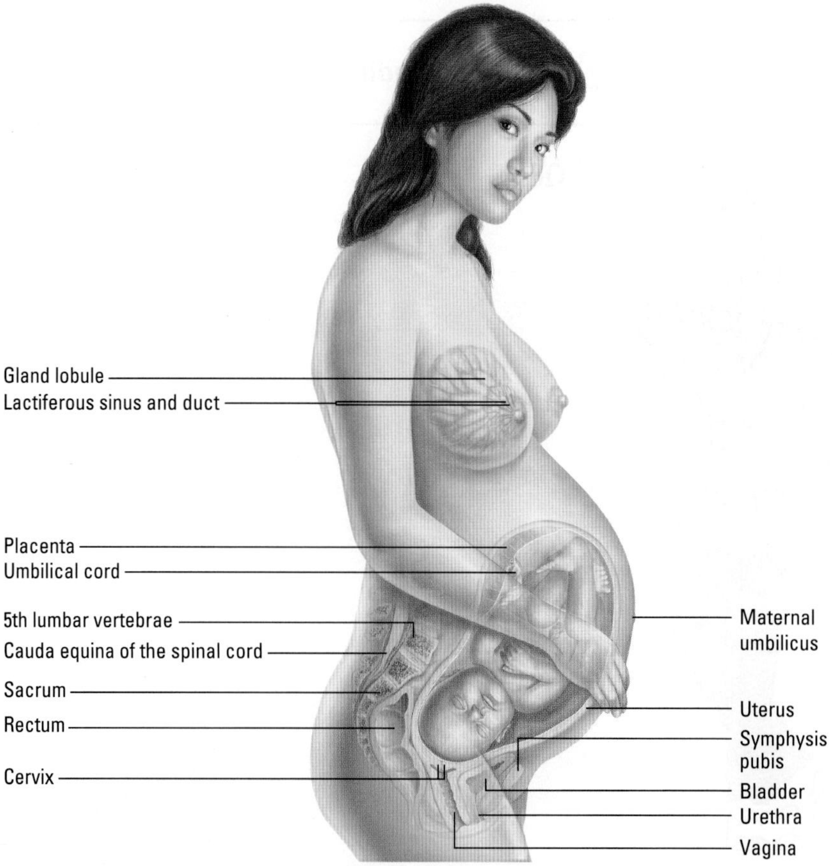
Gland lobule
Lactiferous sinus and duct
Placenta
Umbilical cord
5th lumbar vertebrae
Cauda equina of the spinal cord
Sacrum
Rectum
Cervix
Maternal umbilicus
Uterus
Symphysis pubis
Bladder
Urethra
Vagina

Prenatal assessment

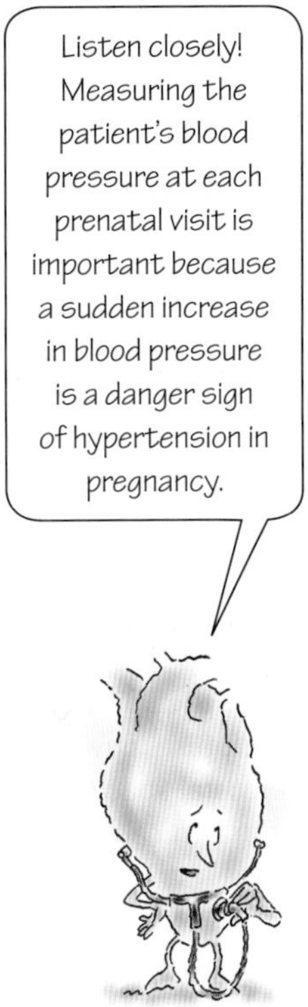
Listen closely! Measuring the patient's blood pressure at each prenatal visit is important because a sudden increase in blood pressure is a danger sign of hypertension in pregnancy.

The prenatal assessment should include the physical, psychosocial, and any specific cultural factors that may impact the pregnancy or maternal health. These assessments should continue throughout pregnancy, starting with the first prenatal visit and continuing through labor, delivery, and the postpartum period. The psychosocial and cultural assessment should include the maternal outlook on the childbearing experience, spiritual needs, religious practices, and any cultural aspects that may affect this experience. A therapeutic relationship should be established on this first maternal prenatal visit.

Physical assessment

The first prenatal visit includes a baseline assessment of vital signs that includes a blood pressure, height, and weight. Gloves should be worn during the exam, the patient should empty her bladder prior to the exam, and a pelvic exam is completed at the end of the assessment by the Health Care Provider.

Estimated date of birth

The most common way to calculate the estimated date of birth (EDB) is the Naegele rule:

- Ask the patient the first day of her LMP (last menstrual period)
- Subtract 3 months from the first day.
- Add 7 days to find the EDB.

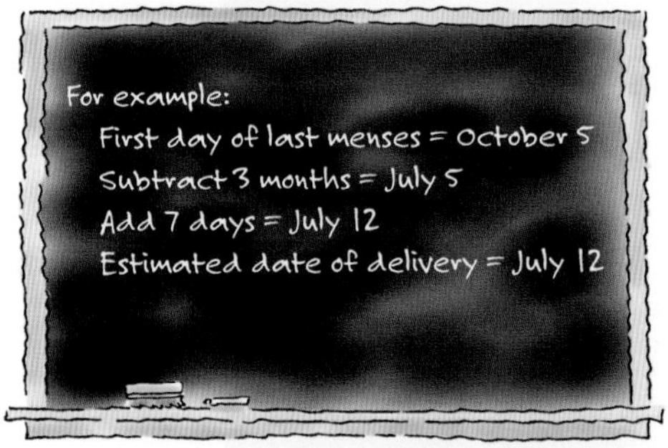
For example:
First day of last menses = October 5
Subtract 3 months = July 5
Add 7 days = July 12
Estimated date of delivery = July 12

Measuring blood pressure

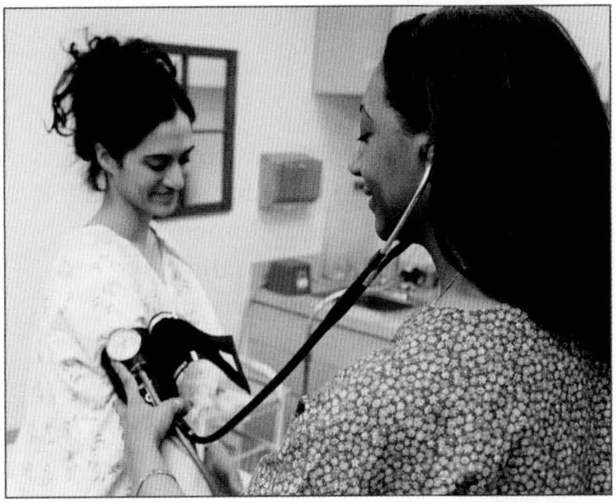

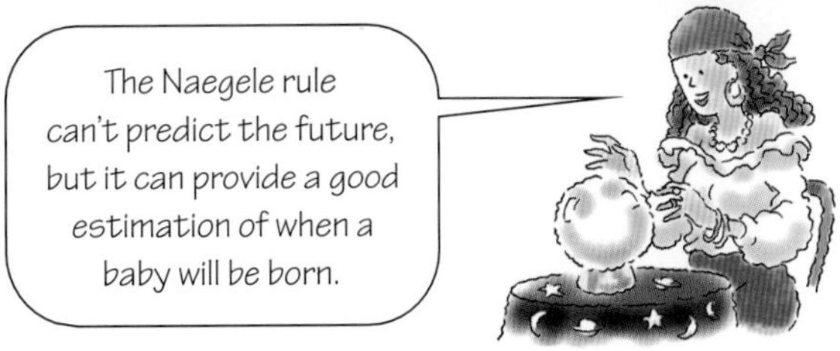
The Naegele rule can't predict the future, but it can provide a good estimation of when a baby will be born.

Breasts

Examine the breasts. In pregnancy superficial veins appear more prominent and the areolae around the nipples become a darker color. Many women may also develop striae, which are red color stretch marks that change to silver after the pregnancy. Montgomery tubercles may be visible on the areolae and may begin to express colostrum during the last trimester. Also palpate the breasts to detect abnormalities.

Breast palpation

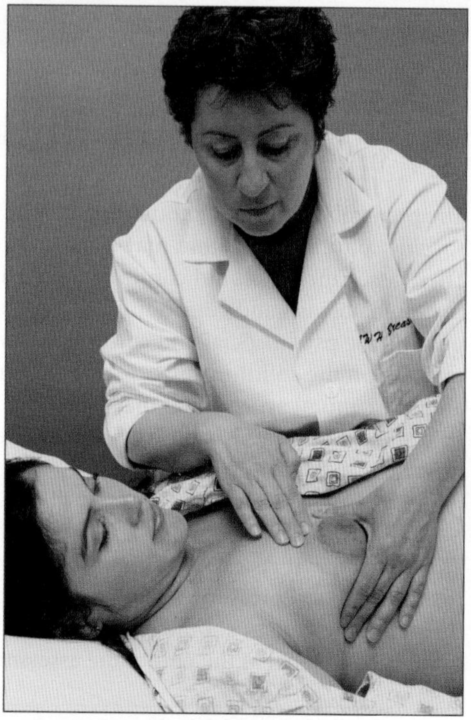

Heart and lungs

Palpate the apical pulse. As the pregnancy advances, the apical pulse may be found slightly higher than the fourth intercostal space because uterine displacement of the diaphragm causes transverse and leftward rotation of the heart.

Abdomen

Observe for a linea nigra, purple-red striae, and scars from previous cesarean births. Palpate the abdomen for the shape and size of the fetus. The abdomen may be flat to round depending on the gestation of the pregnancy. Fetal movement may be felt by a health care provider after the 18th week of gestation.

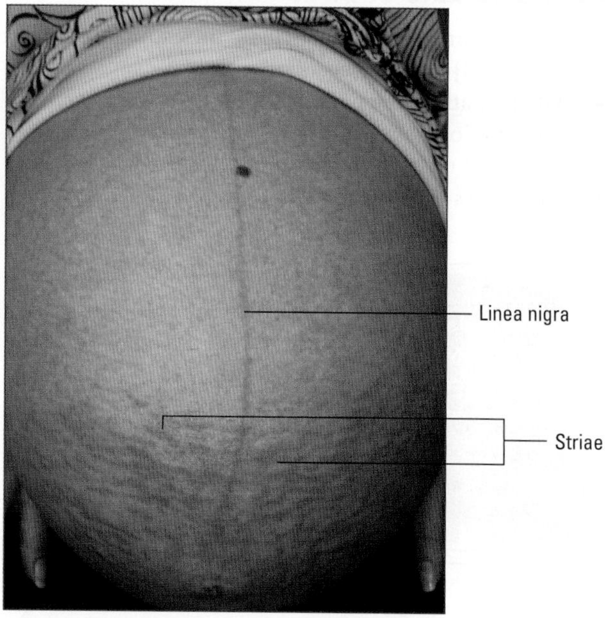
Linea nigra
Striae

Fundal height

At about 12 to 14 weeks' gestation, the uterus is palpable over the symphysis pubis as a firm, globular sphere. It reaches the umbilicus at 20 to 22 weeks, reaches the xiphoid at 36 weeks, and then, in many cases, returns to about 4 cm below the xiphoid process at 40 weeks due to lightening.

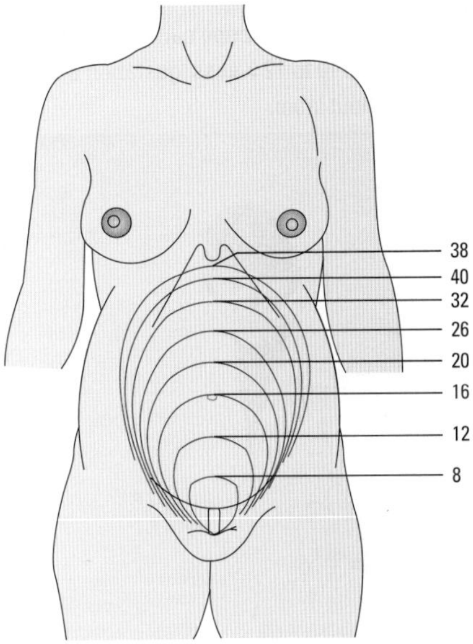
38
40
32
26
20
16
12
8

Skill check

Measuring fundal height

Use a pliable but nonstretchable tape measure to measure from the notch of the symphysis pubis to the top of the fundus, without tipping back the corpus.

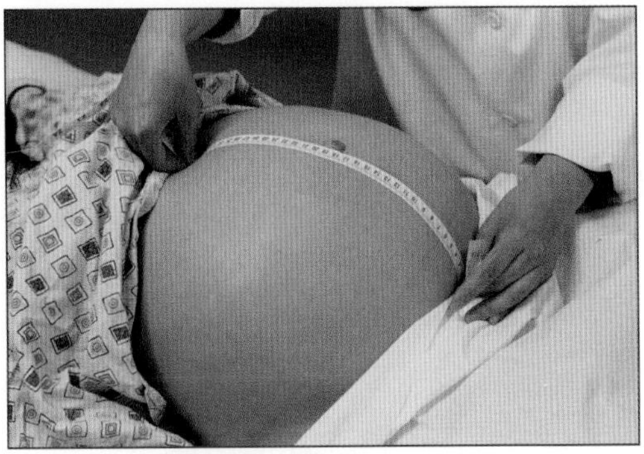

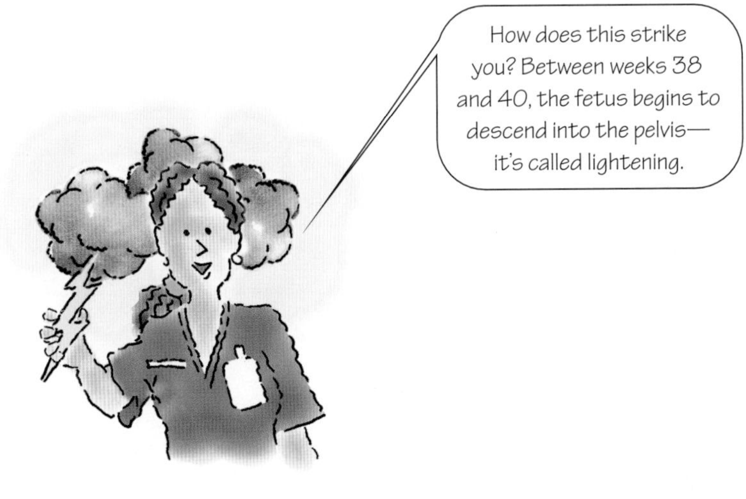
How does this strike you? Between weeks 38 and 40, the fetus begins to descend into the pelvis—it's called lightening.

Fetal heart rate

Place a fetoscope or Doppler stethoscope on the mother's abdomen and count the fetal heartbeats.

- After the 20th week of pregnancy, when fetal position can be determined, palpate for the back of the fetal thorax and position the instrument directly over it. Locate the loudest heartbeats and palpate the maternal pulse. Count fetal heartbeats for at least one full minute while monitoring maternal pulse.

Fetoscope

A fetoscope can detect fetal heartbeats as early as 18 to 20 weeks' gestation.

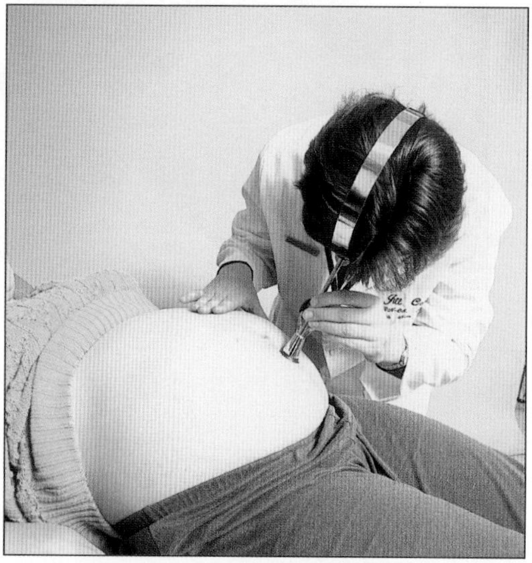

Doppler ultrasound stethoscope

The Doppler ultrasound stethoscope can detect fetal heartbeats as early as 10 to 12 weeks' gestation and is a useful tool throughout labor.

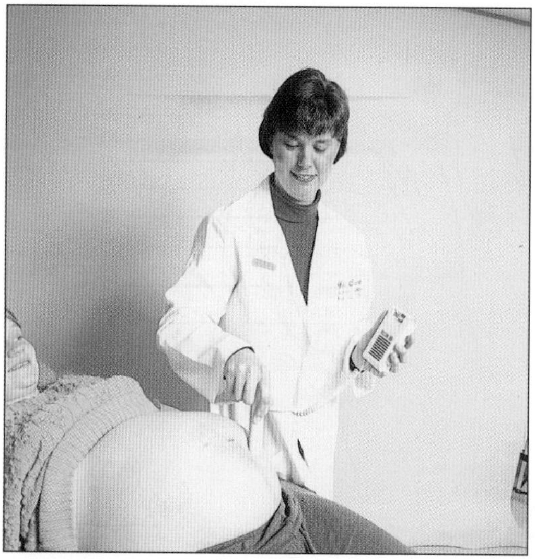

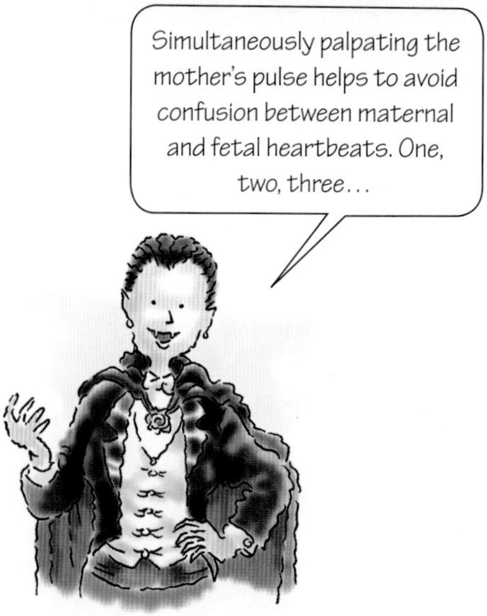
Simultaneously palpating the mother's pulse helps to avoid confusion between maternal and fetal heartbeats. One, two, three...

Skill check

Performing Leopold maneuvers

Use Leopold maneuvers to determine fetal position, presentation, and attitude.

First maneuver

- Place your hands over the patient's abdomen and curl your fingers around the fundus.
- When the fetus is in the vertex position (head first), the buttocks should feel irregularly shaped and firm.
- When the fetus is in the breech position (feet first), the head should feel hard, round, and completely moveable.

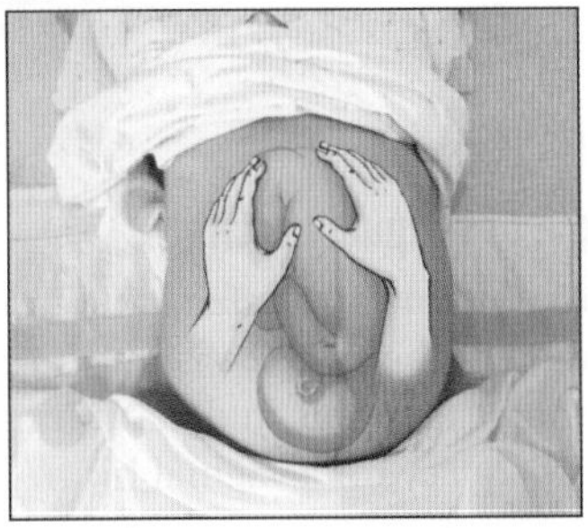

Second maneuver

- Move your hands down the side of the abdomen, applying gentle pressure.
- If the fetus is in the vertex position, you'll feel a smooth, hard surface on one side—the fetal back.
- Opposite, you'll feel lumps and knobs—the knees, hands, feet, and elbows.
- If the fetus is in the breech position, you may not feel the back at all.

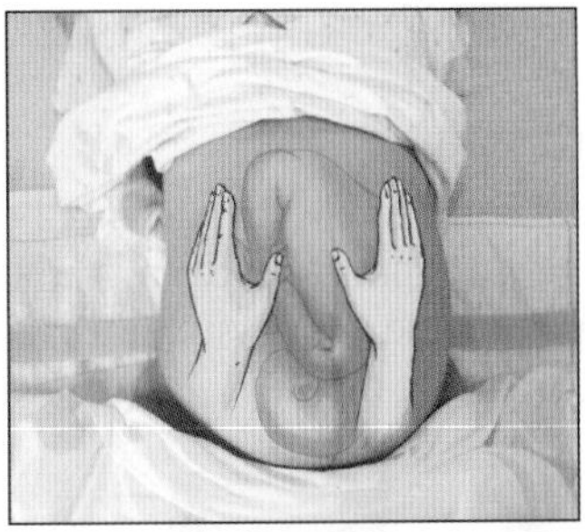

Third maneuver

- Spread your thumb and fingers of one hand, place them just above the patient's symphysis pubis, and then bring your fingers together.
- If the fetus is in the vertex position and hasn't descended, you'll feel the head.
- If the fetus is in the vertex position and has descended, you'll feel a less distinct mass.
- If the fetus is in the breech position, you'll feel a less distinct mass, which could be the feet or knees.

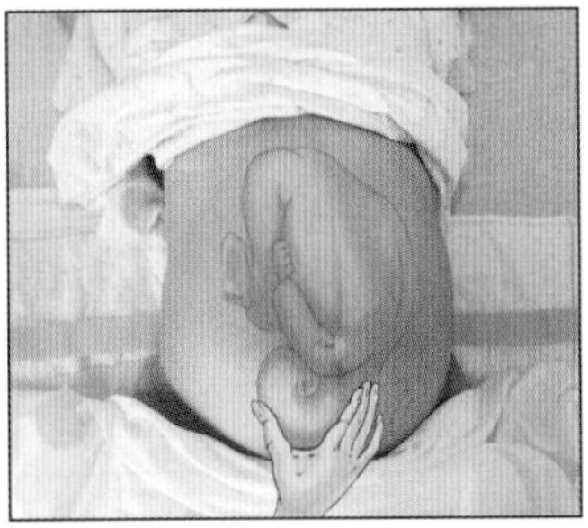

Fourth maneuver

- Use the fourth maneuver to determine flexion or extension of the fetal head and neck.
- Place your hands on both sides of the lower abdomen.
- Gently apply pressure with your fingers as you slide downward toward the symphysis pubis.
- If the head is the presenting part, one of your hands will be stopped by the cephalic prominence.
- If the fetus is in the vertex position, you'll feel the cephalic prominence on the same side as the back.

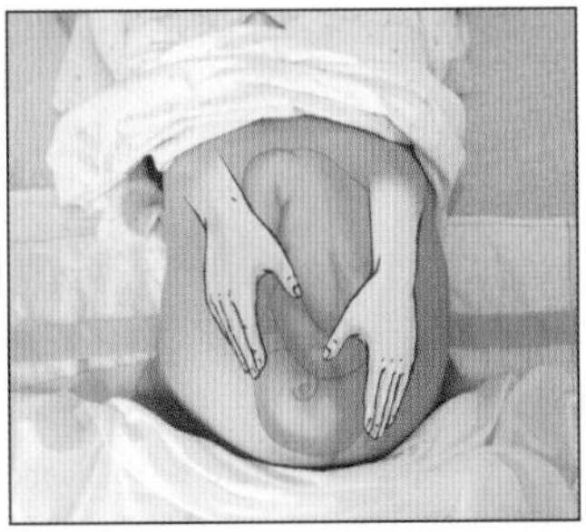

Pelvic measurements

The female pelvis protects and supports the reproductive organs and other pelvic structures. Pelvic measurements can help determine whether a woman will be able to deliver a neonate vaginally and aren't necessary if a woman has previously given birth vaginally. They may be taken at the initial visit or at a visit later in the pregnancy, when the woman's pelvic muscles are more relaxed.

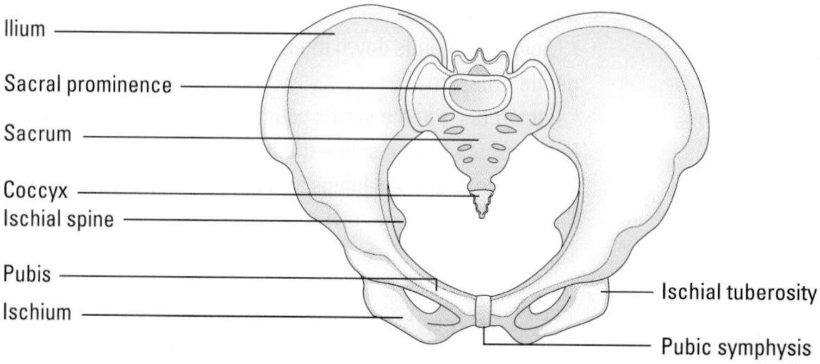
Ilium
Sacral prominence
Sacrum
Coccyx
Ischial spine
Pubis
Ischium
Ischial tuberosity
Pubic symphysis

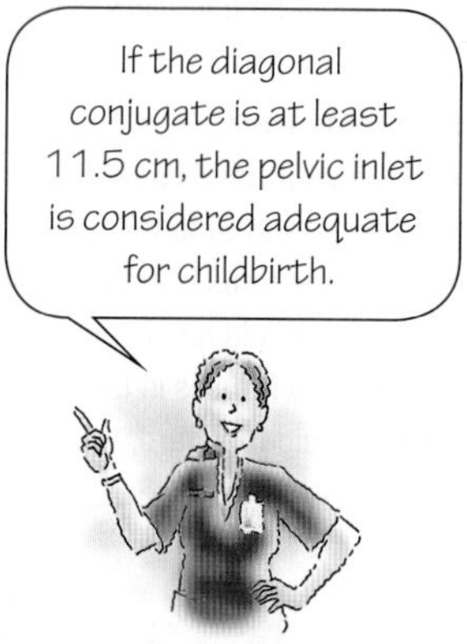
If the diagonal conjugate is at least 11.5 cm, the pelvic inlet is considered adequate for childbirth.

Diagonal conjugate

The diagonal conjugate is the distance between the anterior surface of the sacral prominence and the anterior surface of the inferior margin of the symphysis pubis. It indicates the anteroposterior diameter of the pelvic inlet, the narrower diameter.

Angle of subpubic arch

The subpubic arch refers to the inferior margin of the symphysis pubis. Estimating the angle also aids in determining the pelvic adequacy for a vaginal birth.

Skill check

Measuring the diagonal conjugate

- Place two fingers of your gloved examining hand in the vagina and press inward until the middle finger touches the sacral prominence.
- Use your other hand to mark the location where your examining hand touches the symphysis pubis.
- Withdraw your examining hand, and then measure the distance between the tip of the middle finger and the marked point with a ruler or pelvimeter.

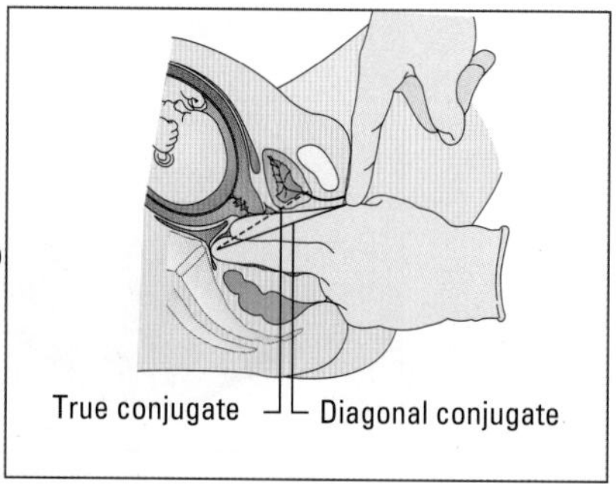
True conjugate
Diagonal conjugate

Skill check

Measuring the subpubic arch

- Place your thumbs at the inferior margin of the symphysis pubis in the perineum (they should be touching).
- Both hands should fit comfortably and form an angle that's greater than 90 degrees.

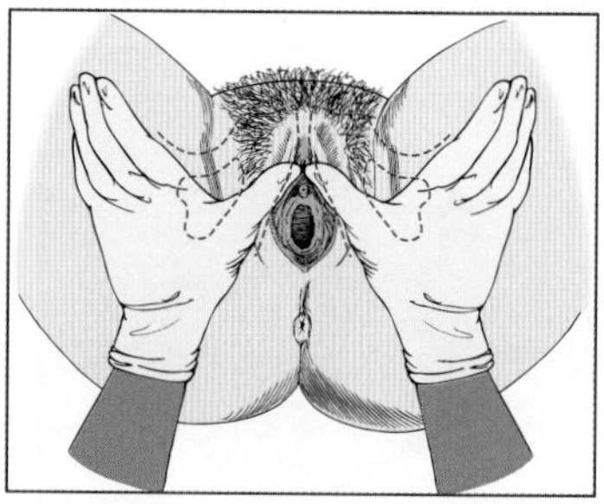

Transverse diameter

The transverse diameter, also known as the *ischial tuberosity diameter,* is the distance between the ischial tuberosities. It's the one diameter that commonly leads to problems with delivery.

Skill check

Measuring the transverse diameter

- Using a clenched fist, measure the width of the knuckles (span of the fist) to get a baseline for comparison.
- Insert the clenched fist between the ischial tuberosities at the level of the anus.
- If the knuckles are a width of 10 cm or more, the pelvic outlet is considered adequate to allow the widest part of the fetal head to pass through.

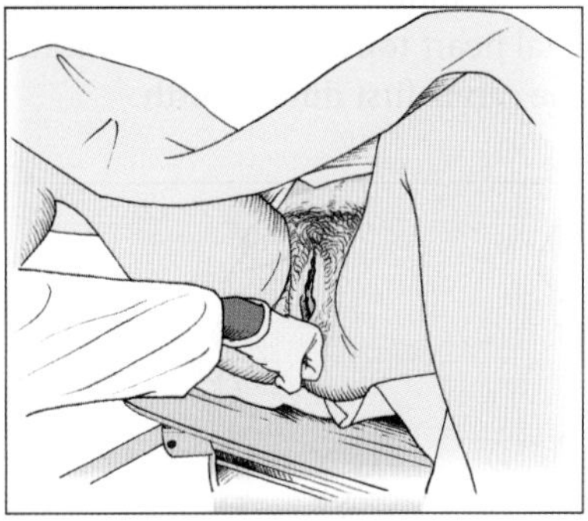

Pelvic shapes and potential problems

Gynecoid pelvis
- Characterized by well-rounded inlets and wide forward and backward diameters and pubic arch and outlet adequate
- Favorable for childbirth

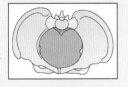

Android pelvis
- Characterized by extremely narrow lower dimensions of the pelvis (the pelvic arch forms an acute triangle) and outlet capacity reduced
- Most common in males but can occur in females
- Not favorable for delivering a fetus

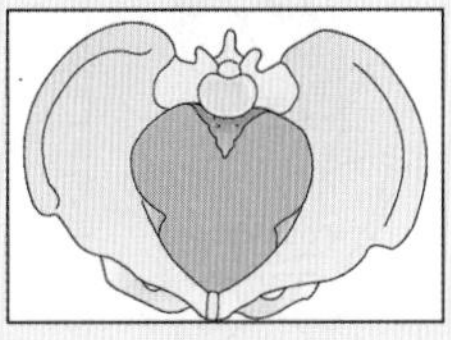

Anthropoid pelvis
- Also known as *apelike pelvis*
- Characterized by narrow transverse diameter and a longer-than-normal inlet anteroposterior diameter and outlet adequate
- Favorable for childbirth

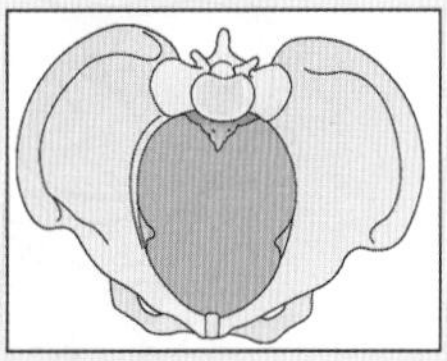

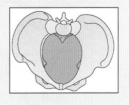

Platypelloid pelvis
- Also known as *flattened pelvis*
- Oval, smoothly curved inlet but a longer-than-normal transverse diameter and outlet capacity inadequate
- Can cause problems during childbirth with rotation of the fetal head
- Not favorable for childbirth

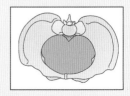

Intrapartum assessment

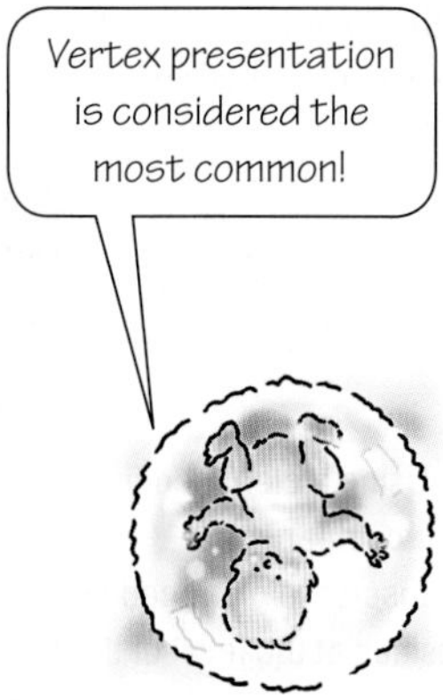
Vertex presentation is considered the most common!

Fetal presentation

Fetal presentation refers to the relationship of the fetus to the cervix. Assessed through vaginal examination, abdominal inspection and palpation, sonography, or auscultation of fetal heart tones (FHTs), it indicates which part of the fetus will pass through the cervix first during birth.

Cephalic

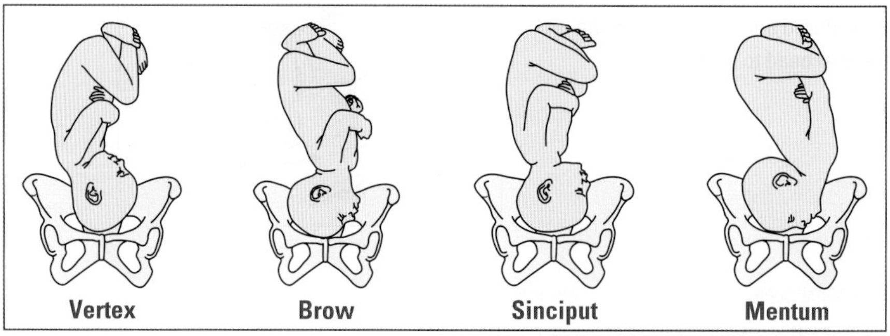
Vertex
Brow
Sinciput
Mentum

Breech

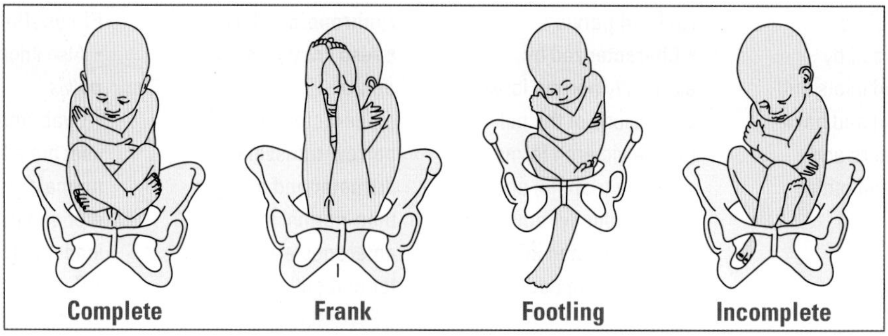
Complete
Frank
Footling
Incomplete

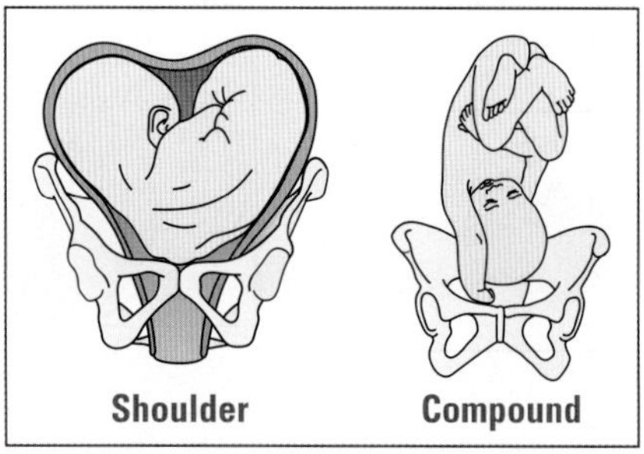
Shoulder
Compound

Fetal position

Fetal position is the relationship of the presenting part of the fetus to a specific quadrant of the mother's pelvis. It influences the progression of labor and helps determine whether surgical intervention is needed.

- Fetal position is defined using three letters:
- The first letter designates whether the presenting part is facing the mother's right (R) or left (L) side.
- The second letter or letters refer to the presenting part of the fetus: the occiput (O), mentum (M), sacrum (Sa), or scapula or acromion process (A).
- The third letter designates whether the presenting part is pointing to the anterior (A), posterior (P), or transverse (T) section of the mother's pelvis.

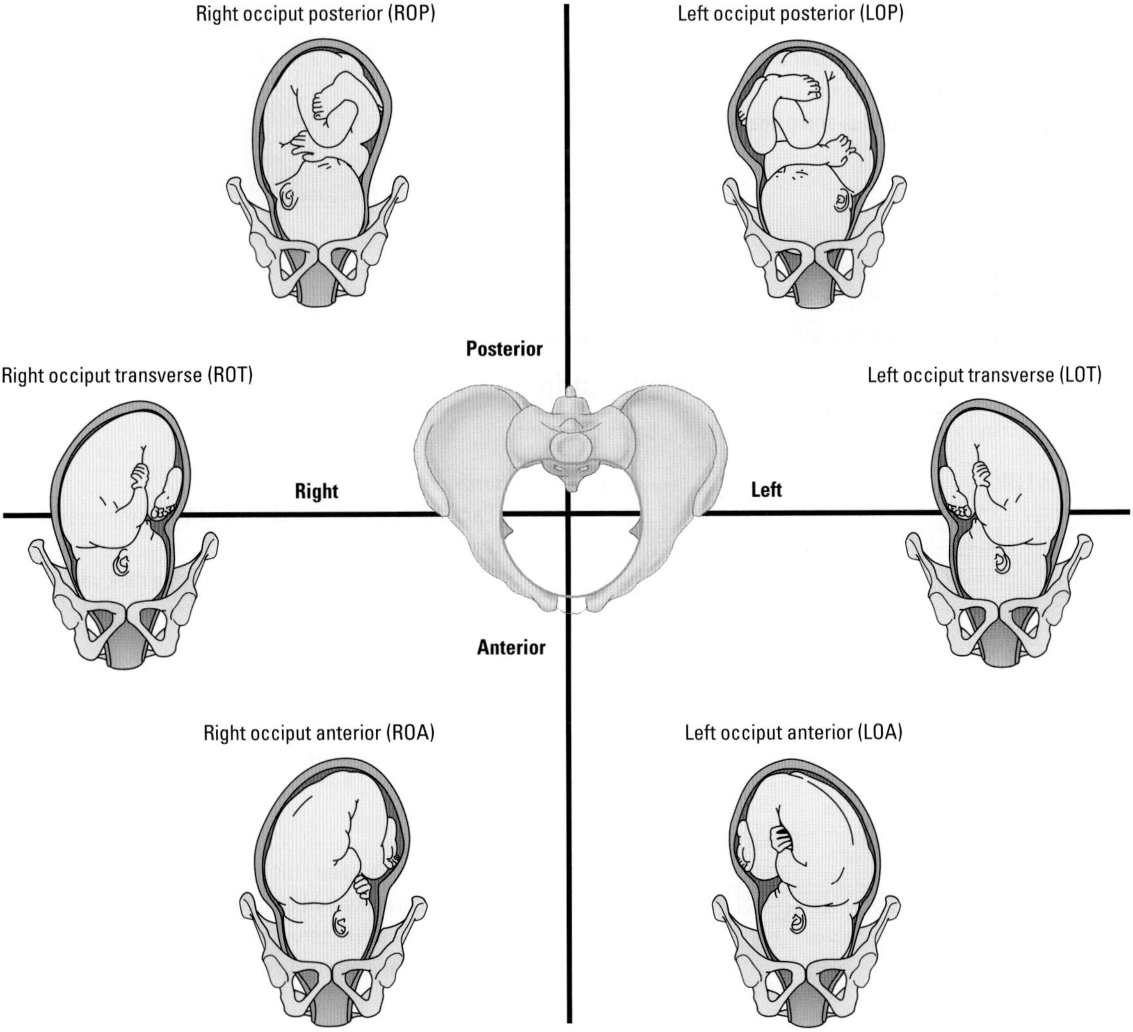
Right occiput posterior (ROP)
Left occiput posterior (LOP)
Posterior
Right occiput transverse (ROT)
Left occiput transverse (LOT)
Right
Left
Anterior
Right occiput anterior (ROA)
Left occiput anterior (LOA)

Fetal heart rate and uterine contractions

Assessment of fetal heart rate and uterine contractions can be accomplished by performing external fetal monitoring.

Skill check

Performing external monitoring

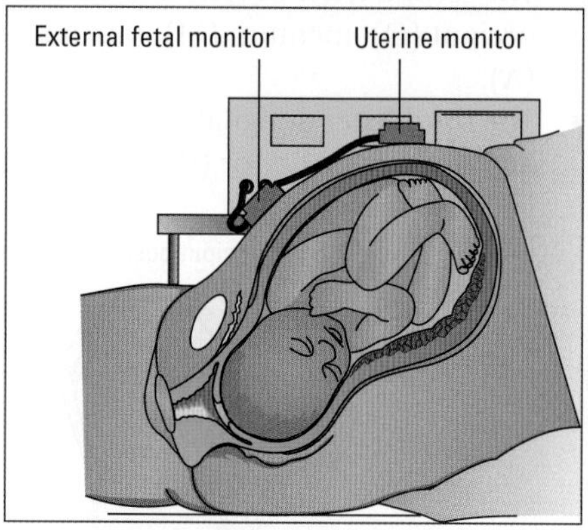
External fetal monitor
Uterine monitor

- Palpate the uterus to locate the fetus's back.
- Place the ultrasound transducer, which reads the fetal heart rate, over the site where the fetal heartbeat sounds the loudest.
- Use the tracing on the monitor strip to confirm the transducer's placement.
- Then place the tocotransducer over the uterine fundus where it contracts, either midline or slightly to one side.
- Place your hand on the fundus and palpate a contraction to verify proper placement.

Skill check

Reading a fetal monitor strip

The top recording shows the fetal heart rate (FHR) in beats per minute.

Baseline FHR

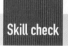

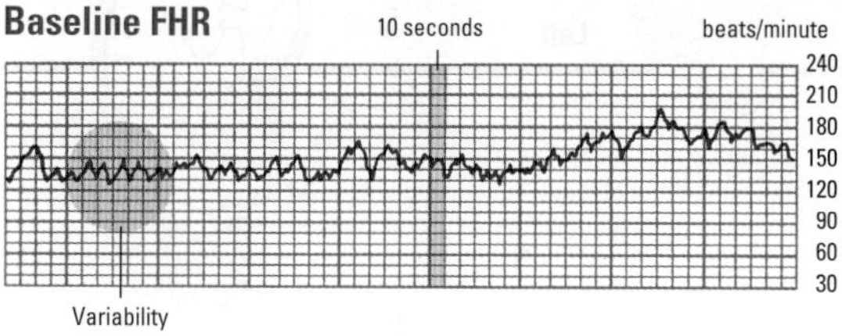
10 seconds
beats/minute
240
210
180
150
120
90
60
30
Variability

The bottom recording shows uterine activity (UA) in millimeters of mercury (mm Hg).

Uterine activity

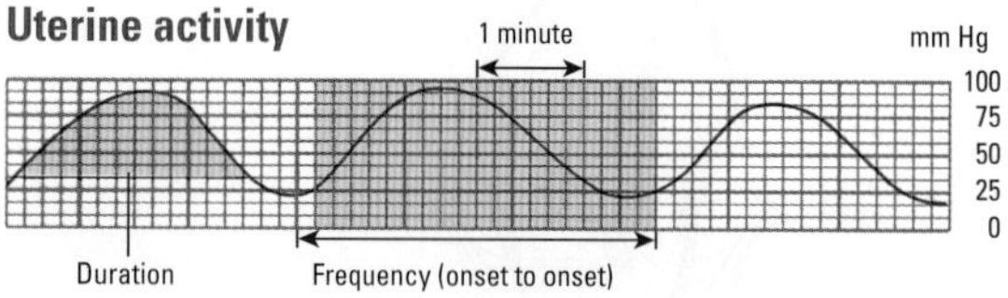
1 minute
mm Hg
100
75
50
25
0
Duration
Frequency (onset to onset)

Horizontally

- Each small block on the FHR or UA strip represents 10 seconds.
- Six consecutive blocks separated by a dark vertical line represent 1 minute.

Vertically

- Each block on the FHR strip represents an amplitude of 10 beats/minute.
- Each block on the UA strip represents 5 mm Hg of pressure.

What to do

- Assess the baseline FHR (the resting rate) between uterine contractions when fetal movement diminishes.
- This baseline FHR serves as a reference for subsequent FHR tracings produced during contractions.

Locating fetal heart sounds

LOA

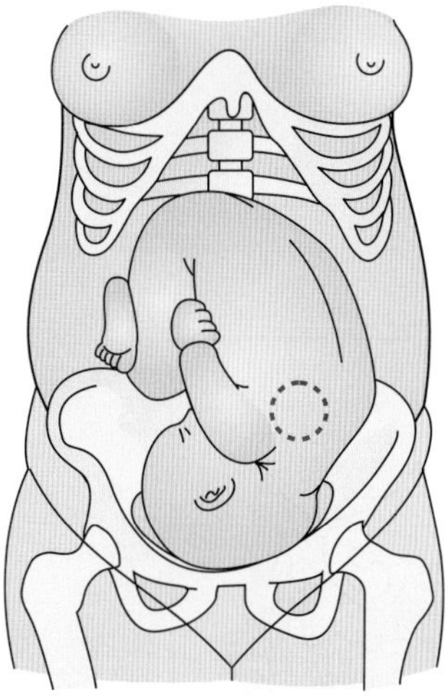

ROA

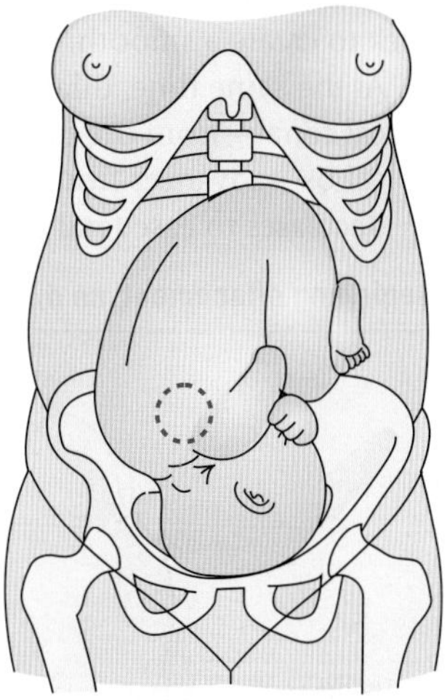

LOP

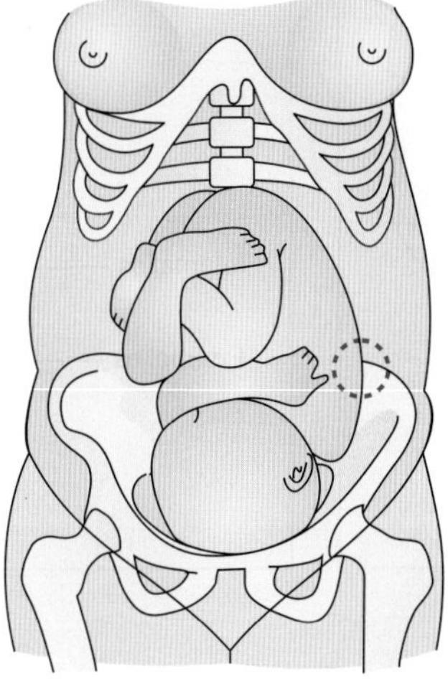

ROP

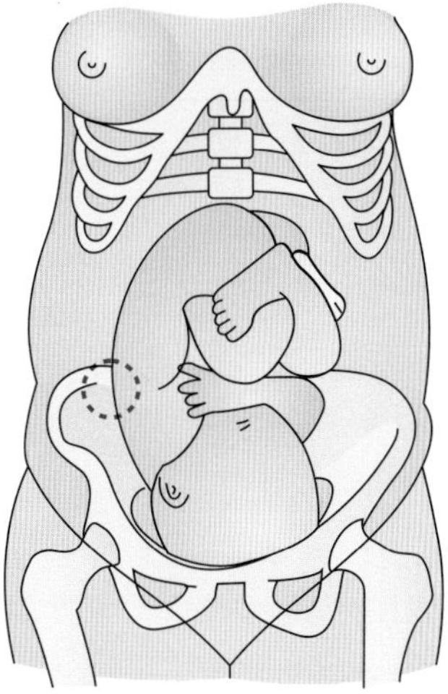

LSA

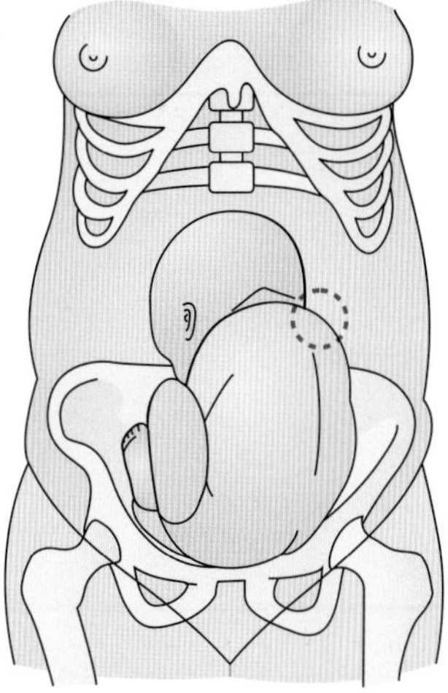

Cervical effacement and dilation

During effacement, the cervix shortens and its walls become thin, progressing from 0% effacement (palpable and thick) to 100% effacement (fully indistinct or effaced and paper-thin). Full effacement obliterates the constrictive uterine neck to create a smooth, unobstructed passageway for the fetus.

- At the same time, dilation occurs. This progressive widening of the cervical canal—from the upper internal cervical os to the lower external cervical os—advances from 0 to 10 cm. As the cervical canal opens, resistance decreases to ease fetal descent.

Beginning effacement; no dilation

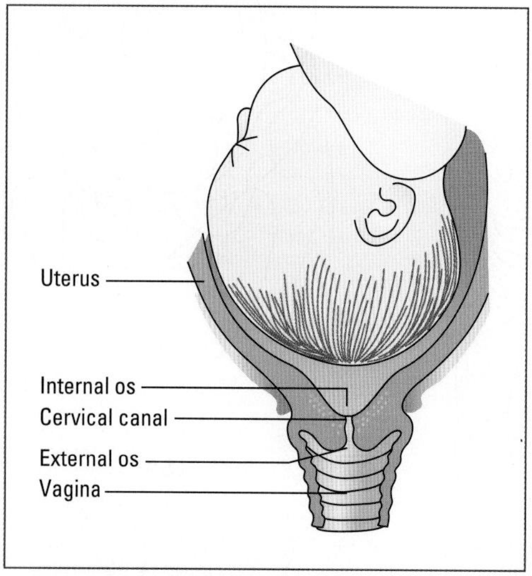
Uterus
Internal os
Cervical canal
External os
Vagina

Full effacement and dilation

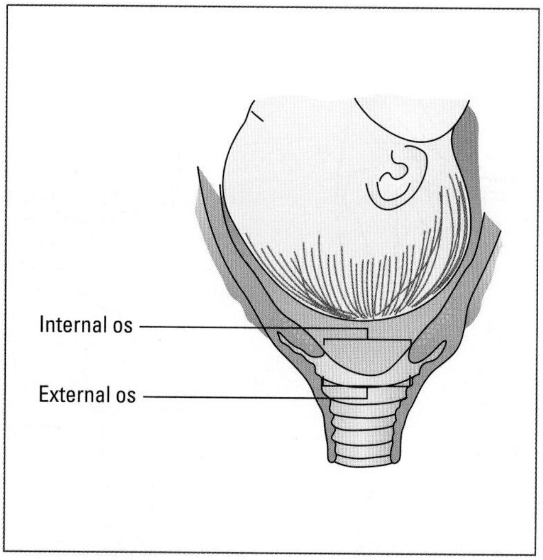
Internal os
External os

Fetal engagement and station

Assess for fetal engagement (the point at which the fetal presenting part advances into the pelvis) during cervical examination. After you have determined fetal engagement, palpate the presenting part and grade the fetal station (where the presenting part lies in relation to the ischial spines of the maternal pelvis).

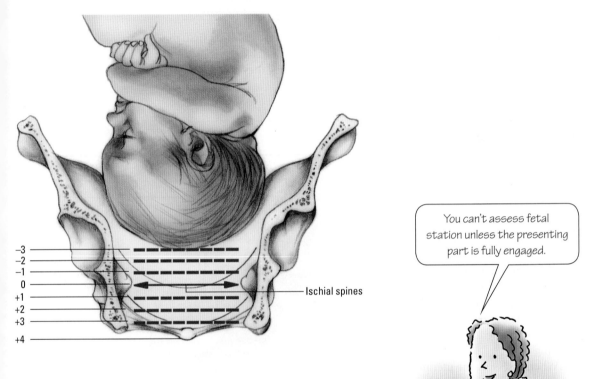

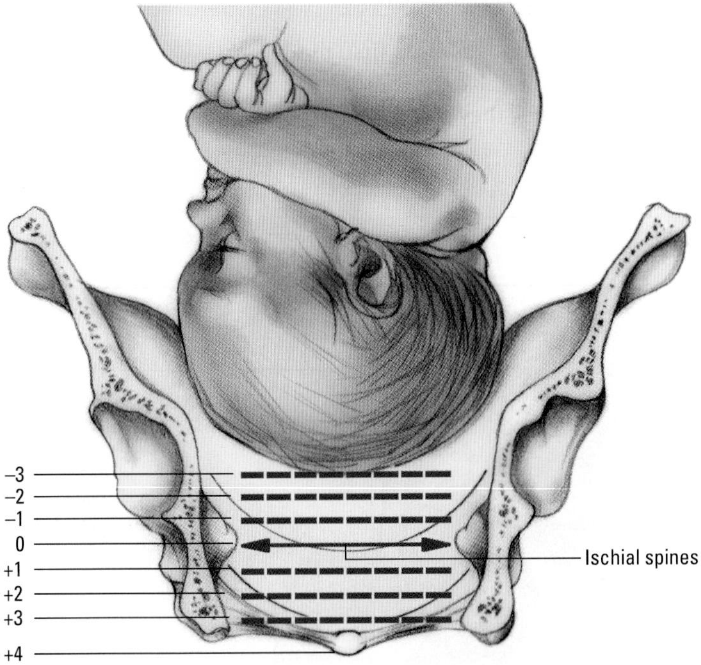
–3
–2
–1
0
+1
+2
+3
+4
Ischial spines

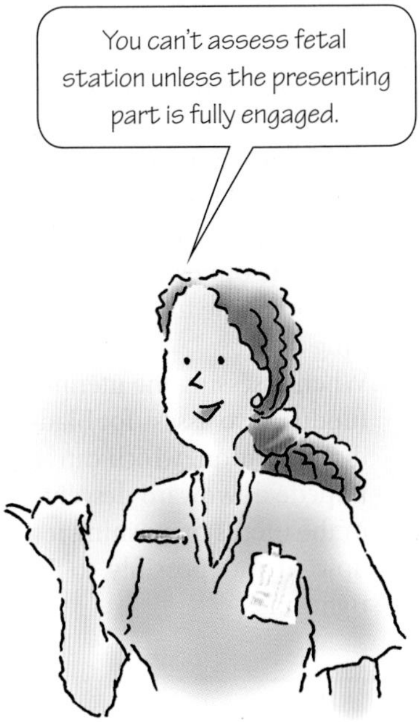
You can't assess fetal station unless the presenting part is fully engaged.

Postpartum assessment

Breasts

Inspect and palpate the breasts, noting their size, shape, and color. At first, the breasts should feel soft and secrete thin, yellow fluid called *colostrum*. As they fill with milk—usually around the third postpartum day—they should begin to feel firm and warm.

Fundal assessment

Pregnancy stretches the ligaments that support the uterus, placing it at risk for inversion during palpation. To guard against this:

- Place one hand against the abdomen at the symphysis pubis level to steady the fundus and prevent downward displacement.
- Place the opposite hand at the top of the fundus, cupping it.
- When assessing the uterine fundus, also assess for bladder distention, which can impede downward descent of the uterus by pushing it upward and, possibly, to the right side.

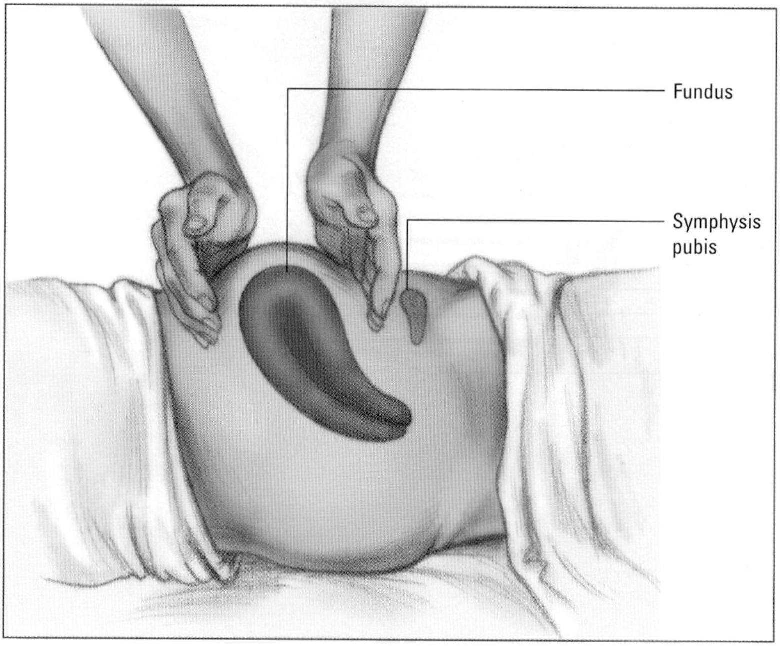
Fundus
Symphysis pubis

Uterine involution

After birth, the uterus begins its descent back into the pelvic cavity. After delivery is complete, the top of the fundus lies midline and halfway in between the symphysis pubis and the umbilicus. Assessment of the fundus 6 to 12 hours later should locate the top of the fundus approximately at the umbilicus level. The uterus continues to descend 1 cm/day until it isn't palpable above the symphysis pubis, at about 9 days after birth.

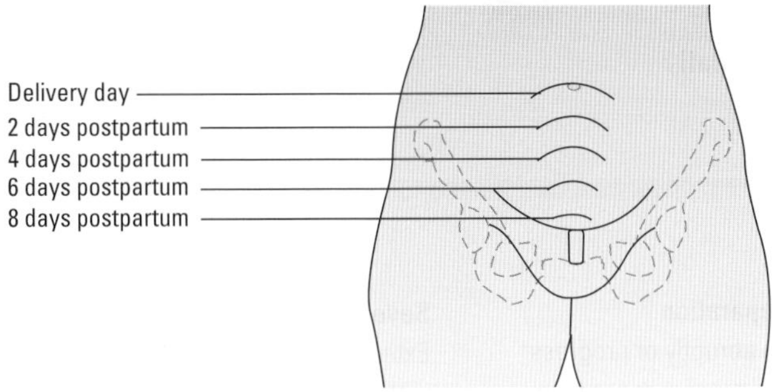
Delivery day
2 days postpartum
4 days postpartum
6 days postpartum
8 days postpartum

Lochia

After birth, the outermost layer of the uterus becomes necrotic and is expelled. This vaginal discharge—called lochia—is similar to menstrual flow and consists of blood, fragments of the decidua, white blood cells, mucus, and some bacteria.

- Assess lochia flow for amount, color, odor, and consistency. A foul or offensive odor may indicate infection. Evidence of large or numerous clots indicates poor uterine contraction and requires further assessment.

Lochia rubra

Red, vaginal discharge that occurs from approximately postpartum days 1 to 3. This may contain clots. Passing a few small clots no bigger than a nickel is normal during this time. If the clots are bigger, the health care provider should be notified.

Lochia serosa

Pinkish or brownish discharge that occurs from approximately postpartum days 3 to 10

Lochia alba

Creamy white or colorless vaginal discharge that occurs from approximately postpartum days 10 to 14 (may continue for up to 6 weeks)

Perineum and rectum

Assess the perineum and rectum when you assess the lochia. Observe for intactness of skin, positioning of the episiotomy (if one was performed), and appearance of sutures (from episiotomy or laceration repair) and the surrounding rectal area. Note ecchymosis, hematoma, erythema, edema, drainage, or bleeding from sutures; a foul odor; or signs of infection. Also observe for hemorrhoids.

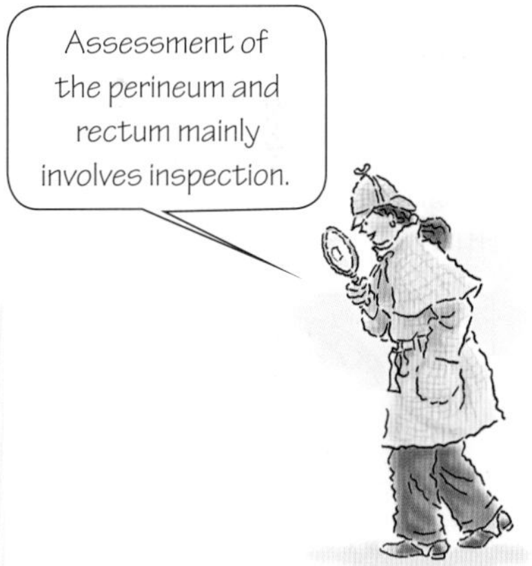
Assessment of the perineum and rectum mainly involves inspection.

Abnormal findings

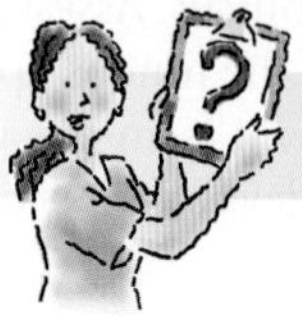

Outside the norm

Abruptio placenta

Abruptio placenta is premature separation of a normally implanted placenta from the uterine wall.

Types of abruptio placentae

Mild separation

Begins with small areas of separation and internal bleeding (concealed hemorrhage) between the placenta and uterine wall

Signs and symptoms

- Gradual onset
- Mild to moderate bleeding
- Vague lower abdominal discomfort
- Mild to moderate abdominal tenderness and uterine irritability
- Strong, regular fetal heart tones (FHTs)

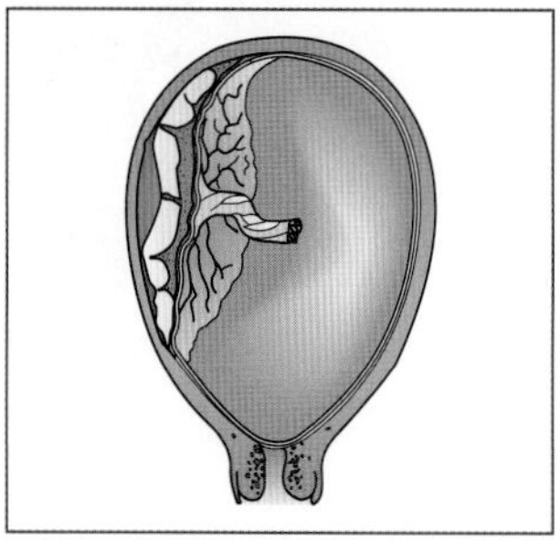

Moderate separation

May develop abruptly or progress from mild to extensive separation with external hemorrhage

Signs and symptoms

- Gradual or abrupt onset
- Moderate, dark red vaginal bleeding
- Continuous abdominal pain
- Tender uterus that remains firm between contractions
- Barely audible or irregular and bradycardic FHTs
- Possible signs of shock

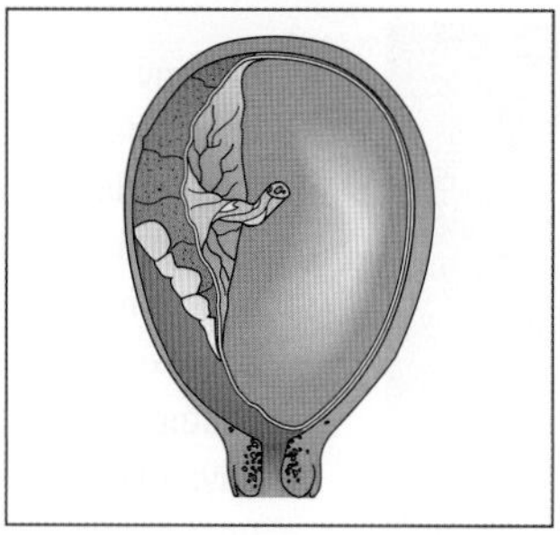

Severe separation

External hemorrhage occurs, along with shock and possible fetal cardiac distress

Signs and symptoms

- Abrupt onset of agonizing, unremitting uterine pain
- Moderate vaginal bleeding
- Boardlike, tender uterus
- Absence of FHTs
- Rapidly progressive shock

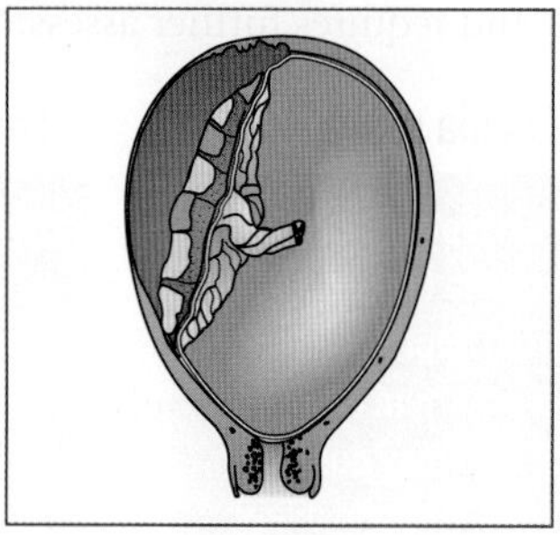

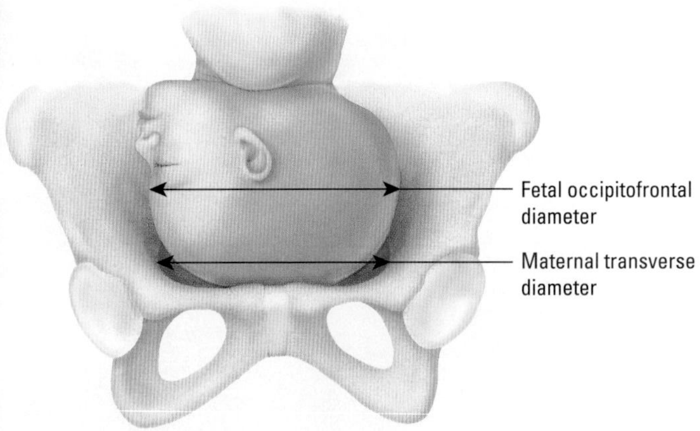
Fetal occipitofrontal diameter
Maternal transverse diameter

Cephalopelvic disproportion

Narrowing of the birth canal at the inlet, midpelvis, or outlet causes a disproportion between the size of the fetal head and the pelvic diameters, or cephalopelvic disproportion (CPD). CPD results in failure of labor to progress.

Ectopic pregnancy

Ectopic pregnancy occurs when a fertilized ovum implants outside the uterine cavity, most commonly in a fallopian tube. Mild abdominal pain may occur. Typically, the patient reports amenorrhea or abnormal menses (fallopian tube implantation), followed by slight vaginal bleeding and unilateral pelvic pain over the mass. The uterus feels boggy and is tender. The patient may report extreme pain when the cervix is moved.

Sites of ectopic pregnancy

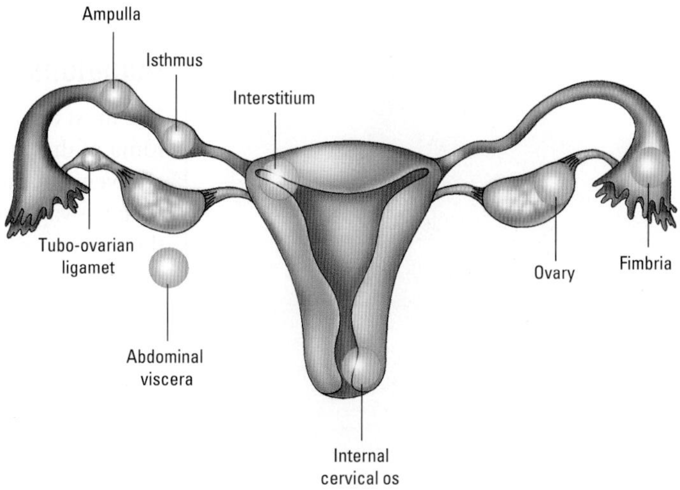
Ampulla
Isthmus
Interstitium
Tubo-ovarian ligamet
Abdominal viscera
Internal cervical os
Ovary
Fimbria

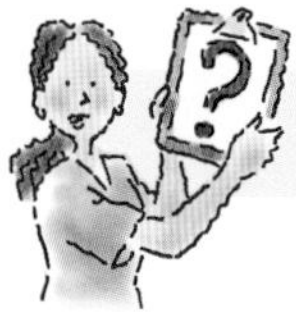

Outside the norm

Gestational trophoblastic disease

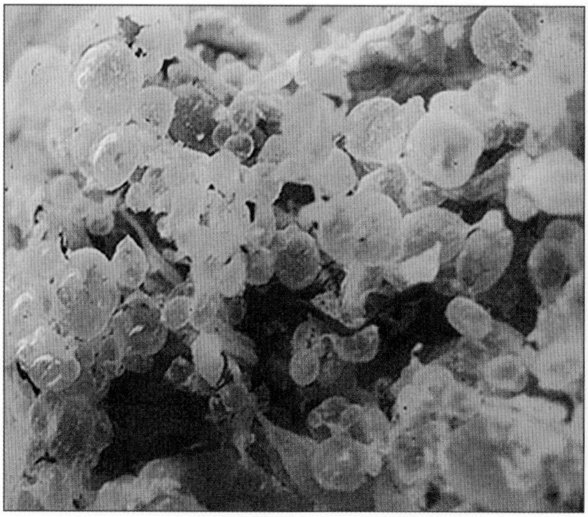

Gestational trophoblastic disease, or molar pregnancy, is the rapid deterioration of trophoblastic villi cells. As a result of this cell abnormality, the embryo fails to develop.

- Signs and symptoms include mild vaginal bleeding, ranging from brownish red spotting to bright red hemorrhaging. The patient may report passing tissue that resembles grape clusters. Her history may also include hyperemesis, lower abdominal cramps, and signs and symptoms of preeclampsia.

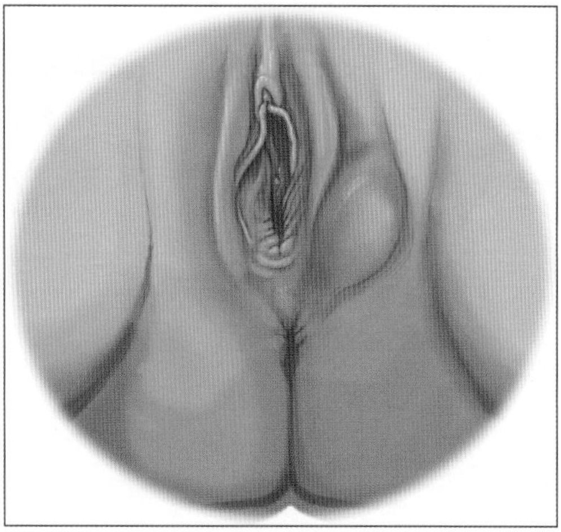

Hematoma

The most common hematoma following birth is a hematoma of the vulva, which results from ruptured arteries and veins in the superficial fascia that seep into nearby tissue. A vaginal hematoma may result after trauma to the soft tissue of the vagina after birth. It can obstruct the urethra, making urination difficult.

Hypertension in pregnancy

Hypertension in pregnancy is defined as a blood pressure greater than 140 mm Hg systolic and greater than 90 mm Hg diastolic on two occasions at least 6 hours apart.

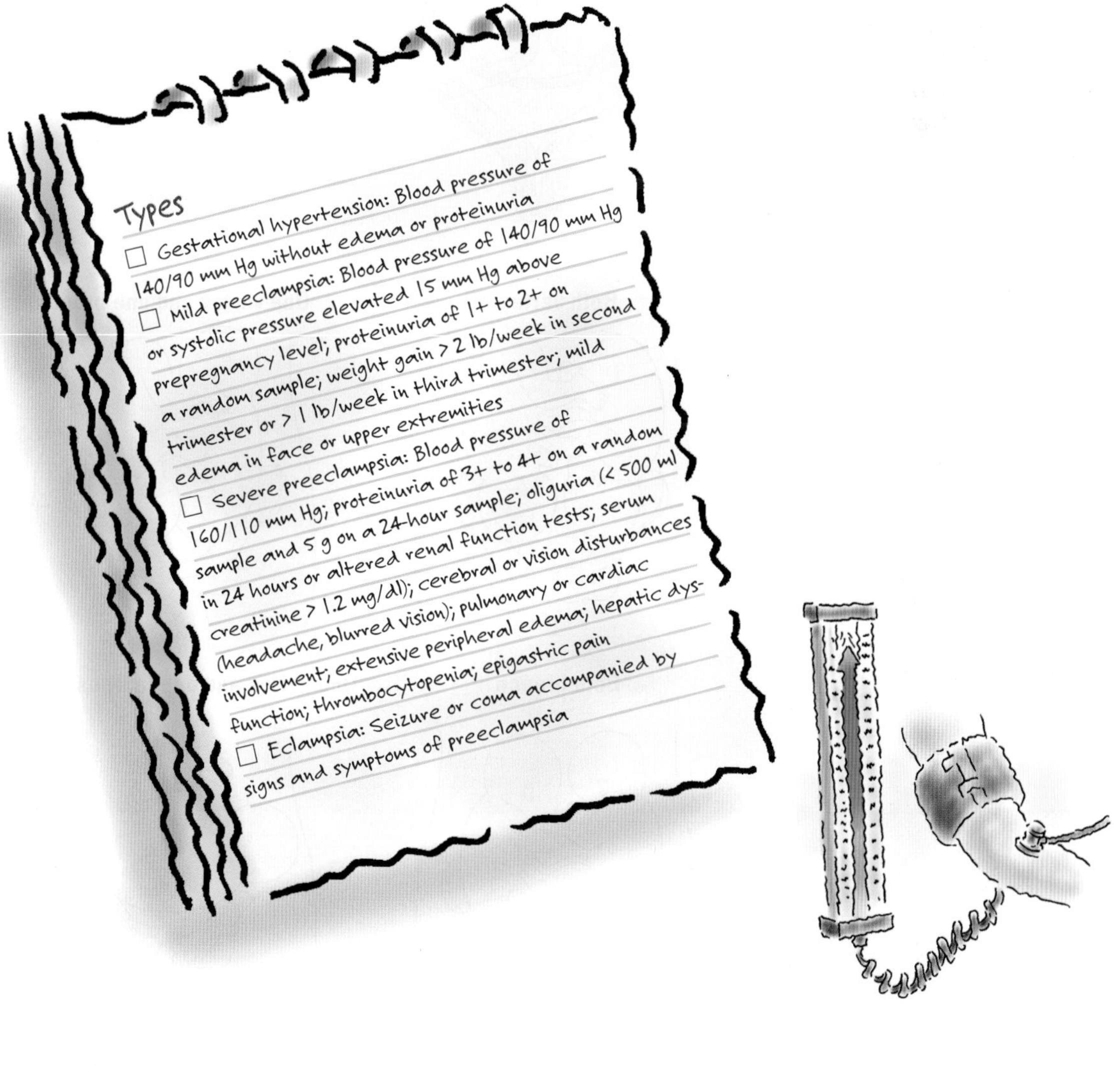
Types
☐ Gestational hypertension: Blood pressure of 140/90 mm Hg without edema or proteinuria
☐ Mild preeclampsia: Blood pressure of 140/90 mm Hg or systolic pressure elevated 15 mm Hg above prepregnancy level; proteinuria of 1+ to 2+ on a random sample; weight gain > 2 lb/week in second trimester or > 1 lb/week in third trimester; mild edema in face or upper extremities
☐ Severe preeclampsia: Blood pressure of 160/110 mm Hg; proteinuria of 3+ to 4+ on a random sample and 5 g on a 24-hour sample; oliguria (< 500 ml in 24 hours or altered renal function tests; serum creatinine > 1.2 mg/dl); cerebral or vision disturbances (headache, blurred vision); pulmonary or cardiac involvement; extensive peripheral edema; hepatic dysfunction; thrombocytopenia; epigastric pain
☐ Eclampsia: Seizure or coma accompanied by signs and symptoms of preeclampsia

Multiple pregnancy

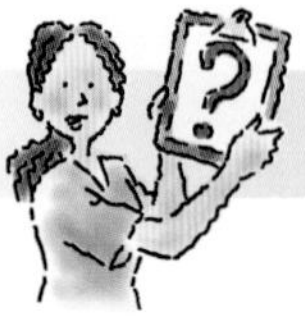

Outside the norm

Multiple pregnancy, **or** ***multiple gestation,*** refers to a pregnancy involving more than one fetus. It's considered a complication of pregnancy because the woman's body must adjust to the effects of carrying multiple fetuses.

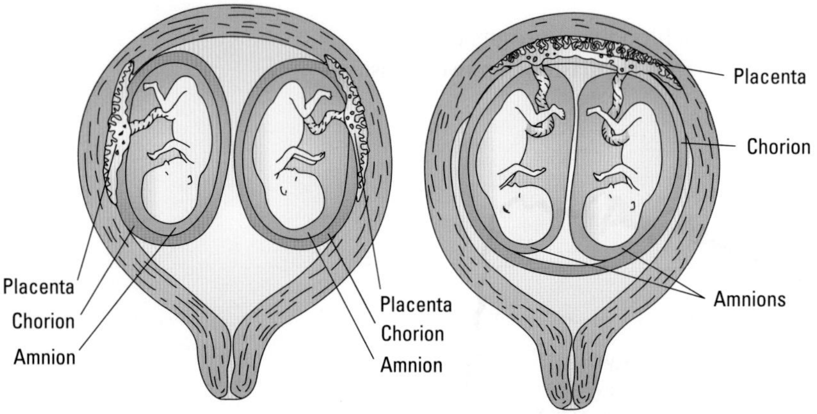
Placenta
Chorion
Amnion
Placenta
Chorion
Amnion
Placenta
Chorion
Amnions

Twin pregnancy presentations

With a twin or other multiple pregnancy, the fetuses can be in several presentation combinations.

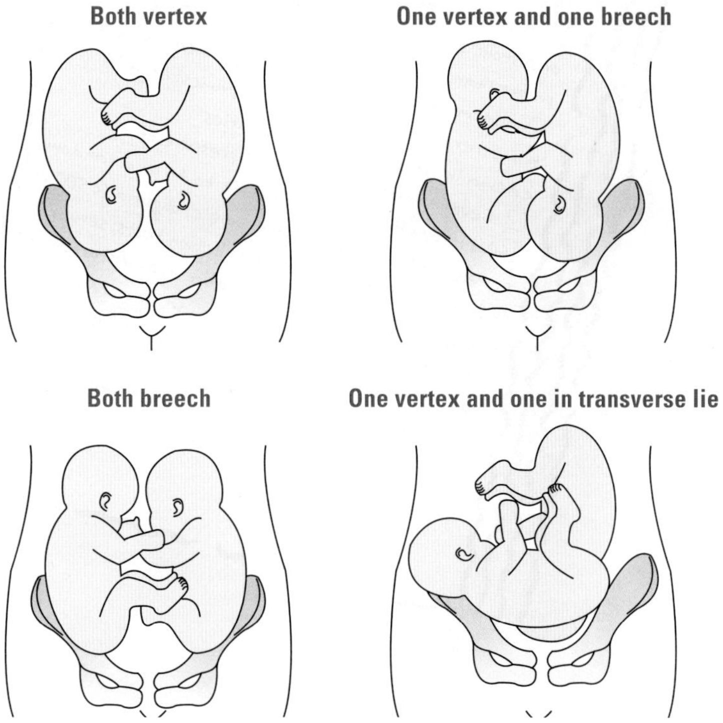
Both vertex
One vertex and one breech
Both breech
One vertex and one in transverse lie

Placenta previa

Placenta previa occurs when the placenta implants in the lower uterine segment, where it encroaches on the internal cervical os. It causes painless, bright red, usually episodic vaginal bleeding after the 20th week of pregnancy. Malpresentation is possible because the placenta's abnormal location interferes with descent of the fetal head.

Types of placenta previa

Low implantation
The placenta implants in the lower uterine segment.

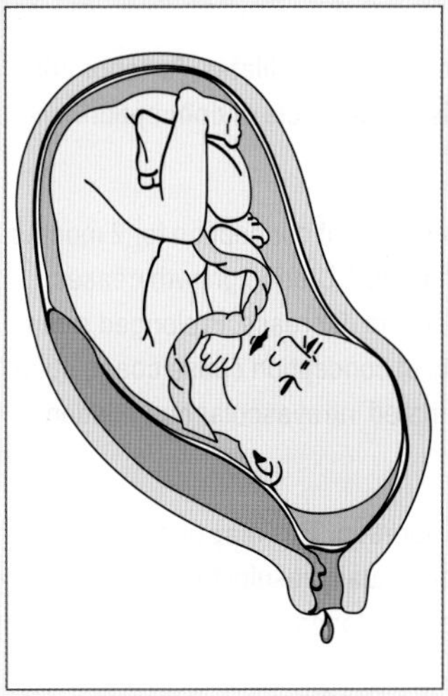

Partial placenta previa
The placenta partially occludes the cervical os.

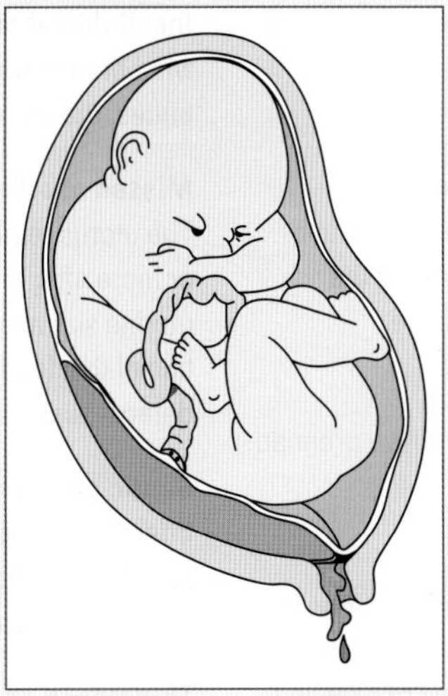

Total placenta previa
The placenta totally occludes the cervical os.

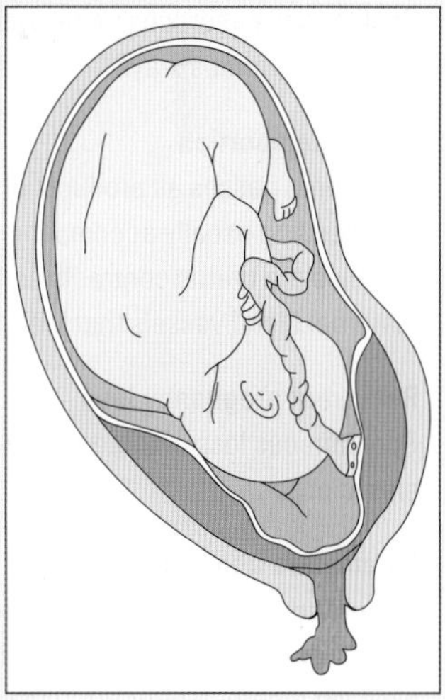

Postpartum hemorrhage

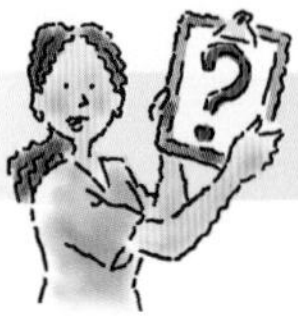

Outside the norm

Postpartum hemorrhage is any blood loss from the uterus that exceeds 500 ml during a 24-hour period. It's a major cause of maternal mortality.

Causes of postpartum hemorrhage

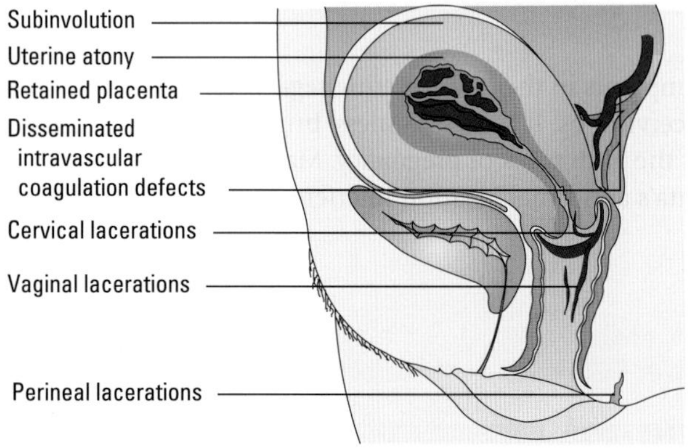
Subinvolution
Uterine atony
Retained placenta
Disseminated intravascular coagulation defects
Cervical lacerations
Vaginal lacerations
Perineal lacerations

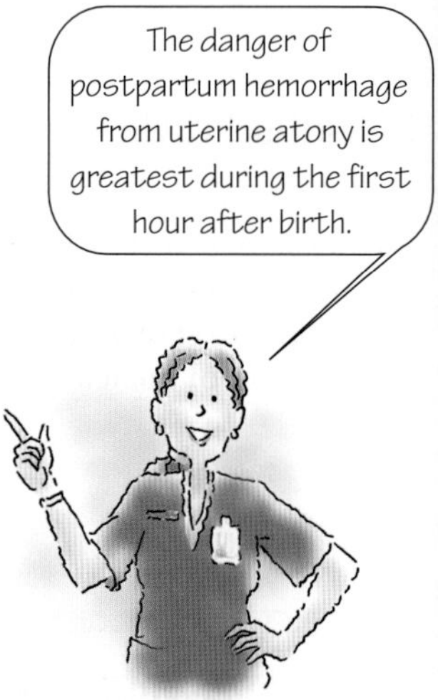
The danger of postpartum hemorrhage from uterine atony is greatest during the first hour after birth.

Spontaneous abortion

Types of spontaneous abortion

Spontaneous abortions occur without medical intervention and in various ways.

Complete abortion
The uterus passes all products of conception. Minimal bleeding usually accompanies complete abortion because the uterus contracts and compresses the maternal blood vessels that feed the placenta.

Recurrent pregnancy loss
Spontaneous loss of three or more consecutive pregnancies in order.

Incomplete abortion
The uterus retains part or all of the placenta. Before 10 weeks' gestation, the fetus and placenta are usually expelled together; after the 10th week, they're expelled separately. Because part of the placenta may adhere to the uterine wall, bleeding continues. Hemorrhage is possible because the uterus doesn't contract and seal the large vessels that feed the placenta.

Inevitable abortion
Membranes rupture, and the cervix dilates. As labor continues, the uterus expels the products of conception.

Missed abortion
The uterus retains the products of conception for 2 months or more after the fetus has died. Uterine growth ceases; uterine size may even seem to decrease. Prolonged retention of the dead products of conception cause coagulation defects such as disseminated intravascular coagulation.

Septic abortion
Infection accompanies abortion. This may occur with spontaneous abortion but usually results from a lapse in sterile technique during threatened abortion.

Threatened abortion
Bloody vaginal discharge occurs during the first half of pregnancy. About 20% of pregnant women have vaginal spotting or actual bleeding early in pregnancy. Of these, about 50% abort.

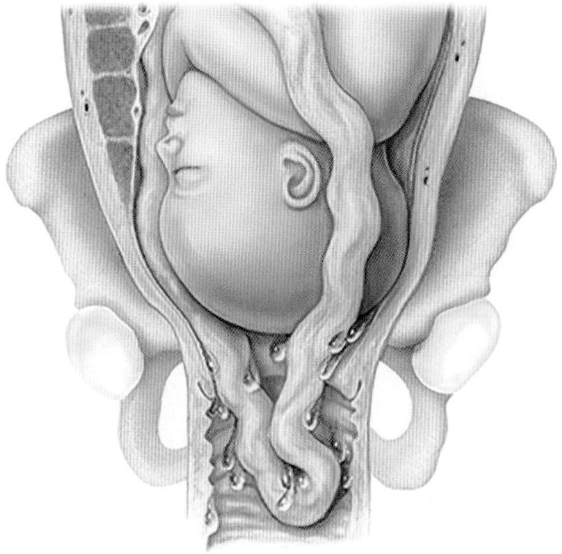

Umbilical cord prolapse

In umbilical cord prolapse, a loop of the umbilical cord slips in front of the fetal presenting part. It can occur at any time after the membranes rupture, especially if the presenting part isn't firmly engaged in the cervix.

Other abnormal findings

Bleeding
Vaginal bleeding at any time during a pregnancy is a potential danger sign that requires further investigation. It can range from slight spotting to frank bleeding and may or may not be accompanied by pain.

Premature cervical dilation
In premature cervical dilation, the cervix dilates prematurely and can't hold the fetus until term. Often the first sign is a pink-stained vaginal discharge or increased pelvic pressure, which may be followed by rupture of the amniotic fluid membranes.

Premature rupture of membranes
A sudden gush of clear vaginal fluid suggests rupture of the membranes and onset of labor, which typically occurs at term. Before term (before 37 weeks), it's called preterm premature rupture of membranes (PPROM) and predisposes the mother and fetus to infection. Additionally, PROM can lead to inadequate nutritional supply to the fetus and possible prolapse of the umbilical cord.

Preterm labor
Preterm labor is the onset of rhythmic contractions that produce cervical changes after fetal viability but before fetal maturity. It usually occurs between 20 and 37 weeks' gestation.

Q&A

Able to label?

Identify the anatomic structures of pregnancy indicated on this illustration.

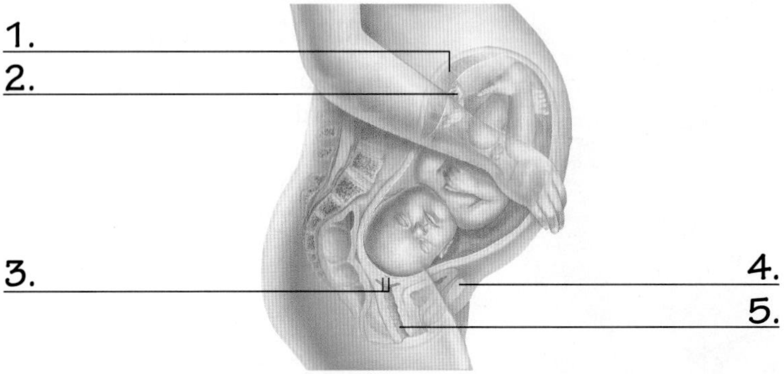
1.
2.
3.
4.
5.

Matchmaker

Match the abnormal pregnancy findings shown with their correct names.

1. ______

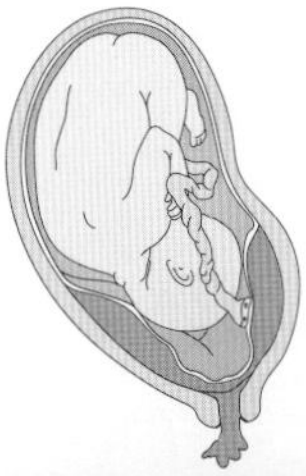

2. ______

3. ______

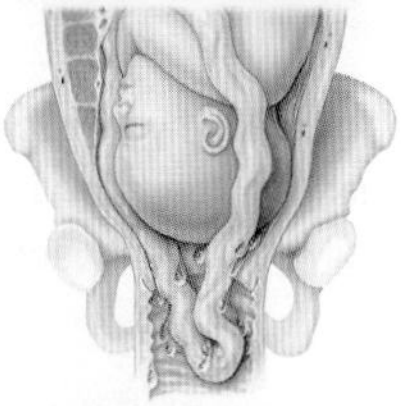

4. ______

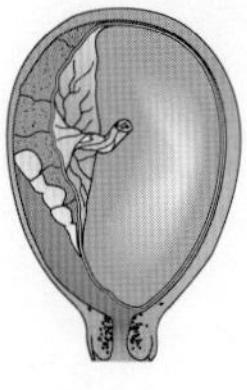

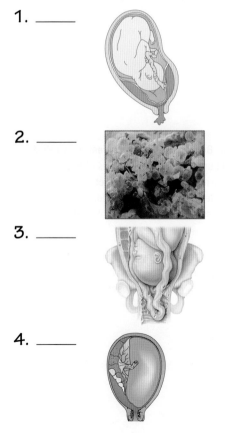

A. Umbilical cord prolapse

B. Abruptio placentae

C. Placenta previa

D. Gestational trophoblastic disease

Answers: Able to label? 1. Placenta, 2. Umbilical cord, 3. Cervix, 4. Symphysis pubis, 5. Vagina; Matchmaker 1. C, 2. D, 3. A, 4. B.

Selected References

London, M. L., Ladewig, P. W., Ball, J. W., Bindler, R. C., & Cowen, K. J. (2014). *Maternal & child nursing care* (4th ed.). New York, NY: Pearson.

Perry, S. E., Hockenberry, M. J., Lowdermilk, D. L., & Wilson, D. (2014). *Maternal child nursing care* (5th ed.). St. Louis, MO: Elsevier.

Index

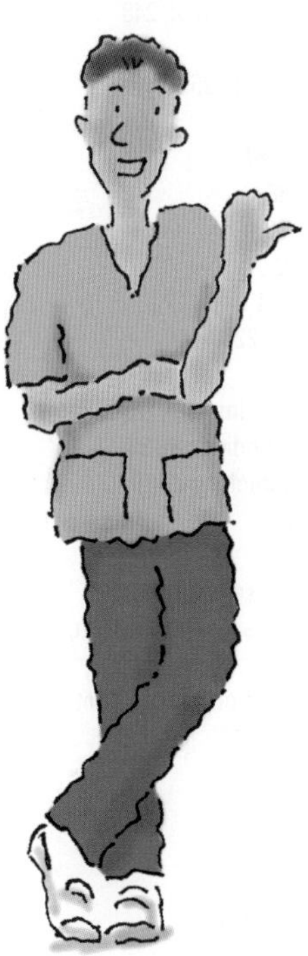

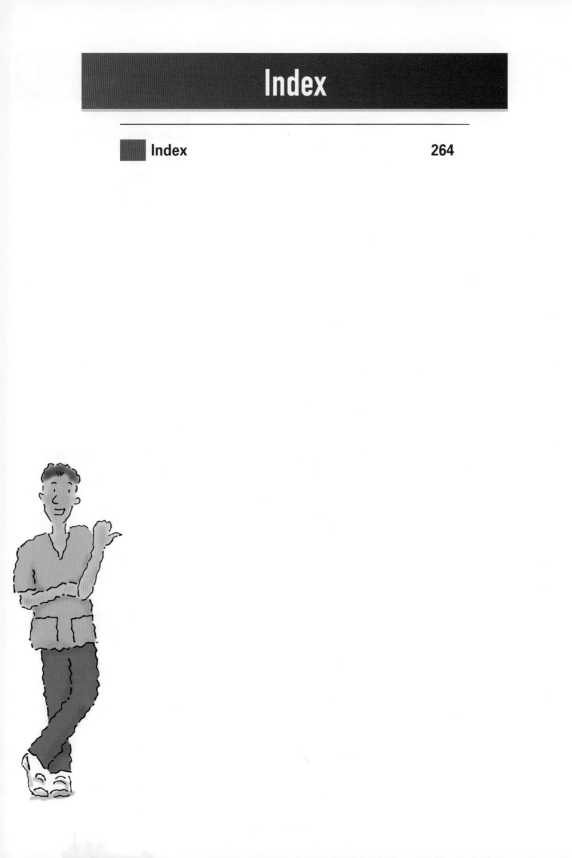

Index